In memory of Andreas R. Grüntzig

Thomas Ischinger

Practice of Coronary Angioplasty

With Contributions by
U.T. Aker P.C. Block B.R. Chaitman T. Corcos
M. Cowley P.R. David G. Dorros H.M. Goodgold
G.O. Hartzler J. Hollman T. Ischinger G.C. Kaiser
L.R. McBride B. Meier J. Meyer R. Roth
M. Vandormael P. Zack

With 129 Figures

Springer-Verlag
Berlin Heidelberg New York Tokyo

THOMAS ISCHINGER, M.D.
Division of Cardiology
Hospital München-Bogenhausen
Englschalkinger Straße 77
D-8000 München 81

Library of Congress Cataloging-in-Publication Data. Ischinger, T. (Thomas) Practice of coronary angioplasty. Includes index. 1. Transluminal angioplasty. I. Aker, U.T. (Umit T.) II. Title. [DNLM: 1. Angioplasty, Transluminal – methods. 2. Coronary Disease – surgery. WG 300 I774p] RD598.5.I83 1985 617'.412 85-26115

ISBN-13: 978-3-642-70817-6 e-ISBN-13: 978-3-642-70815-2
DOI: 10.1007/978-3-642-70815-2

Softcover reprint of the hardcover 1st edition 1986

2127/3130-543210

To Jeannette

Preface

After 7 years of clinical use, percutaneous transluminal coronary angioplasty (PTCA) has now found worldwide acceptance, and its basic techniques are well standardized. A growing number of invasive cardiologists are acquainting themselves with the procedure in order to be in a position to offer new therapeutic options to their patients. However, the transition from the diagnostic to the therapeutic intervention is not always easily accomplished. Certain prerequisites concerning technique, the physician, technical equipment, and program organization are necessary for safe and effective performance.

The consequences of unsuccessful coronary angioplasty range from waste of time and money to severe complications for the patient; the decision to perform PTCA needs to be based on sound indications and techniques according to the best current scientific evidence.

Techniques and technology for coronary angioplasty continue to evolve. Scientific evidence of its short- and long-term value continues to accumulate, and applications of the procedure are still being extended.

This volume is obviously no substitute for well-guided hands-on experience with the procedure; it is intended rather to present current policies of patient selection and patient management; to describe standard techniques (femoral and brachial approaches) and potential applications; to point out problem areas and limitations of the procedure; and to provide tips that may be useful even for the more experienced angioplasty operator.

I believe the aim of presenting different experts' views and practical approaches to PTCA, although unavoidably resulting in some overlap, has helped to create a state-of-the-art report as well as a useful practical reference.

I thank my former colleagues from St. Louis University Division of Cardiology, in particular Harold L. Kennedy (Chief of Division), for their support and their enthusiasm for my work as director of interventional cardiology, which helped encourage me to create this book. I thank my former teacher Andreas R. Grüntzig of Emory University, for sharing with me his outstanding abilities and his experience.

St. Louis/Munich, November 1985 THOMAS ISCHINGER

Contents

List of Contributors

AKER, U.T., Associate Professor of Medicine, St. Louis University School of Medicine, 1325 South Grand Boulevard, St. Louis, MO 63104, U.S.A.

BLOCK, P.C., Associate Professor of Medicine, Cardiac Catheterization Laboratory, Bulfinch I, Massachusetts General Hospital, Boston, MA 02114, U.S.A.

CHAITMAN, B.R., Professor of Medicine, St. Louis University Medical Center, 1325 South Grand Boulevard, St. Louis, MO 63104, U.S.A.

CORCOS, T., M.D., Institute of Cardiology, Montreal Heart Institute, 5000 East Belarger Street, Montreal H1T 1C8, Quebec, Canada

COWLEY, M., Associate Professor, Medical College of Virginia, Box 59, MCV Station, Richmond, VA 23298, U.S.A.

DAVID, R.P., M.D., Institute of Cardiology, Montreal Heart Institute, 5000 East Belarger Street, Montreal H1T 1C8, Quebec, Canada

DORROS, G., Assistant Clinical Professor, Medical College of Wisconsin, 811 East Wisconsin Avenue, Milwaukee, WI 53202, U.S.A.

GOODGOLD, H.M., Assistant Professor of Medicine, St. Louis University Medical Center, 1325 South Grand Boulevard, St. Louis, MO 63104, U.S.A.

HARTZLER, G.O., M.D., Cardiovascular Consultants, Inc., Medical Plaza II-20, 4320 Wornall Road, Kansas City, MO 64111, U.S.A.

HOLLMAN, J., M.D., Cleveland Clinic Foundation, Cleveland, OH 44106, U.S.A.

ISCHINGER, T., M.D., Division of Cardiology, Hospital München-Bogenhausen, Englschalkinger Str. 77, 8000 München 81, FRG

KAISER, G.C., Professor of Surgery, St. Louis University School of Medicine, 1325 South Grand Boulevard, St. Louis, MO 63104, U.S.A.

McBRIDE, L.R., Assistant Professor of Surgery, St. Louis University School of Medicine, 1325 South Grand Boulevard, St. Louis, MO 63104, U.S.A.

MEIER, B., M.D., Cardiology Center, University Hospital, 1211 Geneva 4, Switzerland

MEYER, J., Professor of Medicine, II. Medical University Clinic Johannes Gutenberg University, Langenbeckstr. 1, 6500 Mainz, FRG

ROTH, R., Cardiovascular Nurse/Technician, St. Louis University Medical Center, 1325 South Grand Boulevard, St. Louis, MO 63104, U.S.A.

VANDORMAEL, M., Assistant Professor of Medicine, St. Louis University Medical Center, 1325 South Grand Boulevard, St. Louis, MO 63104, U.S.A.

ZACK, P.M., Assistant Professor of Medicine, St. Louis University School of Medicine, Division of Cardiology, 1325 South Grand Boulevard, St. Louis, MO 63104, U.S.A.

Chapter 1. Introduction and Historical Background

THOMAS ISCHINGER

The feasibility of percutaneous transluminal balloon dilatation of coronary stenoses was not an accidental finding such as often do occur in medicine, but the result of several years of dedicated work: inspired by the telescope-like catheter system introduced by Charles Dotter and Melvin Judkins in 1964 [1, 2], in the early 1970s Dr. Andreas Gruentzig developed an inflatable balloon for dilatation of localized atherosclerotic obstructions in human peripheral arteries [3]. While gathering experience and learning from the results of peripheral angioplasty in a large number of patients, Gruentzig worked toward the goal of modifying the technique for intracoronary use. Animal experiments, postmortem studies, and intraoperative dilatations were performed [4, 5] before the dream came true on 16 September 1977 in the catheterization laboratory at the University Hospital of Zürich, Switzerland, when he tackled the LAD stenosis of his first PTCA patient:

> ... "The dilatation catheter was advanced through the stenosis with no difficulties. The stenosis was severe but the catheter slipped through it without resistance. The catheter wedged the stenosis and the distal coronary pressure was very low. To the surprise of all of us, no ST elevation, ventricular fibrillation or even extra-systole occurred and the patient had no chest pain. At this moment I decided not to start coronary perfusion with the roller pump. After the first balloon inflation the distal coronary pressure rose nicely. Encouraged by this positive response I inflated the balloon a second time to relieve the residual gradient ... I removed the catheter and immediate angiography in several oblique projections revealed a marked reduction of the LAD stenosis. There was no peripheral spasm or embolization. We therefore declared success."

This is part of the account of the first percutaneous transluminal coronary angioplasty (PTCA) performed by Dr. Andreas Gruentzig [6]. Not until 5 months later, in February 1978, were the results obtained in the first 5 patients published in *The Lancet* [7]. The results in a larger series of 50 patients treated with coronary angioplasty were published in 1979 in the *New England Journal of Medicine* [8]. By then, the potential of this new treatment was more widely recognized, and the success story of PTCA took its course. To date, some centers have treated more than 4000 patients with PTCA. Only recently, the results obtained with coronary angioplasty in 3079 patients enrolled in the National Heart Lung and Blood Institute's PTCA Registry were analyzed and published in a special issue of the *American Journal of Cardiology* [9]. There is no doubt that current results have met – if not exceeded – the expections and hopes stimulated by Gruentzig's original report.

Yet, we still share some of Gruentzig's original concerns: Complications of PTCA do occur, and we do not yet have a safe means of preventing myocardial infarction should dilatation result in irreversible coronary occlusion. Gruentzig's original concept of perfusing the distal coronary artery through the dilatation catheter is attracting increasing interest.

On the other hand, the relative ease with which successful PTCA can be carried out is often surprising and may seduce us into too uncritical use of the technique, as Gruentzig describes in his report, when he – "seduced by the enthusiasm" of his colleagues – recrossed the successfully dilated LAD stenosis for dilatation of an insignificant stenosis in a diagonal branch.

The procedure has remained essentially unchanged, and it is amazing how similar Gruentzig's first report is to a PTCA report prepared in 1985. However, there has been no stagnation in techniques and catheter technology. Catheters of the latest generation are becoming consistently smaller (low-profile balloon catheters), more versatile (steerable balloon catheter systems) [10], and stronger (balloons tolerating more than 12 atm). Other improvements include larger central lumina of the dilatation catheters for improved pressure recordings and/or dye injection, more flexible yet steerable guidewires [11], and guide catheters with better torque control. Some procedural modifications have been developed, such as longer inflation times [12] and higher dilatation pressures [13] to give greater initial dilatation and a better long-term outcome [14, 15]. High-resolution fluoroscopy and still-frame disk capacity have further improved the procedure.

Analyses of the vast experiences from large centers and from the NHLBI PTCA Registry have provided us with the necessary feedback: We have learned how to select patients more individually and how to interpret the results of PTCA. Good results have encouraged us to extend the applications of PTCA, but we have been held back by the low but constant incidence of complications. There is still no way of definitely predicting the outcome of PTCA, but we are better at calculating the risks. Today coronary angioplasty is considered the method of choice in some patients with coronary artery disease, and an equal alternative to coronary artery bypass surgery in others.

After its introduction into clinical practice the greatest improvement in PTCA technology was the development of the so-called steerable dilatation catheters. These catheters marked the beginning of a new era and are responsible for the still expanding potential of the procedure. Passage of tight, distal, or diffuse stenoses could not have been safely accomplished without these catheters. "Kissing balloon" techniques and complex procedures [16] involving multiple dilatations in multiple vessels in a single session have become feasible due to these technological advances. Coronary angioplasty now seems ready to accept a major challenge: comparison with coronary bypass surgery in patients with multiple vessel disease.

Whatever the outcome of this comparison, PTCA will remain a desirable palliative measure, one that can help many patients at various stages of their disease process. Furthermore, coronary angioplasty has taught us that it is possible to work successfully inside the human coronary artery. Coronary angioplasty has given birth to the field of interventional cardiology and continues to stimulate the search for new methods of arterial revascularization using techniques other than mechanical stenosis dilatation.

References

1. Dotter CT, Judkins MP (1964) Transluminal treatment of arteriosclerotic obstruction: description of a new technique and preliminary report of its application. Circulation 30:654
2. Dotter CT (1980) Transluminal angioplasty: a long view. Radiology 135:561
3. Gruentzig AR (1976) Die perkutane Rekanalisierung chronischer arterieller Verschlüsse (Dotter-Prinzip) mit einem neuen doppellumigen Dilatationskatheter. Fortschr Röntgenstr 125:80
4. Gruentzig AR, Turina MI, Schneider JA (1976) Experimental percutaneous dilatation of coronary artery stenosis. Circulation 54:81
5. Gruentzig AR, Schneider HJ (1977) Die perkutane Dilatation chronischer Koronarstenosen: Experiment und Morphologie. Schweiz Med Wochenschr 107:1588
6. Willis Hurst J (1985) History of cardiac catheterization. In: King SB, Douglas JS (eds) Coronary arteriography and angioplasty. McGraw Hill, New York, p 7
7. Gruentzig AR (1978) Transluminal dilatation of coronary artery stenosis. Lancet I:263
8. Gruentzig AR, Senning A, Siegenthaler WE (1979) Non-operative dilatation of coronary artery stenosis: percutaneous transluminal coronary angioplasty. N Engl J Med 301:61–68
9. Mock MB (1984) Acute and chronic outcome of percutaneous transluminal coronary angioplasty. Am J Cardiol 53:67 C
10. Simpson JB, Baim DS, Robert EW, Harrison DC (1982) A new catheter system for coronary angioplasty. Am J Cardiol 49:1217
11. Gruentzig AR, Hollman J (1982) Improved primary success rate in transluminal coronary angioplasty using a steerable guidance system. Circulation 66:11 (abstract)
12. Kaltenbach M, Kober G (1982) Can prolonged application of pressure improve the results of coronary angioplasty (PTCA)? Circulation 66:123 (abstract)
13. Meier B, Gruentzig A, King SB, Douglas JS, Hollman J, Ischinger T, Galan K (1984) Higher balloon dilatation pressure in coronary angioplasty. Am Heart J 107:619
14. Schmitz HJ, Meyer J, Kiesslich T, Effert S (1982) Greater initial dilatation gives better late angiographic results in percutaneous coronary angioplasty (PTCA). Circulation 66:123 (abstract)
15. Leimgruber PP, Roubin GS, Rice CR, Tate JM, Gruentzig AR (1984) Influence of intinal dissection after coronary angioplasty (PTCA) on restenosis rate. Circulation 70:174 (abstract)
16. Zack P, Ischinger T (1984) Experience with a technique for coronary angioplasty of bifurcational lesions. Cathet Cardiovasc Diagn 10:433

Chapter 2. The Mechanism of Transluminal Angioplasty Pathology of the Arterial Stenoses that Are Most Amenable to PTCA

PETER C. BLOCK

Normal coronary arteries are compliant, and their lumens can be easily stretched. They have considerable reactivity, and variations in coronary artery lumen size are common due to changes in coronary vascular tone. Microscopically, there are three distinct layers in the coronary arteries: the intima, consisting of endothelial cells attached to a thin layer of extracellular matrix; the media, which is made up of variable layers of circumferentially oriented smooth muscle cells with surrounding elastin and collagen; and the adventitia, which consists of loosely arranged connective tissue, fibroblasts, and a few muscle cells. The internal elastic lamina separates the intima from the media.

There are two major types of atherosclerotic plaques which can cause stenoses of the coronary arteries: fibromuscular plaques and complicated plaques. Fibromuscular plaques are formed when medial smooth muscle cells proliferate, probably in response to focal injury, and variable amounts of intracellular and extracellular lipid are deposited. Any atherosclerotic plaque can produce a loss of normal arterial wall elasticity and reactivity because of a splinting action of the abnormal intima and media on the artery. Though the plaque itself may infringe upon the lumen by virtue of its volume, it has been shown that in arterial segments with experimentally induced fibromuscular plaques, less than 10% of the stenosis is due to the actual volume of the plaque. The remaining stenosis is due mainly to a splinting action and contraction of the underlying arterial wall [11].

A complicated plaque is most likely to be a degenerated fibromuscular plaque altered by necrosis, more lipid infiltration, hemorrhage, and finally calcification. A complicated plaque is usually surrounded by a thin, fibrous cap on the luminal surface, which surrounds a core of necrotic debris and lipid. The media is frequently fragmented, and there may be fraying of the internal elastic membrane with medial destruction. Calcium deposits are common. It is this kind of atherosclerotic plaque that is most often responsible for the clinical manifestations of atherosclerotic coronary artery disease in man. Mural thrombus, which may be formed due to exposure to circulating blood of thrombogenic material secondary to ulceration of the fibrous cap, may become organized and be incorporated further into the plaque. This results in a thicker and more fibrous cap, which compromises the lumen further and increases coronary insufficiency. Ultimately, this type of plaque may ulcerate or rupture due to intraplaque hemorrhage. Sudden mural thrombus formation over the exposed plaque elements leads to vascular thrombosis and possibly to myocardial infarction.

The nature of the atherosclerotic plaque undergoing transluminal angioplasty almost certainly has a direct bearing on the pathophysiologic response of the artery to balloon inflation. For example, passage of a guidewire and a dilating catheter through a long, ulcerated plaque could theoretically involve a high chance of microembolism of loose plaque material distally. Conversely, dilation of a "young" fibromuscular plaque would be less likely to have the same consequences.

Atherosclerotic plaques are mostly focal and produce localized stenoses only. In fact, most stenoses occur in the more proximal segments of muscular arteries. About 70% of coronary atherosclerotic lesions occur within the first 4-cm section of one of the three major coronary arteries [14]. This anatomic distribution favors the use of transluminal angioplasty for the treatment of coronary stenoses, since it is technically easier to reach stenoses that are in the proximal portions of the coronary vasculature.

Experimental Data Concerning the Mechanism of Angioplasty

The mechanism of transluminal angioplasty has been elucidated from four major sources:

1. Angioplasty performed experimentally in autopsied human hearts [1].
2. The study of pathological specimens studied after transluminal angioplasty in normal dog coronary arteries [2, 5, 8, 9, 18].
3. Pathological study of transluminal angioplasty performed in atherosclerotic rabbit models [4, 5, 12, 20].
4. Pathological specimens studied after successful transluminal angioplasty both in femoral vessels and in coronary arteries in humans [6, 21].

Studies of Angioplasty Performed in Autopsied Human Hearts

Transluminal angioplasty performed in vitro in autopsied human hearts shows that the atheromatous plaque is split, usually at its thinnest point. The splits frequently extend from the intima down to the internal elastic membrane. These findings do not support the concept that atheromas are compressed by the expanding angioplasty balloon. Rather, they show that successful angioplasty involves splitting of the plaque, resulting in a larger lumen [1, 5]. These findings initially raised fears that angioplasty might be associated with the high incidence of coronary artery rupture. Since in vitro studies on autopsied arteries are necessarily done using nonviable tissue, the early reports raised questions as to whether their findings could be extrapolated to the effect of angioplasty in man.

Studies in Normal Dog Coronary Arteries

Electron microscopic studies of normal dog coronary arteries after angioplasty do not show as much disruption of the arterial wall as is found in autopsied human hearts. However, a normal dog coronary artery and the size of the inflated angioplasty balloon are approximately equal – a situation not found during

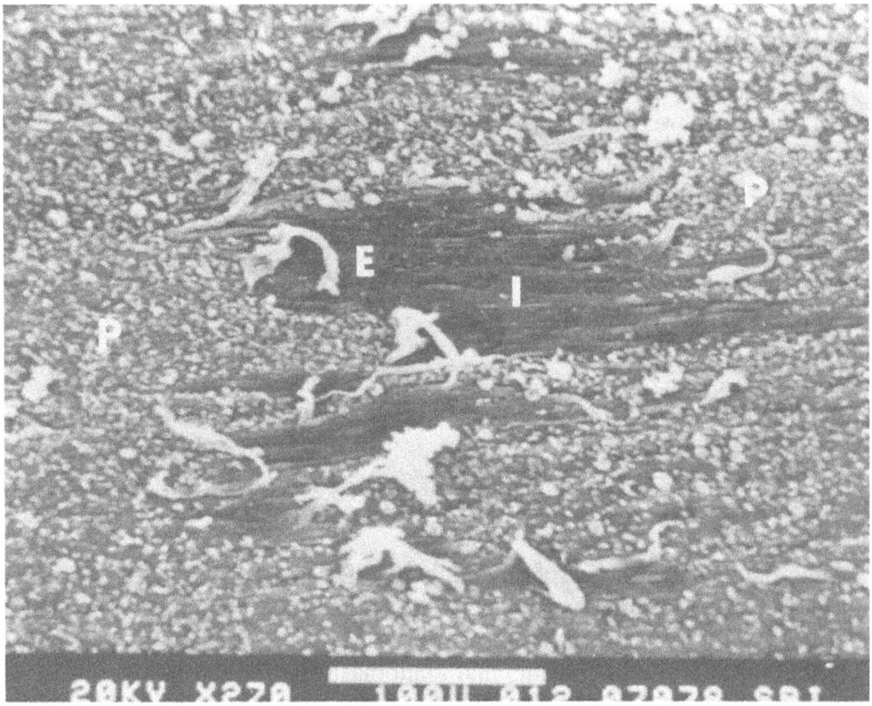

Fig. 1. Electron micrograph of a normal dog coronary artery after angioplasty. Partially adherent endothelial cells (*E*) lie adjacent to small islands of normal endothelium (*I*). A carpet of platelets (*P*) covers all areas denuded of endothelial cells

angioplasty of tightly stenosed coronary arteries in vitro or clinically in man. In the normal dog coronary artery, inflation of the balloon stretches the outer arterial wall only slightly. Contact of the endothelial cells with the inflated angioplasty balloon produces severe desquamation of endothelial cells and platelet deposition in the area of angioplasty. Superfical shearing of endothelial elements enlarges the arterial lumen only slightly. However, the demonstration by these studies that the inflated balloon causes severe desquamation of endothelial cells in the area of angioplasty is important. This highlights the marked platelet deposition that always occurs in the area of angioplasty (Fig. 1) [17, 18]. In the dog, the use of "antiplatelet" agents such as aspirin or low-molecular-weight dextran does not inhibit platelet deposition in the area of angioplasty. Segments of the arteries adjacent to the dilated segment show no endothelial disruption.

Studies in Atherosclerotic Rabbits

An animal model of atherosclerosis can be produced in rabbits by feeding them a 2% cholesterol diet and injuring the arterial endothelium. Arterial lesions pro-

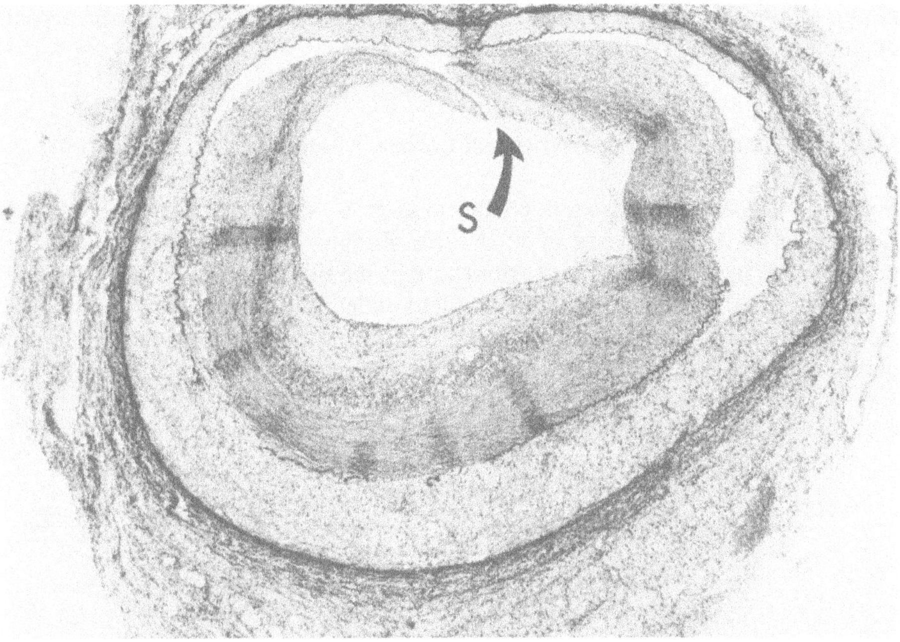

Fig. 2. Section of an atherosclerotic iliac artery of a rabbit after transluminal angioplasty. A split (*S, arrow*) extends through the plaque and continues circumferentially at the internal elastic lamina. X55 [4]. (By permission of the American Heart Association, Inc.)

duced in rabbits tend to be rich in cholesterol-laden macrophages, unlike the fibromuscular plaques seen in man. The response of these plaques to angioplasty may be different than that of the atherosclerotic plaques in man. Studies of angioplasty in this experimental model give clues to the mechanism of angioplasty in human atherosclerosis, since in both instances the size of the constricted atherosclerotic lumen and the size of the inflated angioplasty balloon are quite disparate. This is the situation which is common in angioplasty of human coronary arteries in vivo. The rabbit model for atherosclerosis also produces focal encroachment on the arterial lumen, which allows both angiographic and pathological study of the effects of angioplasty. Angiographic studies in atherosclerotic rabbits show that in areas where the balloon is inflated there is an increase in lumen size as evaluated by measurement of the width of the contrast column before and after angioplasty [4]. Some arteries also show an irregularity of the edge of the contrast medium, a finding frequently seen in human coronary arteries after successful angioplasty. This is most probably due to splitting of the atherosclerotic plaque (see below). Pathological study of the same arteries shows severe endothelial desquamation. A carpet of platelets adheres to the subendothelial collagen matrix, just as in the dog studies. In addition, in almost all instances, the atheromatous plaque splits at its thinnest point. Such splits frequently reach the internal elastic membrane and are very similar to the splits in atheromatous plaques that are seen in human coronary arteries subjected to experimental angioplasty at autopsy (Fig. 2).

Studies of Human Femoral Arteries and Coronary Arteries

Sections of human atherosclerotic femoral arteries and of coronary arteries that have undergone angioplasty in vivo show findings almost identical with the changes seen in human coronary arteries subjected to angioplasty at autopsy and in arteries of atherosclerotic rabbits that had undergone angioplasty. The atherosclerotic plaque splits at its weakest point, the split extending down to the internal elastic membrane (Fig. 3). The outer layers of the artery are stretched by the ex-

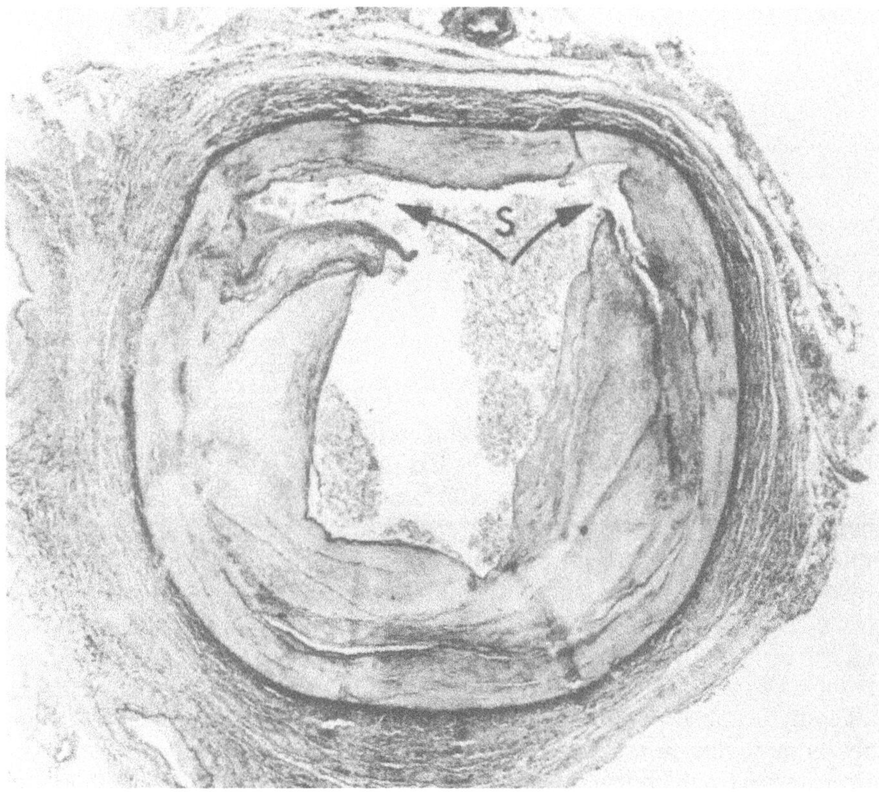

A

Fig. 3. A Section of femoral artery at site of angioplasty, revealing splits (*S*) of the fibrous intimal plaque extending to the internal elastic lamina and following its circumference (*arrows*). The original lume has been enlarged considerably by the splits in the plaque [6]. (Reprinted by permission of the New England Journal of Medicine) **B** Section of left anterior descending coronary artery at site of angioplasty, showing a split (*arrow*) in the thinnest portion of a fibrous atherosclerotic plaque. The split extends into the media with circumferential extension. The lumen is partly occluded by a small thrombus (*dark area*). [6] (Reprinted by permission of the New England Journal of Medicine)

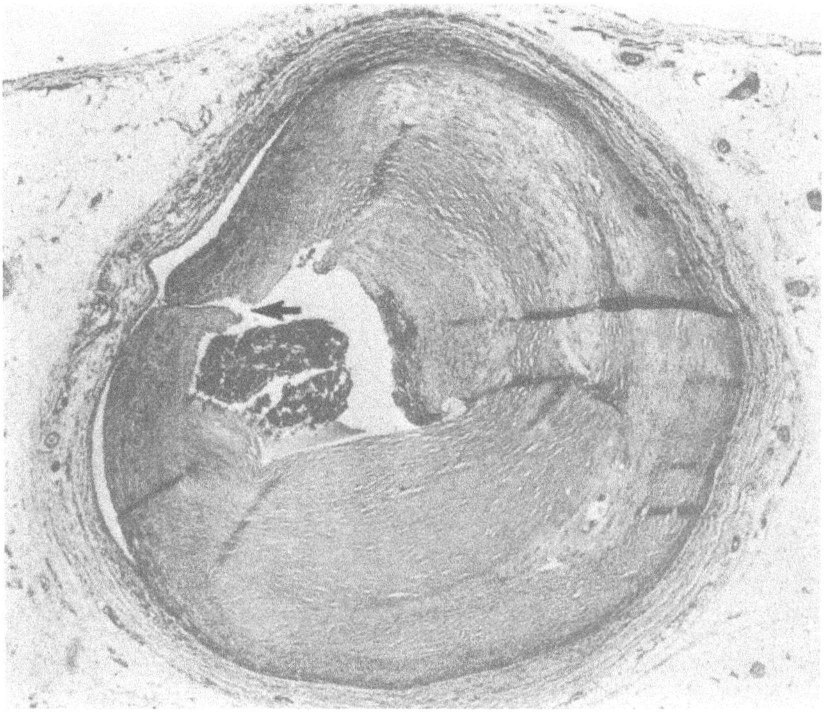

B

Fig. 3B

panding angioplasty balloon. Thus, the lumen is widened by a combination of splitting of the plaque and stretching of the outer media and adventitia of the artery [2].

The pathology of the atherosclerotic lesions mentioned above suggests that splitting of the atheromatous plaque should be expected after angioplasty. Since the plaque is composed of material that is nondistensible, the plaque itself resists stretching by the expanding angioplasty balloon. The outer media and adventitia, on the other hand, distend easily as the angioplasty balloon is fully inflated within the vessel. Thus, as the dilating angioplasty balloon is inflated within the arterial atherosclerotic segment, a progressive expansile force is applied to the plaque as pressure mounts within the balloon segment. The intima may undergo some compression with extrusion of liquid. As pressure mounts in the balloon, the expansile force of the balloon exceeds the tensile strength of the atherosclerotic material, and the plaque splits at its weakest point. Once this occurs, only the elastic media and adventitia are left to resist full circumferential stretching of the vessel to accomodate the size of the angioplasty balloon within it. The final size of the lumen of the artery is reached as the split in the atherosclerotic plaque widens circumferentially and as the media and adventitia are fully stretched over the dilating balloon (Fig. 4). Full dilation of the arterial segment undergoing angioplasty is often not achieved by a single balloon inflation, but multiple inflations of the angioplasty balloon may diminish the elastic recoil of the outer media and ad-

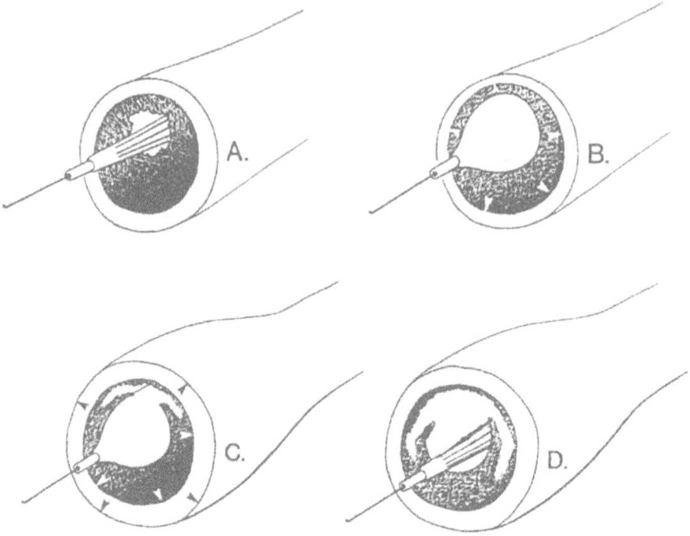

Fig. 4 A–D. Schematic of the mechanism of transluminal angioplasty. The deflated dilating catheter lies within the coronary stenosis (**A**). As the balloon is inflated, the atherosclerotic plaque resists stretching (**B**). With further inflation pressure, the atherosclerotic plaque splits at its weakest point and the elastic outer media and adventitia are stretched; all of this combines to enlarge the lumen (**C**). The balloon is deflated and withdrawn, leaving a stretched, dilated vessel with an enlarged lumen (**D**)

ventitia. Clinically, this is reflected in the fact that the pressure gradient across the arterial stenosis frequently diminishes in a progressive, stepwise fashion as the balloon is inflated and deflated several times sequentially within the atherosclerotic segment (Fig. 5). There must be a progressive loss of elastic recoil of the outer layers of the artery with each balloon inflation, probably due to injury to the medial muscle cells. High balloon inflation pressures [15] may enhance this phenomenon by allowing more complete inflation of the balloon to its predetermined outer diameter and also possibly by causing pressure injury to medial muscle cells. Splitting of the plaque also releases the constricting force produced by the atherosclerotic plaque on the media. Release of this constriction also allows the media to assume its more usual outer diameter. If, in fact, the inflated angioplasty balloon is slightly larger than the normal coronary lumen, slight aneurysmal dilatation of the artery may persist.

This pathophysiologic mechanism explains why angiography frequently reveals a "shaggy" appearance of the arterial lesion immediately after angioplasty. Passage of angiographic contrast medium into split areas accounts for an irregular border of the column of contrast agent, and for the "ground glass" appearance of the arterial segment due to a diminished density of dye in the dilated region. A careful study of coronary angiograms after most successful coronary angioplasties reveals a linear segment of higher density contrast medium within the area of angioplasty [13]. This may appear as a short, extraluminal defect (Fig. 6), but in reality it is due to the residual, split atherosclerotic plaque viewed from the side, which occupies space in the enlarged lumen (Fig. 7). Such splits

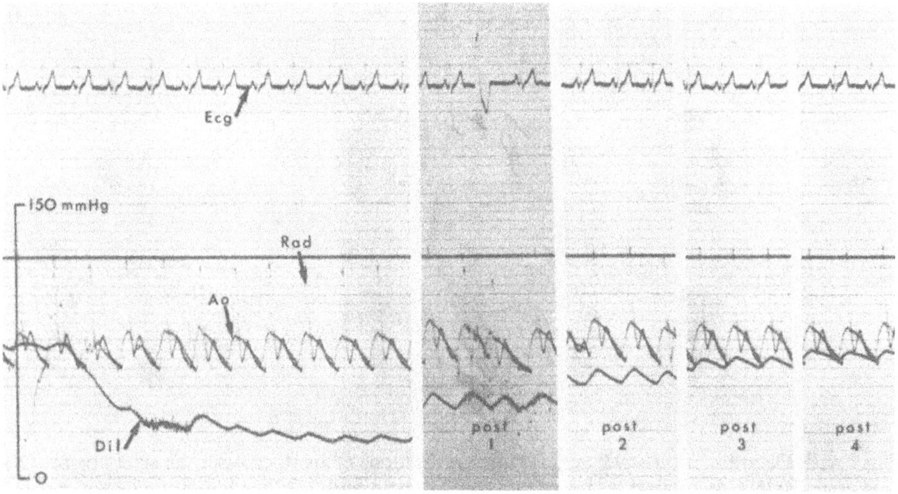

Fig. 5. Pressure recordings from the radial artery (*Rad*), the central aorta (*Ao*), and the tip of the dilating catheter (*Dil*) during PTCA. As the tip of the dilating catheter is advanced through the coronary stenosis, pressure recorded from the tip of the dilating catheter falls. After the first balloon deflation (*post 1*), the gradient across the stenosis is diminished. Three more inflations (*post 2, post 3, post 4*) almost abolish the gradient completely

A 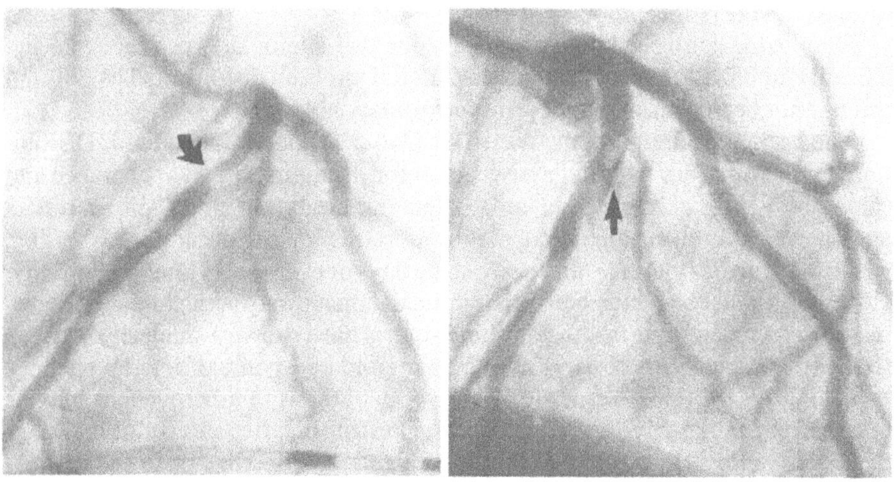 B

Fig. 6. Angiogram of a stenosis of a left anterior descending coronary artery before (**A**) and after (**B**) PTCA. Note the split in the atheromatous plaque, which is seen as a separate area of opacification by angiographic dye (**B** *straight arrow*).[2]

should not be considered complications of angioplasty, but rather a correlate of successful angioplasty. A long split may lead to an intimal flap, which can compromise the arterial lumen, but in most instances the split is relatively short and does not cause complications. True dissecting hematoma is a rare complication of angioplasty [10]. This is probably because the intima adjacent to the angioplasty site is diseased and fibrotic, and resists antegrade or retrograde prop-

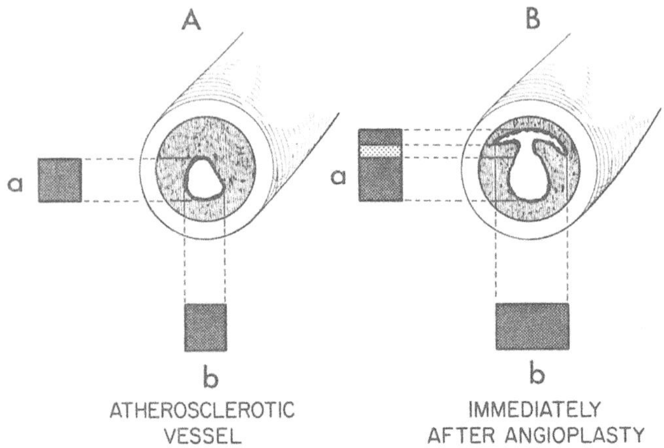

Fig. 7 A, B. Diagram of theoretic angiographic projections of an atherosclerotic artery before (**A**) and after (**B**) PTCA. Intimal splitting produced by successful PTCA enlarges the lumen. Angiographically, the lumen appears enlarged in both projections (**a** and **b**), but only in projection **a** can the split be seen (cf. Fig. 6). [2]

agation of the split. If true antegrade propagation of dissection of the arterial lumen occurs after angioplasty compression of the coronary lumen is a frequent consequence, and immediate bypass graft surgery may be necessary to avoid myocardial damage [10, 22].

Despite the controlled injury to the plaque that angioplasty produces, no significant embolization of atheromatous material has been documented [7, 20], and this has not been clinically important in coronary angioplasty.

The healing of the split atherosclerotic plaque is poorly understood. Dissolution of atheromatous material may account for the more normal appearance and smoother lining of the vessel seen angiographically in areas of successful angioplasty in followup angiograms. Fibrous retraction can occur during healing, which may further increase lumen size some days or even weeks after angioplasty. However, it must be remembered that intimal damage may accelerate the atheromatous process in some instances. Many studies have shown a similarity between the development of atherosclerosis in humans and a response of arteries to endothelial injury [19]. This "response to injury" hypothesis of atherogenesis may be one reason for the 25%–35% incidence of restenosis after successful coronary angioplasty [16]. It is postulated that loss of endothelial cells due to the desquamating injury caused by the inflating angioplasty balloon leads to a large deposition of platelets in the area of endothelial desquamation. The arterial wall can be infiltrated by platelet-derived growth factor released by platelets and other plasma components which activate underlying smooth muscle cells in the media. This produces proliferation of smooth muscle cells and migration of muscle cells into the intima. Once in the intima, the smooth muscle cells proliferate further and deposit a connective tissue matrix, producing a fibromuscular plaque. Although clinical studies suggest that in the majority of patients the improvement in luminal size persists, recurrence of atherosclerotic narrowing may be due partly to this acceleration of the atheromatous process.

There are other mechanisms for restenosis. Since successful angioplasty only splits the atherosclerotic plaque and dilates the outer layers of the affected artery, the total volume of plaque material within the arterial lumen is unchanged; only the adjacent lumen is larger, owing to stretching of the outer media and adventitia. A gradual return to the original lumen size over a period of days or weeks as medial muscle cells regained vasomotor tone while recovering from pressure injury would result in re-establishment of a smaller lumen, which would still contain the original stenosing atherosclerotic plaque.

Lastly, the splits in the atherosclerotic plaque produced by successful angioplasty expose large areas of subendothelial tissue to circulating blood elements. If only a monolayer of platelets is deposited in the splits and reendothelialization occurs, and if the outer layers of the artery remain stretched, an enlarged lumen will persist. However, if a multilayer platelet thrombus fills the splits produced by angioplasty (a factor which may be enhanced owing to diminished blood flow through the angioplasty site, poor runoff, low blood pressure, or low cardiac output) reendothelialization of the area will lead to a smaller lumen than was present immediately after angioplasty.

The pathophysiology of angioplasty raises a number of issues that directly affect patient care before, during, and after the procedure.

Before Angioplasty. Many centers use antiplatelet therapy in patients, beginning the day before, or the day of, coronary angioplasty. Most centers use either aspirin alone or aspirin in combination with dipyridamole. It is felt that pretreatment with such an antiplatelet regimen may minimize platelet deposition in the area of angioplasty at the time of the procedure.

During Angioplasty. To avoid the development of thrombosis in the area of angioplasty during the procedure, all patients who have coronary angioplasty must be given high-dose heparin at the beginning of the procedure. In addition, many centers use low-molecular-weight dextran i.v. at the beginning of the procedure and continue an infusion of 25 cc/h for 12–24 h thereafter in an effort to minimize platelet adhesiveness. Since platelet deposition in an area of connective tissue exposure and thrombus formation are inversely related to blood flow over the injured area, it is important to maximize coronary flow during any coronary angioplasty procedure. Hence, the use of i.v. nitroglycerin during the procedure and pretreatment with calcium channel blockers (such as nifedipine, verapamil, or diltiazem) are probably important. In addition, blood pressure should be maintained and cardiac output kept at an adequate level to maintain normal flow through the coronary arteries throughout the procedure.

After Angioplasty. After the procedure, antiplatelet regimens are usually maintained. Low-molecular-weight dextran can be given for 12–24 h i.v. In addition, most centers continue an antiplatelet regimen of aspirin and dipyridamole. Use of long-acting nitrates and calcium channel blockers also seems prudent.

It is important to emphasize that there is only theoretical justification for the use of any or all of these medications at present. Whether the use of any or all of these agents will affect the complication rate, the long-term patency of the angioplasty site, or the incidence of early restenosis is still unknown. Nevertheless, the relative merit of using these agents seems to outweigh their potential disadvantages at present.

References

1. Baughman KL, Pasternak RC, Fallon JT, Block PC (1978) Coronary transluminal angioplasty in autopsied human hearts. Circulation 58:11–80
2. Block PC (1982) Percutaneous transluminal coronary angioplasty. In: Yu PN, Goodwin JF (eds) Progress in cardiology, vol II. Lea and Febiger, Philadelphia, pp 1–15
3. Block PC (1980) Percutaneous transluminal coronary angioplasty. AJR 135:955–959
4. Block PC, Baughman KL, Pasternak RC, Fallon JT (1980) Transluminal angioplasty: correlation of morphological and angiographic findings in an experimental model. Circulation 61:785–788
5. Block PC, Fallon JT, Elmer D (1980) Experimental angioplasty: lessons from the the laboratory. AJR 135:907–912
6. Block PC, Myler RK, Stertzer S, Fallon JT (1981) Morphology after transluminal angioplasty in human beings. N Engl J Med 305:382–385
7. Block PC, Elmer D, Fallon JT (1982) Release of atherosclerotic debris after transluminal angioplasty. Circulation 65:950–952
8. Castaneda-Zuniga WR, Formanek A, Tadavarthy M, Vlodaver Z, Edwards JR, Zollikofer C, Amplatz K (1980) The mechanism of balloon angioplasty. Radiology 135:565–571
9. Castaneda-Zuniga R, Sibley R, Amplatz K (1984) The pathologic basis of angioplasty. Angiology 35:195–205
10. Dorros G, Cowley M, Simpson J, Bentivoglio L, Block P, Bourasa M, Detre K, Gosselin A, Gruntzig A, Kelsey S, Kent K, Mock M, Mullin S, Myler R, Passamani E, Stertzer S, Williams D (1983) Percutaneous transluminal coronary angioplasty: report of complications from the National Heart, Lung and Blood Institute PTCA registry. Circulation 67:723–730
11. Fallon JT (1980) Pathology of arterial lesions amenable to percutaneous transluminal angioplasty. AJR 135:913–916
12. Faxon DP, Weber VJ, Haudenschild C, Gottsman SB, McGovern WA, Ryan TJ (1982) Acute effects of transluminal angioplasty in three experimental models of atherosclerosis. Arteriosclerosis 2:125–126
13. Holmes DR Jr, Vlietstra RE, Mock MB, Reeder GS, Smith HC, Bove AA, Bresnahan JF, Piehler JM, Schaff HV, Orszulak TA (1983) Angiographic changes produced by percutaneous transluminal coronary angioplasty. Am J Cardiol 51:676
14. McNamara JJ, Norenburg RG, Goebert HW, Soeter JR (1976) Distribution and severity of atherosclerosis in the coronary arteries. J Thorac Cardiovasc Surg 71:637–640
15. Meier B, Gruntzig AR, King SB, Douglas JS, Hollman J, Ischinger T, Galan K (1984) Higher balloon dilatation pressure in coronary angioplasty. Am Heart J 107:619–622
16. National Heart, Lung, and Blood Institute (1984) Proceedings of the NHLBI workshop on PTCA, June, 1983. J Cardiol 53:69–71
17. O'Gara PT, Guerrero JL, Feldman B, Fallon JT, Block PC (to be published) Effect of dextran and aspirin on platelet adherence following transluminal angioplasty of normal canine coronary arteries. Am J Cardiol
18. Pasternak RC, Baughman KL, Fallon JT, Block PC (1980) Scanning electron microscopy after coronary transluminal angioplasty of normal canine coronary arteries. Am J Cardiol 45:591–598
19. Ross R, Glomset JA (1976) The pathogenesis of atherosclerosis. N Engl J Med 285:369–377, 420–425
20. Sanborn TA, Faxon DP, Waugh D, Small DM, Haudenschild C, Gottsman SB, Ryan TJ (1982) Transluminal angioplasty in experimental atherosclerosis: analysis for embolization using an in vivo perfusion system. Circulation 66:917
21. Waller BF (1983) Early and late morphologic changes in human coronary arteries after percutaneous transluminal coronary angioplasty. Clin Cardiol 6:363
22. Zack P, Ischinger T (1985) Late occlusive dissection after successful coronary angioplasty. Cathet Cardiovasc Diagn 11:41

Chapter 3. Clinical Selection Criteria and Role of Noninvasive Testing for PTCA

BERNARD R. CHAITMAN, HENRY M. GOODGOLD, and THOMAS ISCHINGER

Percutaneous transluminal angioplasty is a relatively new revascularization procedure that was first performed humans by Andreas Gruentzig in September 1977. In June 1979, experience collected worldwide in 205 patients was presented at an NIH-sponsored PTCA workshop. Since then, the number of patients who have undergone PTCA has increased markedly; the data collected on 3079 patients from 105 contributing centers was reported at an NIH workshop in June 1983. Increased operator experience, improved catheter design, and the realization that PTCA can be safely performed in high-risk patients (unstable angina, persistent angina following infarction, and poor left ventricular function), together with successful complex coronary angioplasty results in patients with multivessel disease or serial stenoses have brought about a further increase in the number of patients considered for PTCA procedures.

Long-term results following coronary angioplasty are not yet available. Unlike results with coronary bypass surgery, 5-year permeability rates after PTCA in a large series of patients are not available at the time of this report. Therefore, the natural history of angina pectoris, results of recent trials comparing coronary bypass surgery and drug treatment, and advances in noninvasive and invasive diagnostic procedures that might be useful in evaluating PTCA patients before and after a PTCA procedure are presented. The data will be used to formulate guidelines to assist physicians in selecting patients for PTCA and will illustrate how noninvasive test procedures can be used to select and monitor patients considered for this procedure.

Indications for Myocardial Revascularization

Symptomatic ischemic heart disease can become manifest as chronic stable angina, unstable angina, variant angina, myocardial infarction, or congestive heart failure. Occasionally, obstructive coronary disease occurs in asymptomatic individuals, some of whom have silent episodes of myocardial ischemia. The natural history of patients with obstructive coronary disease has been well described [1–9]. Three large randomized trials of patients with chronic stable angina have helped redefine indications for myocardial revascularization. Table 1 reviews the patient entry criteria in each of the three studies, illustrating substantial differences in entry criteria. The Coronary Artery Surgery Study (CASS) included women (10% of total randomized), whereas the other two trials, performed earlier, included only men. In the CASS, the initial operative mortality rate was

Table 1. Entry criteria in randomized studies of coronary bypass surgery

Variable	1975–1979 CASS	1970–1974 VA	1973–1976 ECSS
Men only	No	Yes	Yes
Angina for 3–6 months	No	Yes	Yes
ECG ischemia or MI	No	Yes	No
Angina ≧ class III	No	Yes	Yes
Asymptomatic	Yes	No	No
Single-vessel disease	Yes	Yes	No
Ejection fraction ≧0.50	Yes	Yes	No
Angiographic stenosis	70%	50%	50%

CASS, Coronary Artery Surgery Study; VA, Veterans Administration study; ECSS, European Coronary Surgery Study; MI, Myocardial Infarction

1.4%, versus 3.3% and 5.8% in the European Coronary Surgery Study (ECSS) and the Veterans Administration (VA) study, respectively. The VA study required electrocardiographic evidence of myocardial ischemia, whereas the other studies did not. The VA study included patients of all ages, while the others excluded patients older than 65 years.

Perhaps the most important differences among these studies are those in symptomatic status. The CASS permitted randomization of asymptomatic subjects and did not include patients with angina of functional class III or greater. The ECSS and the VA study contained 42% and 58% of randomized patients who had at least functional class III angina. A luminal narrowing of at least 70% in a major coronary artery was required in CASS, whereas the VA study and ECSS required a 50% narrowing. ECSS contained a larger percentage of patients with proximal left anterior descending coronary disease than did the CASS study. Thus, transient myocardial ischemic episodes were probably more common in patients enrolled in the VA study and ECSS.

The differences in annual mortality rates for patients with one-, two-, and three-vessel disease are shown in Table 2. The 5-year annual mortality rate for medically treated patients was lowest in CASS, intermediate in ECSS, and highest in the VA study. In CASS, no significant differences were observed between medical and surgical therapy in any of the subgroups analyzed at 5 years. Survival in the surgical group was not significantly improved over that for patients treated medically, even when patient subgroups such as those with proximal left anterior descending coronary disease or patients with exercise-induced ST segment depression greater than or equal to 2 mm were examined. However, at 7 years the CASS study shows improved survival following surgery for patients with three-vessel coronary disease who had an ejection fraction of less than 0.50 at entry (88% versus 65%; $P = 0.009$). The difference in survival was even more impressive in patients who had angina during their exercise test at the time of randomization. Of several exercise electrocardiographic parameters measured in patients with three-vessel disease, the presence of angina during the exercise test was the most important exercise parameter in determining 7-year survival following randomization.

Table 2. Annual mortality rates of patients randomized to medical versus surgical therapy

Number of diseased vessels	Therapy received	Annual mortality rate over 5 years		
		CASS	VA	ECSS
One	Med	1.4	2.6	NR
	Surg	0.8	1.4	NR
Two	Med	1.2	2.8	2.6
	Surg	1.0	4.4	1.8
Three	Med	2.2	5.2	3.6 } ★
	Surg	1.2	2.8	1.4 }
Two and prox LAD	Med	1.8	NR	3.6 } ★
	Surg	1.2	NR	2.0 }

Prox LAD, proximal left anterior descending coronary artery; Med, medical; Surg, surgical; CASS, Coronary Artery Surgery Study; VA, Veterans Administration Trial of Coronary Bypass Surgery; ECSS, European Coronary Surgery Study
★ $P<0.05$

The lack of improvement after surgery in patients with three-vessel coronary disease and an ejection fraction greater than 0.50 is a point of difference from ECSS, in which a significant improvement in favor of patients treated surgically was observed in patients who had three-vessel coronary disease. The prognosis of medically assigned patients who had two-vessel coronary disease and at least 50% narrowing in the proximal left anterior descending coronary artery was worse than that of medically assigned patients who had nonproximal left anterior descending coronary disease. The VA study did not show significant differences between medically and surgically treated patients, regardless of the number of diseased vessels. However, when hospitals with an elevated surgical operative mortality were excluded, a significant difference could be demonstrated in patients who had three-vessel coronary disease. Eleven-year follow-up in the VA study shows a significant improvement with surgical therapy in the subgroup of patients with three-vessel coronary disease and impaired left ventricular function.

The effect of symptoms in determining the benefit of coronary bypass surgery has recently been examined by Kaiser et al. [8]. In this CASS registry study, patients with three-vessel coronary disease and class III or IV angina had a significantly better 5-year survival when left ventricular function was normal (92% versus 74%; $P<0.001$) or when left ventricular dysfunction was present (82% versus 52%; $P<0.001$). A similar benefit in favor of surgery was not observed in the patients with three-vessel coronary disease who had less severe angina.

Thus, the results collated from observational data and the three large randomized trials in patients with chronic stable angina show that coronary bypass surgery does not appear to improve survival in patients with mild angina, except for patients who have left main coronary disease or three-vessel coronary disease and an ejection fraction lower than 0.50. The survival benefit of revascularization procedures in patients with mild angina who have two-vessel disease involving the proximal left anterior descending coronary artery is not completely known at the time of this report. In patients with this type of coronary anatomy, we usually recommend a revascularization procedure to those patients in whom myocardial ischemia can be demonstrated at low to moderate exercise workloads.

The randomized studies in patients with chronic stable angina show that a significant number of medically treated patients developed worsening angina and required myocardial revascularization over the followup period. In CASS, the crossover rate to surgical therapy was directly related to the number of diseased vessels. The average numbers of patients requiring surgery each year for worsening symptoms were 2.0%, 4.2%, and 7.6% for patients who had one-, two-, and three-vessel disease, respectively, in CASS.

The role of coronary bypass surgery in patients with unstable angina was examined in a randomized NIH study carried out in nine medical centers in the United States of America [10]. Between 1973 and 1976, 288 patients entered the study, all of whom had transient ST-T wave changes and 90% of whom had pain while at rest. In this randomized trial, the hospital mortality rate in the last 4 years of the study was 3% in the surgical group and 2% in the medical group (not significant). The rates of inhospital myocardial infarction were 13% and 10%, respectively (not significant). No differences were observed in subsets of patients who had one, two, or three vessels affected. The data indicate that patients with unstable angina pectoris can be managed in the short term with intensive medical therapy without an increased risk of early mortality or myocardial infarction.

The role of revascularization therapy following acute myocardial infarction was examined in CASS and also by Norris et al. [5, 6, 11]. In CASS, coronary bypass surgery did not prevent recurrent myocardial infarction or improve survival over 5 years of followup in asymptomatic infarct survivors randomized an average of 9 months after infarction. In the study by Norris et al. 100 patients with few or no symptoms following myocardial infarction were randomized to surgical or medical therapy. Actuarial survival curves indicated an annual mortality rate of 3%–4% per year over 4½ years, with no advantage of surgical therapy over medical therapy.

The patients included in each of the randomized trials do not represent consecutive series of patients undergoing coronary angiography. For example, in CASS only 12.7% of the 16626 patients who underwent angiography and were screened for randomization met the entry criteria. Of this group of patients, only 780 were actually randomized. Older patients ($\geqq 65$ years), those with severe impairment of left ventricular function and an ejection fraction less than 35%, and patients who had undergone previous coronary bypass surgery were excluded. Thus, the results of none of the three randomized trials in patients with chronic stable angina can be applied to all patients undergoing coronary angiography, and indications for myocardial revascularization must be individualized for particular patients. Coronary bypass surgery improves survival in patients who have left main coronary disease greater than or equal to 50%, particularly when the left main coronary narrowing is severe or when associated obstructive right coronary disease or impaired left ventricular function is present [4].

Quality of life can be improved in patients who have mild angina following a myocardial revascularization procedure. As many as 90% of patients are improved by at least one functional class, and many are asymptomatic in the years immediately after the operation. Approximately 5% of patients per year will redevelop angina following coronary bypass surgery. Patients who relapse usually have incomplete revascularization, although postoperative changes in vein grafts or coronary arteries can also determine angina recurrence. Angina can also recur in as many as 20% of patients following coronary angioplasty in the initial 6 months following the procedure. Recurrence of angina following PTCA is usually due to restenosis, although incomplete revascularization may also be an important determinant in some patients.

At the present time, we do not recommend a myocardial revascularization procedure for patients who have mild angina and one- or two-vessel coronary disease, who can lead a relatively active life that is not compromised by the side effects of medication or by angina. We individualize the recommendation for revascularization when specific anatomic findings are present in the coronary arteries. These include left main coronary stenosis greater than 50%, proximal LAD stenosis greater than 70% associated with an obstructed right coronary artery, and severe triple-vessel disease associated with impaired left ventricular function. We tend to recommend coronary revascularization more often when myocardial ischemia occurs with only mild exertion.

In the patients who have more severe angina (class II or greater) and who fail to improve with intensive medical therapy, a revascularization procedure should be recommended. In each case, the angiographic findings should be carefully reviewed to determine to what extent myocardial revascularization can be achieved and what type of symptomatic result can be expected following the procedure. Clearly, the decision about proceeding with revascularization when only one minor artery can be revascularized will be considered on a different basis than when each of the three major arteries which supply viable myocardium can be revascularized.

Almost all patients who have unstable angina should be examined by coronary angiography to determine the coronary artery status. In patients who have left main coronary disease or triple-vessel disease a myocardial revascularization procedure is indicated. The patients who have less severe disease and who respond rapidly to medical therapy with no major evidence of myocardial ischemia on noninvasive testing could be treated with medical therapy alone, although many will ultimately require myocardial revascularization.

Similarly, patients who have variant angina and major ST segment elevation at rest with chest pain should be considered candidates for surgery when extensive coronary disease is present. The medical management of patients with variant angina differs from that of the large subset of patients with unstable angina in that beta blockers should not be given and calcium blocker drugs should be the main form of therapy, along with nitrates. The role of coronary angioplasty in patients with variant angina remains controversial. In a series reported from the Montreal Heart Institute, the 6-month incidence of restenosis or development of severe stenosis adjacent to the site of PTCA in ten patients who had variant angina and who underwent successful coronary angioplasty was 70% [12]. Further studies are required to validate this finding.

Table 3 summarizes a decision algorithm for patients with ischemic heart disease who have mild symptoms and who have already undergone coronary angi-

Table 3. Decision algorithm for patients with ischemic heart disease and mild symptoms who have undergone coronary angiography

Medical therapy	Revascularization procedure
I. Asymptomatic or mild angina and normal or near-normal LV function	
Medical therapy	*Revascularization procedure*
One, two, three vessels affected	Left main coronary disease
Isolated proximal LAD disease	Proximal LAD stenosis $\geqq 70\%$ and 100% RCA
II. Asymptomatic or mild angina and abnormal LV function	
Medical therapy	*Revascularization procedure*
One, two vessels affected	Left main or three vessels affected
Isolated proximal LAD disease	Proximal LAD stenosis $\geqq 70\%$ and 100% RCA

Modifiers: Age, associated medical illness, occupation, tolerance to major stress-induced ischemia, coronary vasospasm, degree of jeopardized myocardium, extent of revascularization
LAD, left anterior descending coronary disease

ography. Indications for medical therapy or a revascularization procedure are modified by age, associated medical illness, occupation, etc. Major stress-induced ischemia with arrhythmias would also be an indication for a revascularization procedure, even in patients who have less extensive coronary disease. Similarly, medical therapy would be the treatment of choice in patients with mild symptoms who have triple-vessel disease and left ventricular dysfunction when only a minor degree of revascularization can be achieved.

The indications for myocardial revascularization are different according as whether the procedure being considered is coronary bypass surgery or coronary angioplasty. Coronary angioplasty does not require general anesthesia, nor is there pain associated with healing or a 2- to 3-month convalescence period following surgery. Thus, some physicians would extend the indications for myocardial revascularization to patients with less severe symptoms, holding that improved revascularization invariably leads to a better prognosis and a reduced incidence of subsequent coronary events (unstable angina, myocardial infarction). At the time of this report, there have been no randomized long-term trials comparing the late results of coronary angioplasty and of medical or surgical therapy. Recent improvements in medical therapy, with favorable survival rates and decreased morbidity, should discourage attempts to perform angioplasty in patients with mild symptoms who are doing well. Coronary angioplasty has not been shown to prevent the progression of atherosclerosis and in some patients may actually result in disease progression.

The role of coronary angioplasty in patients with luminal narrowings of 50% –70% remains controversial [13]. PTCA should not be attempted if myocardial ischemia cannot be easily induced. The PTCA procedure is not innocuous and is associated with a small but fixed percentage of patients who fail the procedure and require emergency coronary bypass surgery and with a >20% incidence of restenosis, which occasionally can be worse than the original stenosis dilated.

The Role of Noninvasive Examinations

The sensitivity of most noninvasive diagnostic procedures in the detection of myocardial ischemia increases with the number of diseased vessels and the severity of the luminal narrowing. Patients with submaximal stress or those with single-vessel disease are the most difficult to assess, particularly when the luminal narrowing is less than 70% and the left circumflex or right coronary artery is the only diseased vessel. Table 4 illustrates noninvasive test results associated with an increased risk of subsequent coronary events. The specificity of electrocardiographic stress test results is decreased in the presence of an abnormal baseline ECG, digitalis, left ventricular hypertrophy, Wolff-Parkinson-White syndrome, hypokalemia, bundle branch block, hyperventilation-induced ST abnormalities, etc.

Comparison of serial noninvasive test results in the same patient over time is a useful followup procedure to determine indications for repeat coronary angiography. When the test results of sequential tests are compared over time, both laboratory conditions and drug therapy and protocol should be standardized before a change is attributed to disease progression or restenosis.

The sensitivity of exercise electrocardiography can be increased by 10%–20% when thallium-201 scintigraphy is performed in conjunction with the test. Thallium-201 scintigraphy is useful in localizing the site of coronary stenosis, whereas the exercise electrocardiogram alone is not a very good predictor of location of coronary disease. The sensitivity of thallium scintigraphy in detecting right coronary, left anterior descending, and left circumflex coronary disease is approximately 80%, 86%, and 60%, respectively. For these reasons, many investigators perform exercise thallium-201 scintigraphy before and after PTCA to monitor patients who have undergone the procedure. Scholl et al. reported the diagnostic value of exercise electrocardiography with 14 leads and thallium-201 scintigraphy in 45 patients who had successful PTCA [14]. Complete noninvasive studies had been performed before and 1 month after PTCA in 36 patients, 33 of whom had no asymptoms. The number of patients with abnormal exercise ECGs decreased from 20 to 7 ($P<0.01$) and the number with abnormal thallium-201 scintigrams, from 21 to 6 ($P<0.01$). Treadmill work time was substantially increased follow-

Table 4. Noninvasive stress test results associated with an increased risk of subsequent coronary events

ST depression >2 mm at low workloads (<5 mets)
Prolonged ST depression (>5 min) in recovery
Flat or fall in systolic blood pressure >10 mmHg with progressive exercise
Poor exercise tolerance (<5 mets)
Complex ventricular arrhythmias at low workloads
Downsloping ST segment depression
Multiple ECG leads (≧5) with ST depression ≧1 mm
Multiple or extensive thallium-201 perfusions defects
Increased lung uptake of thallium-201 after exercise
Marked exercise-induced regional left ventricular dysfunction or marked fall (>10%) in ejection fraction on radionuclide ventriculography

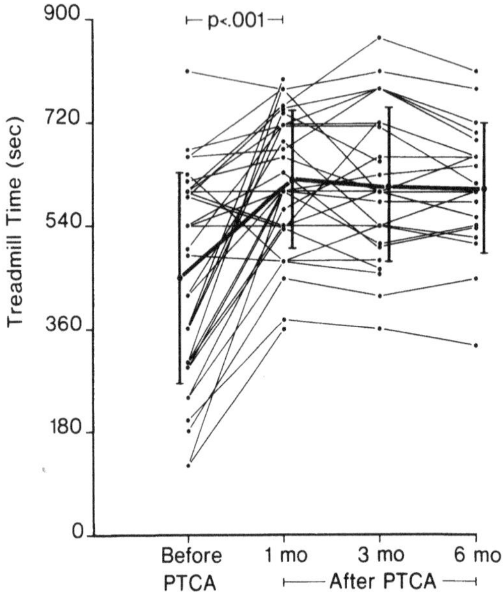

Fig. 1. Treadmill worktime before and after PTCA in patients symptom free at 1, 3, and 6 months after the procedure. (Reproduced with permission from the American Heart Association [14])

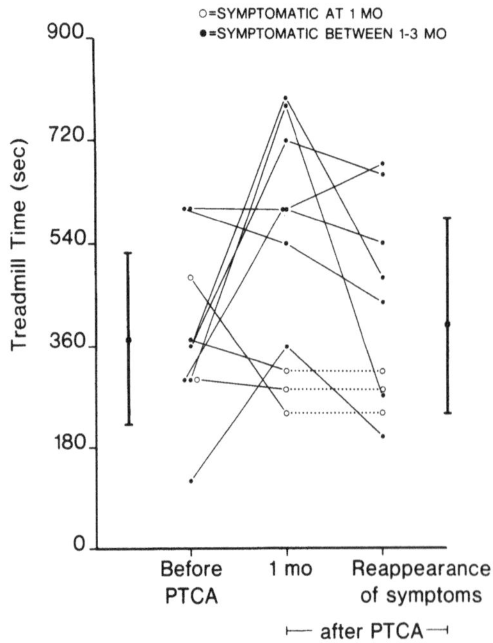

Fig. 2. Treadmill worktime before and after PTCA in patients who redeveloped anginal symptoms. Treadmill times at recurrence of symptoms were similar to those pre- and postangioplasty. At 1 month, five patients had a marked improvement in treadmill time compared with before angioplasty, but when symptoms reappeared, exercise time decreased in all patients, in some to the level achieved before PTCA, and in others to a lesser degree. (Reproduced with permission from the American Heart Association [14])

ing PTCA and was still improved 6 months after PTCA (Fig. 1). The number of symptomatic patients in whom at least one of the two tests was positive decreased from 26 to 10. Of the 10 patients with an abnormal test, 2 had a partial restenosis in excess of 50% but less than 70% at the 6-month control angiogram; two had a residual stenosis greater than 50% and a vessel that could not be dilated; and

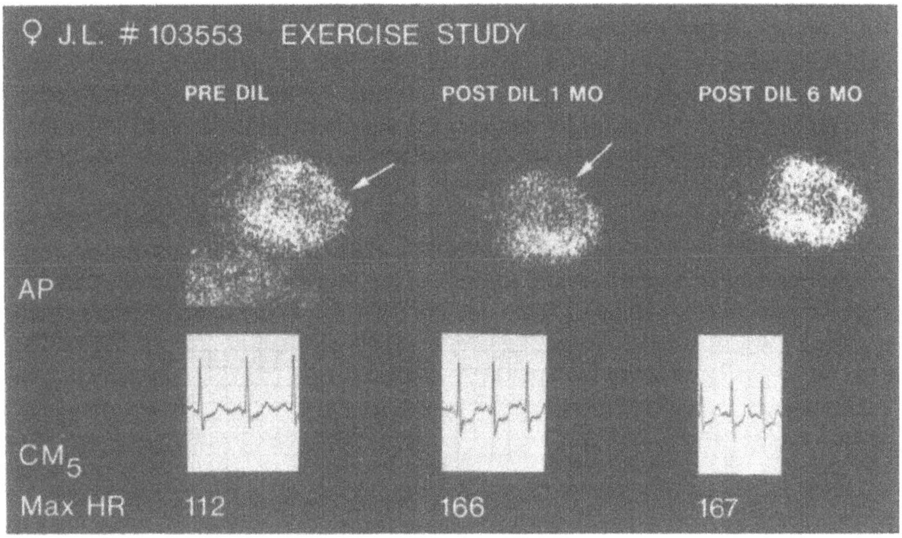

Fig. 3. An isolated LAD stenosis of 80% was dilated, reducing it to 25% in this 51-year-old woman who was in angina class III before PTCA. Following the procedure she was asymptomatic. The exercise ECG was abnormal before and at 1 and 6 months after PTCA, although the maximum heart rate achieved was substantially higher after angioplasty than before. The scintigram was abnormal before and 1 month after PTCA, but became normal 6 months later. The 6-month control angiogram revealed the same 25% stenosis in the LAD. (Reproduced with permission from the American Heart Association [14])

3 had an abnormal scintigram before and 1 month after PTCA, which subsequently became negative at 6 months. Of 10 patients who redeveloped angina within 3 months of PTCA, 9 had a restenosis in excess of 60% and 1 patient had a 90% left circumflex stenosis that could not be dilated or grafted. Treadmill time in the patients who became symptomatic following PTCA are illustrated in Fig. 2.

At 1 month after PTCA, treadmill time was markedly improved in 5 patients compared with that before angioplasty, but decreased to the level recorded before PTCA when symptoms reappeared. The difference in treadmill time before and after PTCA in the asymptomatic group (Fig. 1) is even more impressive when it is borne in mind that before PTCA the majority of patients were receiving antianginal medication, whereas few were receiving therapy following PTCA. The majority of patients in this series had single-vessel disease (Fig. 3). With the advent of complex coronary angioplasty and multiple dilatations performed during the same procedure, the evaluation of patients following PTCA is even more complex. Other investigators have reported on the diagnostic utility of exercise thallium scintigraphy and exercise testing alone to assess and follow patients after PTCA [15–20].

Intravenous dipyridamole and thallium studies can also be performed to assess PTCA results, particularly in patients unable to exercise. Dipyridamole i.v. increases coronary blood flow to three to five times that at rest. A decrease in the

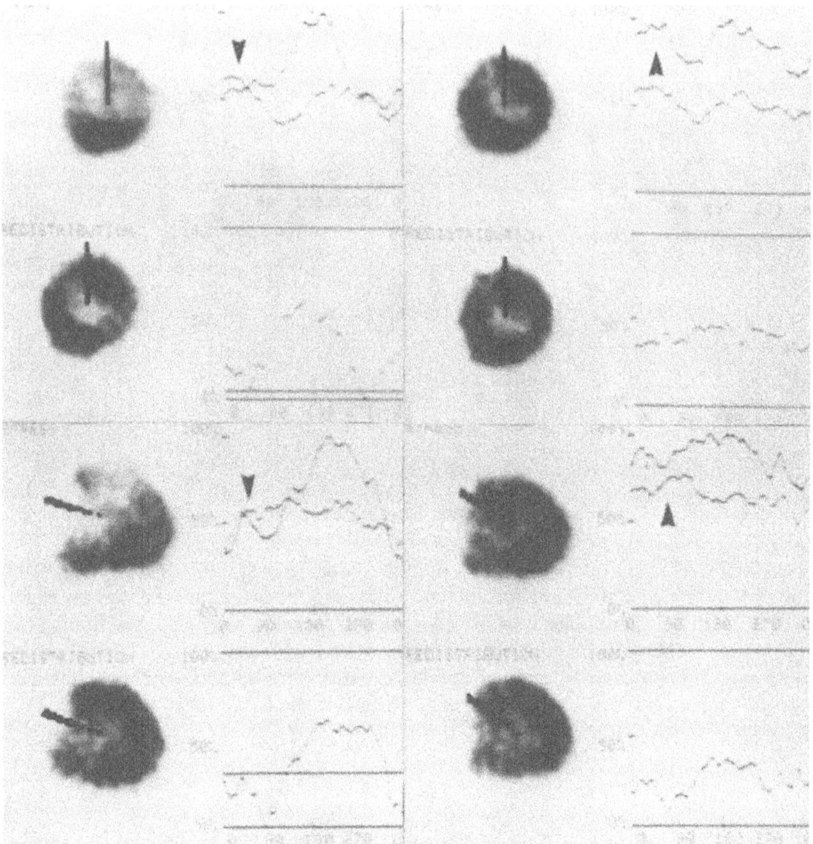

Fig. 4. i.v. dipyridamole study before PTCA: *Left upper panel,* 45° left anterior oblique (LAO) view. *Left lower panel,* anterior view; and after PTCA: *right upper panel,* 45° LAO view; *right lower panel,* anterior view. Improved myocardial perfusion to the posterolateral region (*arrow*) and septum followed successful PTCA of a 90% stenosis in a large diagonal branch and an 80% stenosis at the anastomotic site of the right coronary graft (see text)

coronary hyperemic response distal to the significant stenoses creates a relative hypoperfusion defect, which can be useful in assessing underlying coronary disease. Figure 4 illustrates the case of a 64-year-old man with class II angina 6 years after coronary bypass surgery. Coronary anatomy before PTCA showed an 80% stenosis at the site of anastomosis of the right coronary graft (trans-stenotic pressure gradient 52 mmHg), 90% proximal diagonal stenosis, and occlusion of the left circumflex coronary artery. Following PTCA, the graft stenosis was dilated to 20% with a reduction in trans-stenotic gradient to 7 mmHg. The diagonal stenosis was dilated to 20%. The occluded left circumflex vessel could not be crossed. Improved myocardial perfusion following the multivessel PTCA procedure is demonstrated by this i.v. dipyridamole thallium-201 study. The quantitative thallium-201 scans were obtained using an Elsinct 215 Apex gamma camera.

Exercise radionuclide ventriculography can also be used to assess cardiac functional status following PTCA. In a series reported by Rosing et al., 29 patients who had abnormal test results at baseline underwent a successful PTCA procedure, with supine radionuclide cineangiographic studies at rest and during exercise before and 8 months after the procedure [21]. After successful PTCA in 16 patients (52%) the positive result persisted. In 10 patients there was at least one area of regional contraction abnormality during exercise, and in 15 the ejection fraction response to exercise was abnormal. The data from this and other studies indicate that an abnormal radionuclide cineangiography study after PTCA does not necessarily indicate restenosis or a failed result [21–24]. Although Rosing's group [21–23] concluded that the abnormal results after PTCA most probably indicated subclinical ischemia, exercise radionuclide cineangiography is not as specific a test for myocardial ischemia as thallium-201 scintigraphy, and their results most probably indicate a false-positive result for restenosis.

All patients who are considered candidates for coronary angioplasty should have objective evidence of myocardial ischemia confirmed before the procedure. In patients with chronic stable angina, an exercise test without radionuclide cineangiography would suffice for most patients. However, in patients in whom complex coronary angioplasty is considered, exercise electrocardiography with thallium-201 scintigraphy will provide a more useful evaluation of angioplasty results. If only a single vessel, can be dilated, the functional importance of the remaining coronary disease and its contribution to ischemic abnormalities can best be demonstrated.

Following coronary angioplasty, exercise thallium-201 scintigraphy should be performed at 1–2 months to defect early restenosis and to serve as a baseline for subsequent followup. The test should be performed while patients are not taking any medication and during maximal stress. In the 20%–30% of patients who develop restenosis, the symptomatic status will usually suggest that restenosis has occurred. However, in patients with atypical symptoms, the exercise thallium study will often determine whether or not restenosis is present.

The assessment of successful angioplasty results 3–5 years after the procedure is complicated by the fact that disease progression in other arteries that were not dilated may cause myocardial ischemia. Restenosis is an uncommon event in patients who have a successful 1-year post-PTCA result. The presence of a markedly abnormal stress test result should be an indication for coronary angiography (Table 4), whereas excellent exercise tolerance in the absence of stress-induced ischemia should negate the need for repeat study.

Summary

The indications for coronary angioplasty in patients with mild angina pectoris embrace only those patients who are unable to tolerate medical therapy or who have an occupation which would prevent them from working even after adequate medical therapy. Whereas coronary bypass surgery has been shown to improve survival in patients with mild angina who have abnormal left ventricular function and triple-vessel coronary disease, coronary angioplasty has not, and studies are required in this patient subgroup to determine whether coronary angioplasty can improve survival in patients with triple-vessel coronary disease to a greater extent than that which could be obtained in hospitals where excellent coronary bypass surgery is performed.

In patients with more severe angina or unstable angina, coronary angioplasty is an excellent means of ameliorating symptoms, and may obviate the need for coronary bypass surgery even in patients with more extensive coronary disease. Exercise thallium-201 scintigraphy before and after coronary angioplasty is a useful procedure to assess the results of therapy and follow the patient serially over time to determine the presence or absence of a new stenosis or disease progression. Exercise electrocardiography alone and exercise radionuclide cineangiography alone are less specific tests in the followup of patients who have undergone coronary angioplasty.

References

1. Mock MB, Ringqvist I, Fisher LD et al. (1982) Survival of medically treated patients in the coronary artery surgery study (CASS) registry. Circulation 66:562
2. Ringqvist I, Fisher I, Mock M (1983) Prognostic value of angiographic indices of coronary artery disease from the coronary artery surgery study (CASS). J Clin Invest 71:1985
3. Chaitman BR, Davis K, Fisher LD (1983) A life table and Cox regression analysis of patients with combined proximal left anterior descending and proximal left circumflex coronary artery disease: non-left main equivalent lesions (CASS). Circulation 68:1163
4. Chaitman BR, Fisher LD, Bourassa MG (1981) Effect of coronary bypass surgery on survival patterns in subsets of patients with left main coronary artery disease. Am J Cardiol 48:765
5. CASS Principal Investigators and Their Associates (1984) Myocardial infarction and mortality in the coronary artery surgery study (CASS) randomized trial. N Engl J Med 310:75
6. CASS Principal Investigators and Their Associates (1983) Coronary artery surgery study: a randomized trial of coronary bypass surgery: survival data. Circulation 68:939
7. European Coronary Surgery Study Group (1982) Prospective randomized study of coronary artery bypass surgery in stable angina pectoris: a progress report on survival. Circulation 65 [Suppl II]:67
8. Kaiser GC, Davis KB, Fisher LD (to be published) Survival following CABG in patients with severe angina pectoris (CASS). J Thorac Cardiovasc Surg
9. Murphy ML, Jultgren HN, Detre K (1977) Treatment of chronic stable angina. N Engl J Med 297:621
10. Russel RO, Resnekov L, Wolk M (1978) Unstable angina pectoris: national cooperative study group to compare surgical and medical therapy. II. In-hospital experience and initial follow-up results in patients with one, two and three vessel disease. Am J Cardiol 42:839
11. Norris RM, Agnew TM, Brandt PW (1981) Coronary surgery after recurrent myocardial infarction: progress of a trial comparing surgical with nonsurgical management for asymptomatic patients with advanced coronary disease. Circulation 63:785
12. David PR, Waters DD, Scholl JM (1982) Percutaneous transluminal coronary angioplasty in patients with variant angina. Circulation 66:695
13. Ischinger T, Gruentzig AR, Hollman J (1983) Should coronary arteries with less than 60% diameter stenosis be treated by angioplasty? Circulation 68:149
14. Scholl JM, Chaitman BR, David PR (1982) Exercise electrocardiography and myocardial scintigraphy in the serial evaluation of the results of percutaneous transluminal coronary angioplasty. Circulation 66:380

15. Hirzel HO, Nuesch K, Gruentzig AR, Horst W, Krayenbuehl HP (1980) Thallium^{201} exercise scintigraphy after percutaneous transluminal angioplasty of coronary artery stenoses. Med Clin North Am 64:163
16. Hirzel HO, Nuesch K, Gruentzig AR, Luetolf UM (1981) Short- and long-term changes in myocardial perfusion after percutaneous transluminal coronary angioplasty assessed by Thallium^{201} exercise scintigraphy. Circulation 63:1001
17. Gruntzig AR, Senning A, Siegenthaler WE (1979) Nonoperative dilatation of coronary-artery stenosis. N Engl J Med 301:61
18. Cowley MJ, Vetrovec GW, Wolfgang TC (1981) Efficacy of percutaneous transluminal coronary angioplasty: technique, patient selection, salutary results, limitations and complications. Am Heart J 101:272
19. Rod JL, Foster C, Schmidt DH (1984) Evaluation of percutaneous transluminal coronary angioplasty by symptom-limited graded exercise testing. J Cardiac Rehabil 4:70
20. Meier B, Gruentzig AR, Siegenthaler WE, Schlumpf M (1983) Long-term exercise performance after percutaneous transluminal coronary angioplasty and coronary artery bypass grafting. Circulation 68:796
21. Rosing DR, Van Raden MJ, Mincemoyer RM (1984) Exercise, electrocardiographic and functional responses after percutaneous transluminal coronary angioplasty. Am J Cardiol 53:36C
22. Kent KM, Bonow RO, Rosing DR (1982) Improved myocardial function during exercise after successful percutaneous transluminal coronary angioplasty. N Engl J Med 306:441
23. Bonow RO, Kent KM, Rosing DR (1982) Improved left ventricular diastolic filling in patients with coronary artery disease after percutaneous transluminal coronary angioplasty. Circulation 66:1159
24. Sigwart U, Grbic M, Essinger A, Bischof-Delaloye A, Sadeghi H, Rivier JL (1982) Improvement of left ventricular function after percutaneous transluminal coronary angioplasty. Am J Cardiol 49:651

Chapter 4. Evaluation of the Coronary Arteriogram in Selection of Patients for Coronary Angioplasty

Thomas Ischinger

When coronary arteriograms are evaluated with a view to performing coronary angioplasty, some angiographic features need special attention. As coronary angioplasty is an attempt at "direct" treatment of coronary stenoses through transluminal access, the course and the condition of the coronary vascular bed proximal and distal to the stenosis and the morphology of the coronary stenosis are important for assessment of feasibility of the procedure and the risk of coronary vascular complications. Localization of coronary stenosis and distribution of the PTCA vessel distal to the obstruction largely determine the clinical consequences for the patient should total occlusion of the PTCA vessel occur. Both the presence or absence of angiographically visible collateral flow to or originating from the PTCA vessel and the status of the left ventricle can also influence the selection process with respect to dilatation strategy and patient safety.

Not all these criteria are of similar significance for effective performance of coronary artery bypass graft surgery; surgical accessibility and an adequate condition of the vascular bed receiving the bypass graft are the most important requirements. The operative risk is mainly determined by left ventricular function.

Coronary Anatomy

With the use of steerable and floppy guidewires failure to negotiate tortuous arteries or a single vessel curve has become rare. Tight stenoses right at the takeoff of a coronary vessel (e.g., takeoff of the left circumflex artery from the left main stem), within an acute vessel curve or at a distal location in a tortuous vessel may still represent an obstacle to the safe passage of the dilatation system and may be a potential source of complications (Fig. 1).

Technical maneuvers such as repeated manipulation with the guidewire to negotiate vessel curves or deep engagement of the guide catheter to allow more forceful advancement of the balloon catheter increase the trauma to the vessel intima. Unfortunately, it is not always possible to predict these technical problems by analyzing the coronary arteriogram. However, inability to cross coronary lesions is definitely more frequent with tight and more distal stenoses in tortuous arteries.

Acute angles in the proximal portion of the right coronary artery ("shepherd's crook" configuration) often require very delicate technical maneuvers to keep the guide catheter in a stable position and advance the dilatation system at the same time. Adequate selection and handling of the guide catheters are important and often the key to success.

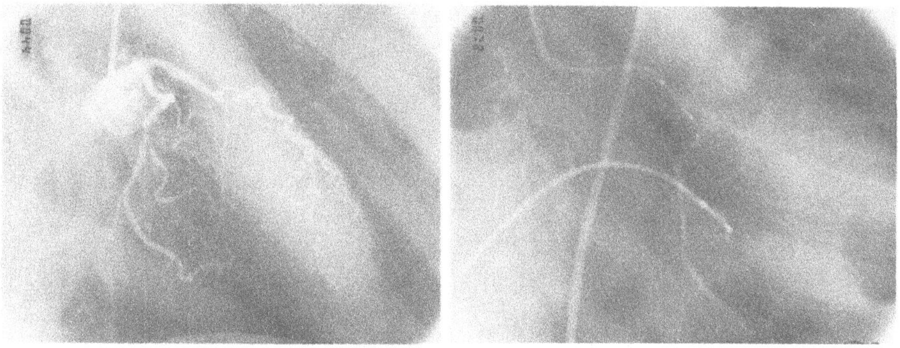

a b

Fig. 1 a, b. Tortuous left circumflex artery (RAO projection) with tight stenosis in the middle segment (**a**). Although the steerable wire was in place, negotiation of the vessel curve with the balloon catheter was impossible with the dilatation system initially chosen (RAO projection with caudal angulation) (**b**). Repeated attempts to pass the balloon catheter through the vessel curve resulted in transient vessel occlusion

Side branches, particularly side branches within vessel curves, may divert the dilatation catheter from its intended course. The availability of steerable guidewires has minimized this problem. However, if the PTCA vessel is tortuous and if many side branches arise proximal and immediately distal to the stenosis, multiple guidewires and more than the average amount of time may be required for crossing the stenosis.

Side branches whose takeoff is involved in the coronary stenosis or which originate from the area of balloon inflation gain a different significance in that they may become acutely obstructed with balloon dilatation of the artery from which they arise (Fig. 2a) [1].

The risk of iatrogenic side branch occlusion may be considerable in the case of side branches that are involved in the stenosis of the PTCA vessel (14%) (Fig. 2b), and almost negligible for nondiseased side branches originating from the area of balloon inflation [1]. Whether or not a side branch can be sacrificed depends on its distribution and functional significance in relation to the significance successful dilatation of the main artery would have for the patient. If the bifurcation of two similarly important vessels is involved (e.g., proximal LAD stenosis involving takeoff of a large diagonal branch) angioplasty may still be attempted using a modification of the "kissing balloon" technique (see chapter: Technique of PTCA – Femoral Approach).

The caliber of the coronary artery proximal and distal to the stenosis is important for selection of an adequate balloon size. The diameter of the inflated balloon should correspond to the smallest vessel diameter within the area of balloon inflation to avoid segmental overdistension. Coronary vessels of small diameter (equal to or less than 2 mm) are generally less suitable for coronary angioplasty, because minor irregularities after PTCA may significantly reduce coronary flow and eventually result in vessel occlusion.

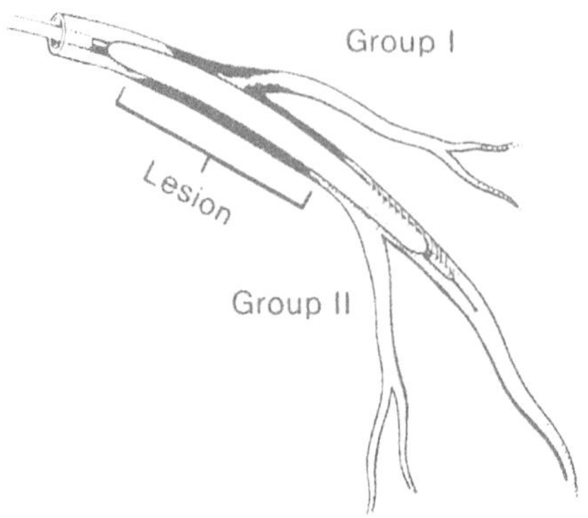

Fig. 2 a. Schematic showing two types of side branches. Group I comprises side branches originating from the lesion itself. Group II comprises side branches originating from the adjacent normal artery but still from the segment encompassed by the balloon. (From reference [1] with permission

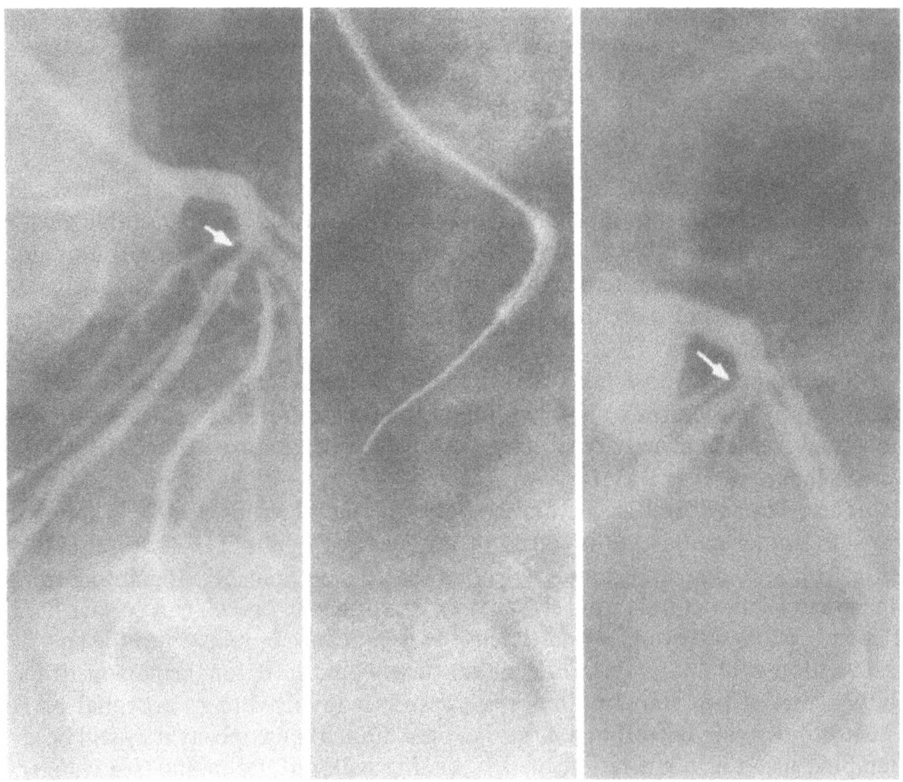

Fig. 2 b. Balloon dilatation of LAD stenosis (LAO projection) with iatrogenic occlusion of diagonal branch. The diagonal branch originates from the stenosed LAD segment and has a significant lesion at its takeoff (*arrows*)

Localization of Coronary Stenosis

With few exceptions, proximal coronary stenoses can be reached more easily with the dilatation system. Proximal stenoses have a greater functional significance and are therefore more often an indication for revascularization.

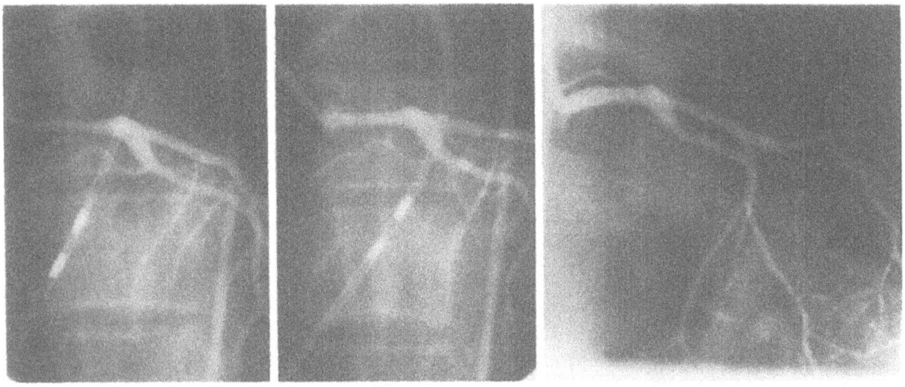

a b c

Fig. 3 a–c. Successful PTCA of left main stenosis. Angiogram before PTCA (**a**), immediately after PTCA (**b**), and at 6 months' followup (**c**)

On the other hand, dilatation of a proximal stenosis may involve a greater risk for the patient should total vessel occlusion occur. Coronary dissection caused by PTCA is usually confined to the segment of balloon inflation, but may also propagate into more proximal or distal segments [2]. Obviously, these events are very rare but not merely theoretical. Thus, dilatation of a proximal LAD stenosis just beyond takeoff of the left circumflex artery carries the potential risk of causing occlusion of the LAD and the circumflex artery at the same time. I have only experienced this once, and it had arisen during PTCA in the setting of acute myocardial infarction. In many cases of dilatation of very proximal LAD stenoses (or left circumflex stenoses) the inflated balloon comes to rest within the left main stem. If this can be anticipated from the diagnostic coronary angiogram one should make sure that the left main stem and the origin of the left circumflex artery (or the LAD) are free of disease. A nondiseased left main stem is usually larger in diameter than the inflated balloon, so that inadvertent dilatation of a nondiseased left main stem can be avoided. Coronary angioplasty for left main stenoses is technically feasible in most cases (Fig. 3). However, it may result in life-threatening situations should a local vascular complication occur, and left main stenosis is therefore not recommended as a routine indication.

Ostial lesions of the right coronary artery may be approached with caution, but technical difficulties are frequent. Stable positioning of the guide catheter for insertion of the dilatation system and during balloon inflation with the balloon across the ostial lesion – which usually requires withdrawal of the guide catheter, so that the balloon can extend into the aorta – may prove to be a difficult maneuver.

Most of the lesions suitable for PTCA that are located in the middle or distal portions of the coronary vessel can be reached and crossed with steerable dilatation systems (Fig. 4).

Coronary stenoses within sharp vessel curves appear to be associated with a higher rate of coronary vascular complications – probably due to increased shearing forces generated by inflation of the balloon within an acute angle [3] (Fig. 5;

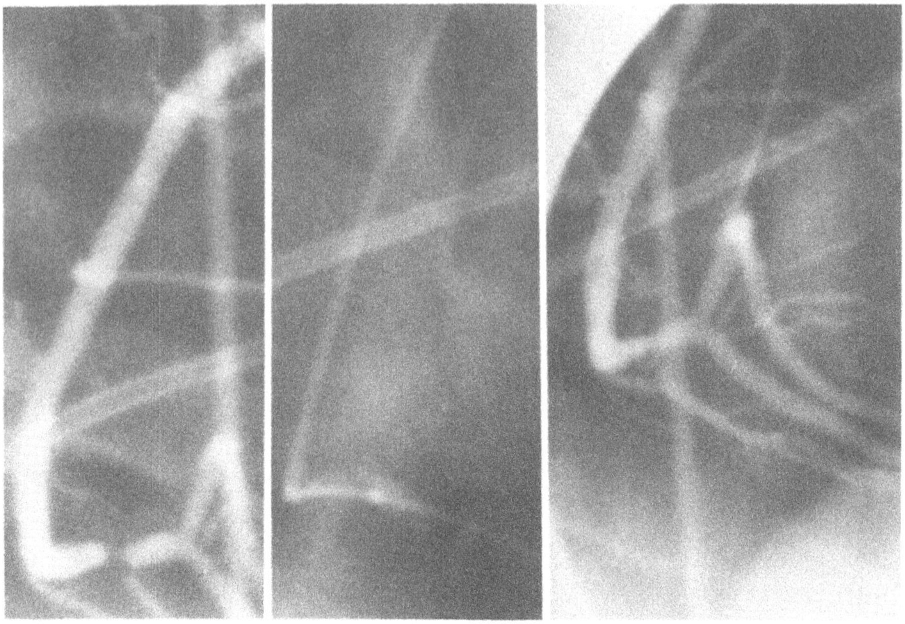

Fig. 4. Localized, concentric lesion in the distal RCA before (*left*), during (*middle*), and after PTCA (*right*)

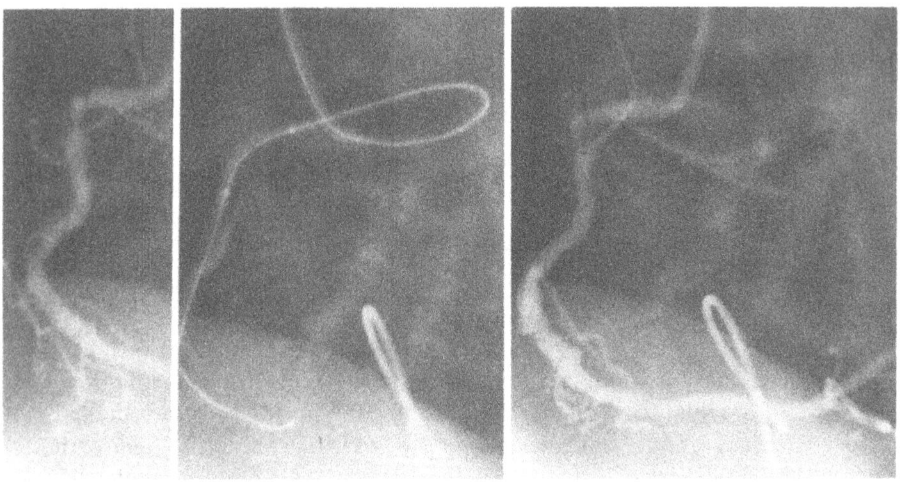

Fig. 5. PTCA of an irregular stenosis in a curve of the proximal RCA. *Left*, angiogram before PTCA; *center*, the dilatation catheter had to be propped against the aortic wall before it could be advanced through the stenosis. *Right*, coronary dissection (resembling a double channel) after PTCA

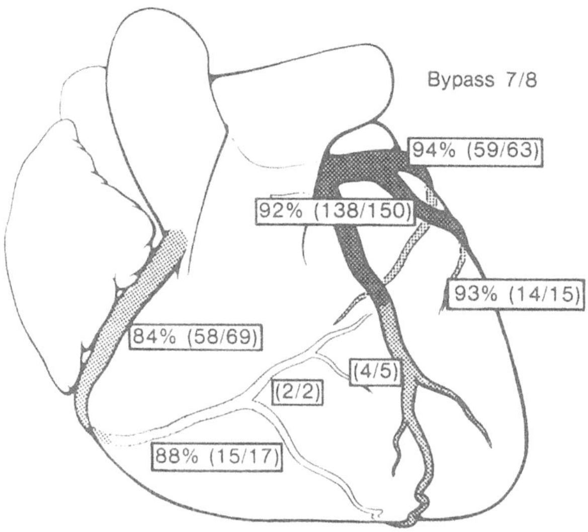

Fig. 6. Primary success rate with stenosis dilatation according to the coronary segment treated. Overall success rate 297/329 = 90%. (St. Louis PTCA results, May 1983 to January 1984)

see also Figs. 10b and 11). These stenoses have to be approached with special caution. Passage of these stenoses, particularly if they are of eccentric or irregular configuration, is best accomplished using the least traumatic soft guidewires available.

The primary success rates obtained with PTCA in the different segments of the coronary circulation have become similar since the introduction of the steerable dilatation system, but somewhat higher primary success rates and lower complication rates are still associated with PTCA in the left coronary circulation than with PTCA in the right coronary artery (Fig. 6). This may be due partly to the tortuosity of the right coronary artery, as both the difficulty of crossing the lesion and the risk of dissection by balloon inflation may be increased with lesions in vessel curves [3].

Significance of Angiographic Morphology of Coronary Stenoses

Coronary dissection and total coronary occlusion are inherent risks of coronary dilatation and account for most of the ischemic complications necessitating emergency coronary bypass surgery. The immediate risk of percutaneous coronary angioplasty is proportionate to the amount of myocardium at risk in the event of coronary occlusion. While the extent of myocardial ischemia resulting from acute coronary obstruction can be predicted from the patient's diagnostic arteriogram, the occurrence of coronary dissection or total occlusion cannot. There is no technical means of safely avoiding coronary dissection. Therefore, efforts have been made to identify angiographic criteria that may help assess the risk of local vascular complications [3–11].

In reviewing coronary arteriograms, focal coronary lesions are usually described in terms of localization and degree of stenosis. Scoring systems for interpretation of coronary arteriograms have not considered other characteristics of the angiographic morphology of the coronary lesion. Yet, atherosclerotic coronary narrowing is a complex process, which may lead to fatty, fibrous or "complicated" types of atherosclerotic plaques [12]. Complicated lesions may be associated with plaque rupture, ulceration, subintimal hemorrhage, or superimposed or recanalized thrombus [13]. These lesions may be more dangerous than fatty or fibrous coronary lesions (uncomplicated lesions) in that they may be more likely to become acutely occluded [14, 15].

It has been shown recently in a pathohistological study that the postmortem angiographic morphology of a complicated coronary lesion correlates well with the suspected histopathologic characteristics [13] (Figs. 7 and 8). Angiographically, complicated morphology of stenoses is defined as irregularity of the stenosis

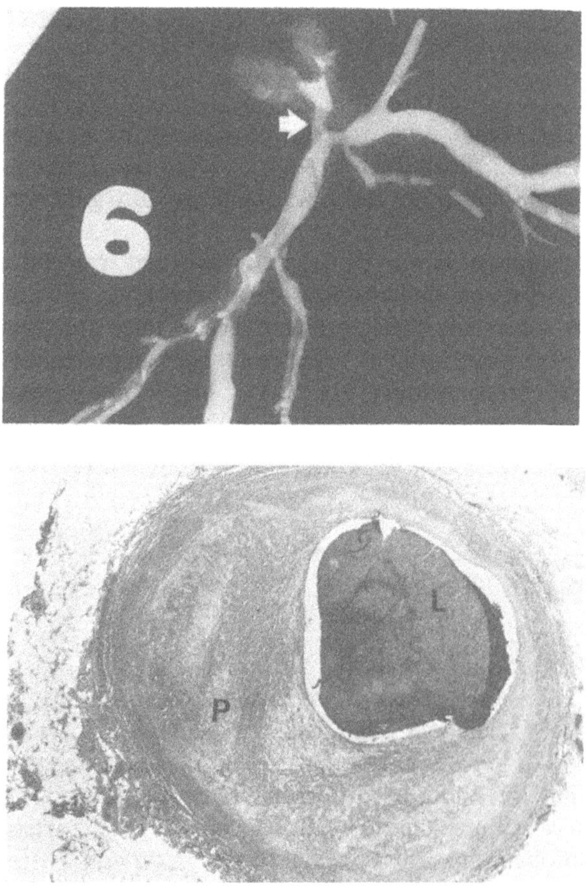

a

b

Fig. 7. a Postmortem angiogram of a smooth hourglass narrowing of the left main coronary artery (*arrow*). There are no intraluminal filling defects or irregularities. **b** The corresponding histological section reveals an eccentric lumen (*L*) resulting from a fibrous, fatty atherosclerotic plaque (*P*), and is typical of uncomplicated lesions. From reference [13] with permission

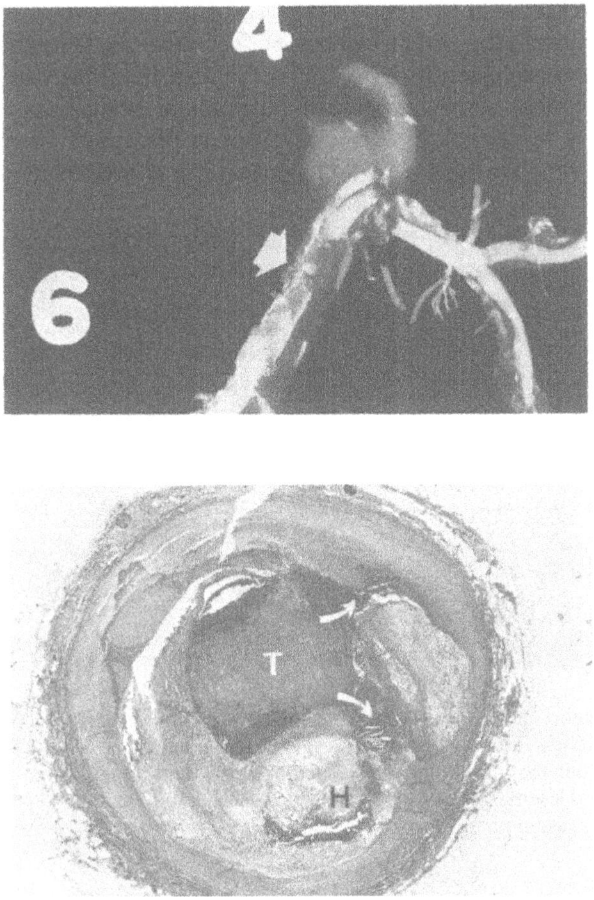

a

b

Fig. 8. a postmortem angiogram of a complicated lesion of the LAD (*arrow*). The borders of the lesion are irregular and there are intraluminal lucencies in the area of the stenosis. **b** The corresponding histologic section shows a complicated atherosclerotic plaque with plaque rupture (*arrows*), intraplaque hemorrhage (*H*) and intraluminal thrombus (*T*). From reference [13] with permission

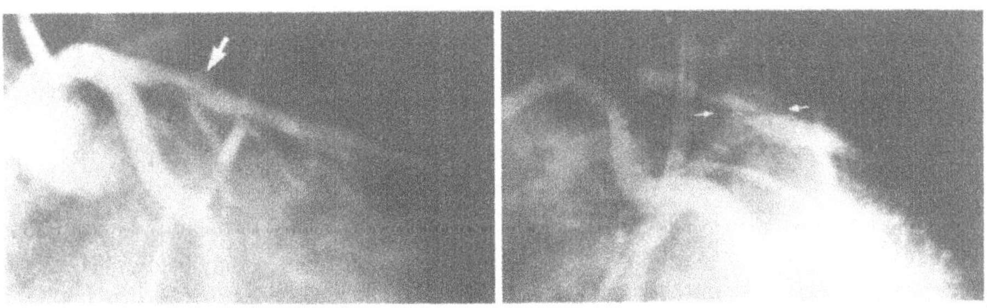

a b

Fig. 9. Angiogram of left anterior descending artery immediately before (**a**) and after (**b**) balloon dilatation. The initial coronary lesion (*arrows* in **a**) exhibits marked luminal irregularities. Balloon inflation resulted in dissection of the artery (dissection line is indicated by *arrows*, **b**) border (Fig. 9) and/or intraluminal lucency (Fig. 10 a, and b) or total disruption of the column of contrast material at the level of stenosis (Fig. 11). We have related complicated stenosis morphology to the incidence of occulsive coronary dissection and/or total coronary occlusion with PTCA [3]. The results of the study indicated that complicated lesions, i.e., stenoses with intraluminal lucencies or irregular borders, may carry a higher risk of occlusive coronary dissection. There are various mechanisms by which dissection or total occlusion may become more

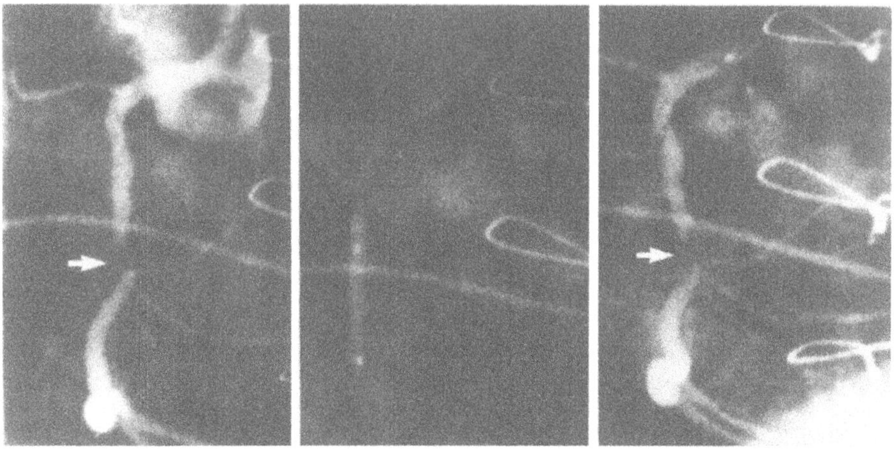

Fig. 10 a. Angiogram of the right coronary artery of a patient with previous bypass surgery before (*left*), during (*middle*), and after (*right*) balloon dilatation. Angiographic evidence of a filling defect is present (*left, arrow*). Balloon dilatation (*middle*) resulted in further compromise of coronary flow at the level of the initial lesion (*right, arrow*). The filling defect is still present and may be consistent with intracoronary thrombus

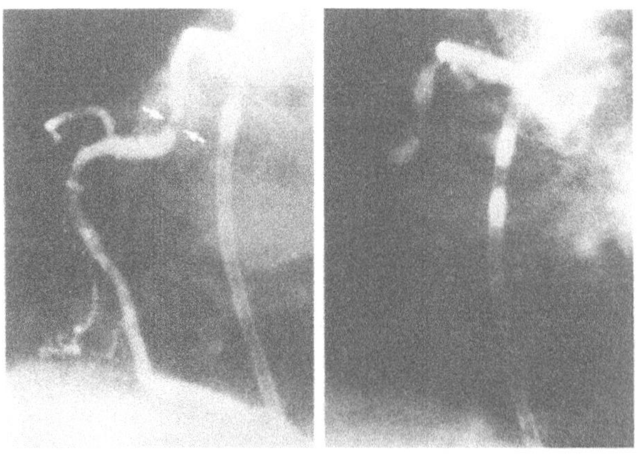

Fig. 10 b. Angiogram of the right coronary artery (*left panel*) immediately before PTCA. The stenosis (*arrows*) shows intraluminal lucency and is localized between two vessel curves. After balloon dilatation (*right panel*) the vessel is totally occluded. A membrane-like transverse disruption of the column of contrast material at the level of the stenosis is visible, possibly representing vessel obstruction by plaque material

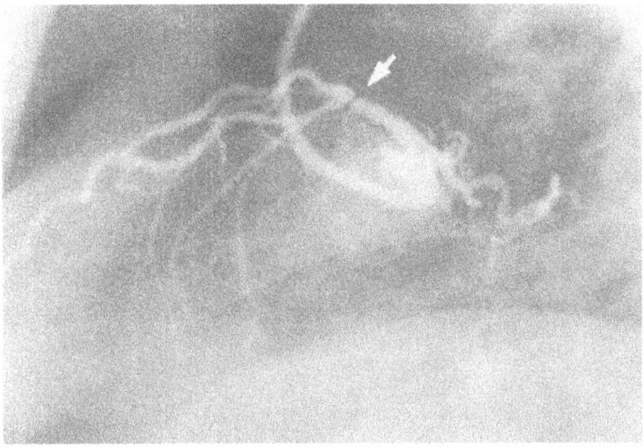

Fig. 10c. A complicated, membranelike, transverse lesion in the proximal LAD (lateral projection). There is an elevated risk of total occlusion of the lumen by these lesions following mechanical irritation of the plaque with the guidewire

likely in complicated lesions. Atherosclerotic or thrombotic material may be more easily dislodged when the stenosis is crossed or during dilatation in the case of complicated lesions. Creation of a false channel with the guidewire or dilatation catheter appears more likely inside an ulcerated lesion than in an hourglass-shaped fibrous plaque with smooth borders (Fig. 5). In my experience, tight and ulcerated lesions, particularly membrane-like transverse lesions (Fig. 10c), also carry a higher risk of total obstruction due to mechanical irritation of the plaque during the attempt to pass the lesion with the steerable guidewire. The use of very soft-tipped (floppy) guidewires is recommended in these situations.

Histologically, plaque ulceration often involves the vessel intima and media, resulting in localized weakness and decreased elasticity of the vessel wall. In these segments local overstretching, occlusive plaque rupture, and intramural hematoma formation on balloon dilatation may be more likely.

In general, eccentricity of stenosis does not have any adverse effect (Fig. 12), but sometimes even repeated dilatations cannot correct a residual narrowing, probably due to the different resistance to balloon distension of the diseased and nondiseased part of the vessel wall or a certain elasticity of the material forming the obstruction (e.g., thrombus, plaque hematoma).

Partial relapse of stenoses immediately after balloon deflation is observed more frequently with complicated or eccentric than with concentric stenoses.

The length of the coronary lesion also influences the outcome of PTCA. Coronary stenoses less than 10 mm in length are more suitable for coronary angioplasty. Longer coronary stenoses may be dilated with acceptable initial success rates [16], while the combination of complicated stenosis morphology with increased lesion length appears to increase the complication rate [7]. There is evidence that intimal tears and recurrence rates tend to be higher with PTCA of longer lesions [16].

In our experience, angioplasty of complicated and longer coronary stenoses more frequently leaves residual stenoses and more or less marked luminal irregu-

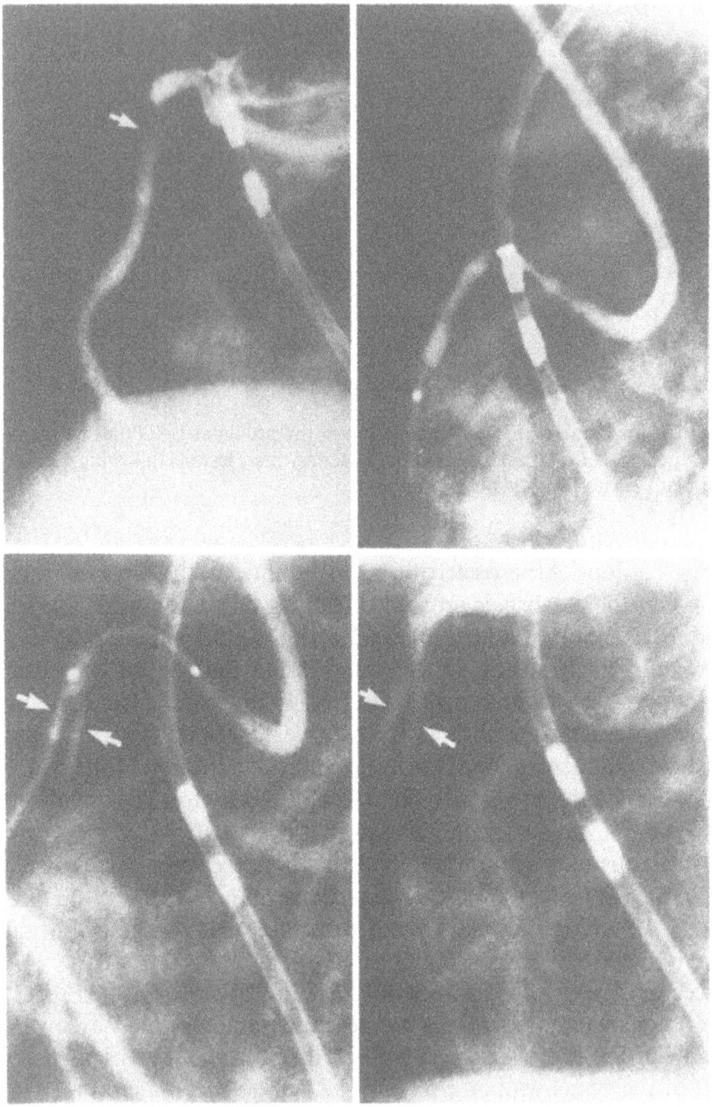

a b c d

Fig. 11. a Angiogram of the right coronary artery immediately before PTCA. Severe lesion (*arrow*) directly after a curve in the artery. Almost total disruption of the column of contrast medium is present (*arrow*). **b** Inflated balloon across stenosis. The balloon is shown to be bent by the curve of the artery. **c** Immediately after inflation of balloon, shown being withdrawn from the lesion. A double contour beginning at the distal marker of the balloon (*arrows*) is visible. **d** Control angiogram after withdrawal of balloon. Total occlusion of the artery due to dissection. The double contour is the characteristic angiographic feature of coronary dissection and is clearly visible (*arrows*)

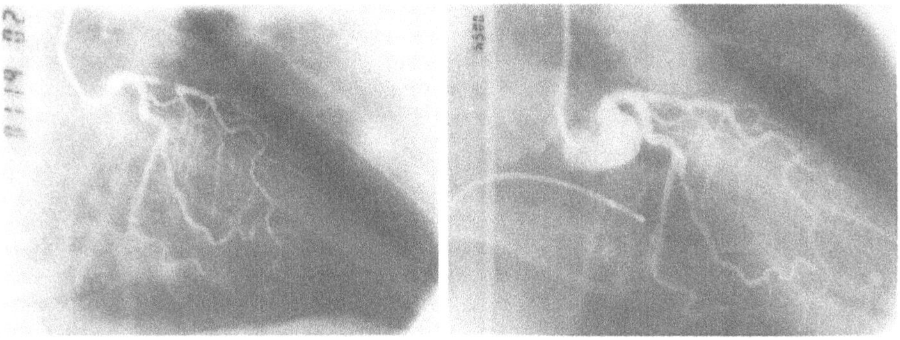

a b

Fig. 12 a, b. Eccentric lesion in the LAD (RAO projection) before (**a**) and after (**b**) successful dilatation

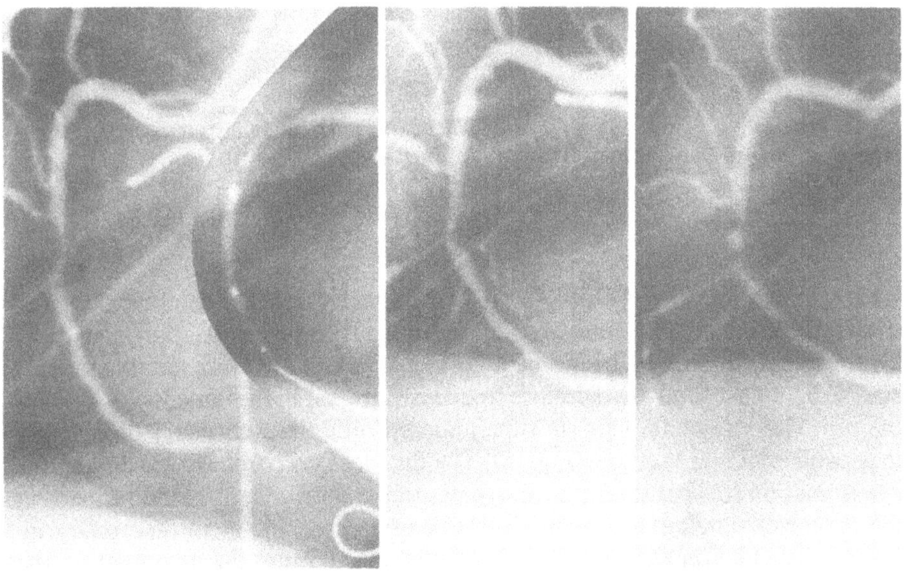

Fig. 13. From left to right: Angiogram of RCA, showing long and irregular lesion; during balloon dilatation; after successful dilatation a residual and irregular stenosis is present, repeat angiography owing to unstable angina pectoris at 6 weeks reveals tight and complicated restenosis

larities at the dilatation site, which compromise long-term vessel patency: Two cases of complicated restenoses with aneurysm formation [17] after PTCA of long and irregular stenoses have occurred in our recent experience (unpublished results from Klinikum Bogenhausen) and are illustrated in Figs. 13 and 14.

Angiographically visible calcifications in tight stenoses may make crossing of the stenoses difficult and require higher inflation pressures for adequate dilatation, but do not have other adverse effects.

In summary, the presence of complicated lesion morphology, including eccentricity and increased length of the lesion, does not constitute a contraindication

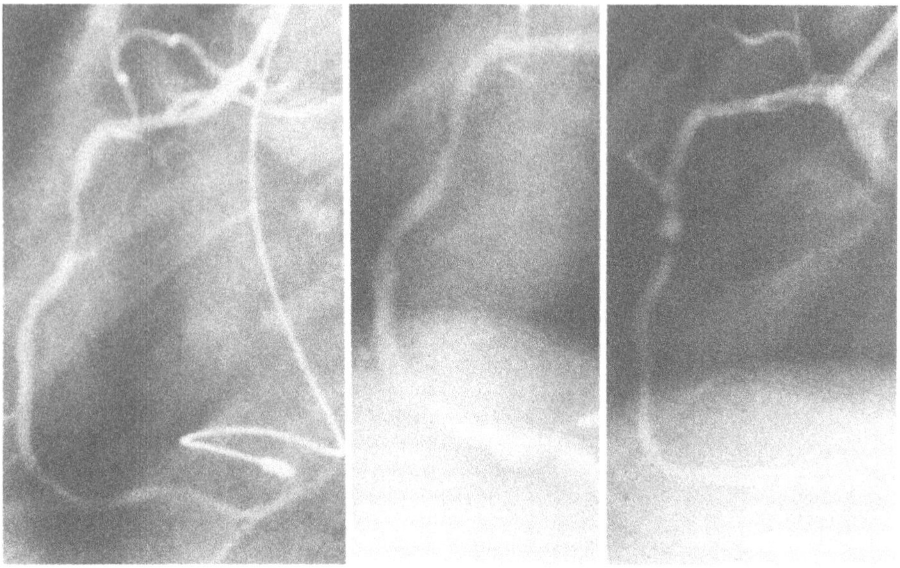

Fig. 14. From left to right: Angiogram of RCA, showing long, subtotal stenosis with total disruption of the column of contrast material; after successful dilatation; recurrent angina prompted repeat angiography at 5 weeks after PTCA, revealing severe complicated restenosis

for PTCA but may involve a higher risk of coronary vascular complication, and should therefore be taken into account when the therapeutic decision is made.

Localized, smooth and concentric coronary lesions are most suitable for coronary angioplasty and are therefore frequently present in the patients selected for the procedure. Coronary spasm superimposed on a fixed coronary obstruction may exhibit similar features (Fig. 18). The diagnosis of coronary spasm and the determination to what extent it contributes to the obstruction should be made at the diagnostic angiograms prior to PTCA using systemic or intracoronary nitrates or calcium antagonists. Coronary angioplasty is not the treatment of first choice for morphologically ideally suited yet "mixed" stenoses that are mainly produced by vasospasm. The rational of performing PTCA in these situations is discussed further in Chap. 18.

Degree of Coronary Stenosis

The minimal luminal diameter and, to a lesser extent, the length of a stenosis determine the hemodynamic significance of a coronary lesion [19–22]. In clinical practice the percentage diameter reduction, with the nondiseased adjacent luminal diameter serving as reference, is used to express lesion severity. In the presence of extensive, diffuse disease and vessel ectasia, the assessment of percentage stenosis becomes a less precise estimate of lesion significance, as the "normal" vessel segments are difficult to identify. The potential of a coronary lesion for decreasing myocardial perfusion depends on the coronary flow rate. Hyperemic coronary flow with fully utilized coronary reserve may be reduced by a stenosis occupying 50% of the luminal diameter, whereas resting coronary flow can remain normal even with an 80% stenosis. Although there is no general agreement on the degree of narrowing that constitutes significant stenosis, a lesion causing a reduction of more than 60% in the luminal diameter (corresponding to a stenosis of more than 84% of the cross section) are considered to represent clinically significant coronary artery disease. Tight stenoses of more than 80%–90% are frequently associated with angina at rest. In such tight stenoses even a minimal increase of the narrowing – due to morphological changes of the stenoses or to vasomotor tone – may result in a marked reduction in coronary blood flow [20]. As the risk of cardiac events and disease progression rises with increasing severity of disease, the degree of stenosis also carries a prognostic significance [23, 24]. Symptomatic patients with tight stenoses should therefore undergo revascularization as quickly as possible.

In rare instances, tight stenoses will not allow passage of the balloon catheter. This is the case especially with tight, calcified, and distal stenoses. Angiographically the residual lumen of a coronary stenosis often appears to be less than the size of the deflated balloon. Yet the catheter can be passed, probably because the material forming the obstruction is giving way. High-grade stenoses alone should not discourage an attempt at PTCA, because passage of the balloon can hardly be predicted.

The average degree of stenosis before PTCA in the Emory patients was 72% ±14% of the diameter, ranging from less than 50% to total occlusion. Analyses of the data of these patients showed that the mean degree of stenosis before PTCA was greater in patients in whom the procedure was unsuccessful and/or complicated than in patients in whom it was successful (76% vs 72% stenosis) [25].

The recent results from the PTCA Registry also indicate a higher rate of coronary vascular events with PTCA in stenoses occupying more than 90% of the lumen [9–11].

Passage of the dilatation system through extremely tight stenoses is a delicate operation, because even minimal mechanical irritations of the atherosclerotic plaque may induce total coronary occlusion. Also, the discrepancy between the minimal lumen at the point of the stenosis and the size of the inflated balloon that fits the nondiseased part of the artery may be pronounced and potentially increase the risk of dissection on balloon dilatation. Therefore to minimize vessel trauma we sometimes tend to choose a smaller balloon than would normally be deemed adequate with reference to the caliber of the arterial segments adjacent to the stenosis. The use of a tandem balloon may also be helpful in these situations.

If residual stenosis is present after PTCA early repeat angiography during followup may be selected.

Mild coronary stenoses (less than 60% diameter reduction) can usually be crossed with ease, and dilatation can be performed with a high primary success rate in such cases [8]. However, complications, including myocardial infarctions, may occur. Also, tight restenosis exceeding the original lesion in severity may de-

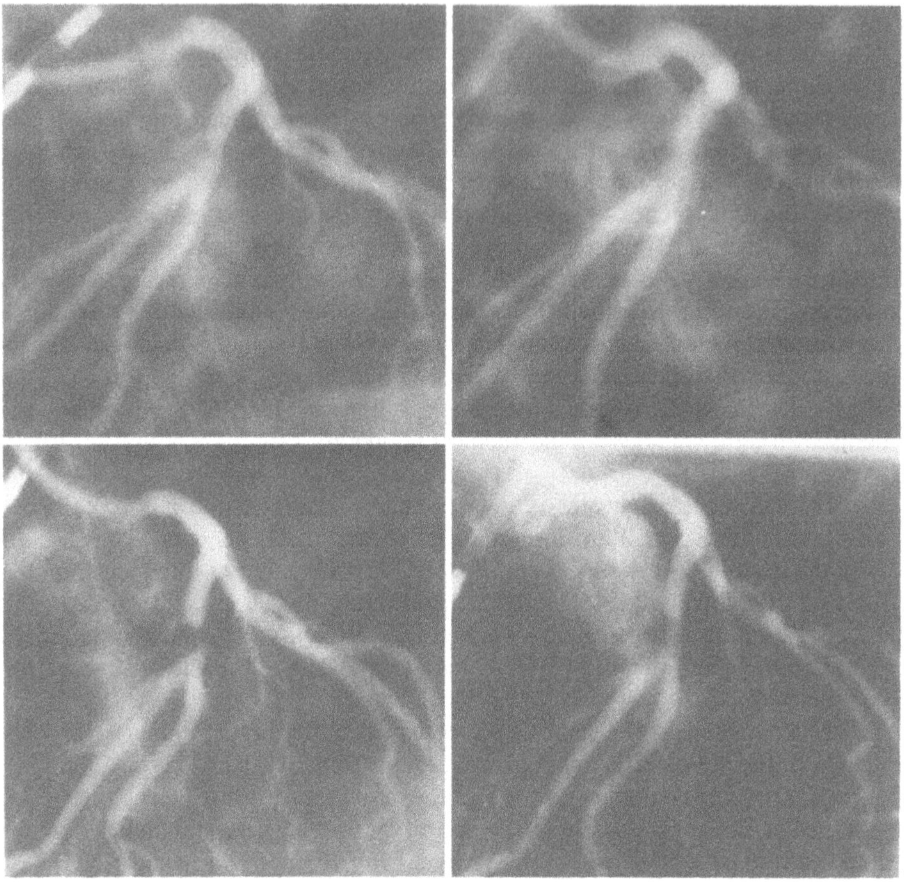

a b c d

Fig. 15 a–d. Coronary angiogram (LAO projection) of LAD. **a** Proximal LAD stenosis of 48% (diameter stenosis, mean of three projections). **b** Stenosis after successful PTCA was 27%. **c** Recurrent angina pectoris 3 months after PTCA prompted repeat angiography revealing subtotal restenosis. **d** Repeat PTCA reduced stenosis to 30%. (From [8] with permission)

velop – possibly reflecting acceleration of the disease process by PTCA (Fig. 15). Therefore PTCA of mild stenoses must not be taken lightly and requires a sound clinical indication.

Chronic total coronary occlusion by itself is not a contraindication for coronary angioplasty. In selected patients whose coronary anatomy suggests success of a recanalization attempt of the occluded vessel, angioplasty may be effective in restoring vessel patency and improving the degree of revascularization of ischemic myocardium [26–28]. If perfusion of ischemic myocardium is not likely to improve recanalization of an occluded vessel is usually not indicated, unless it is part of the strategy during a complex PTCA procedure. The mere prognostic value reopening of occluded vessels could have for patients with progressive coronary artery disease has not yet been determined.

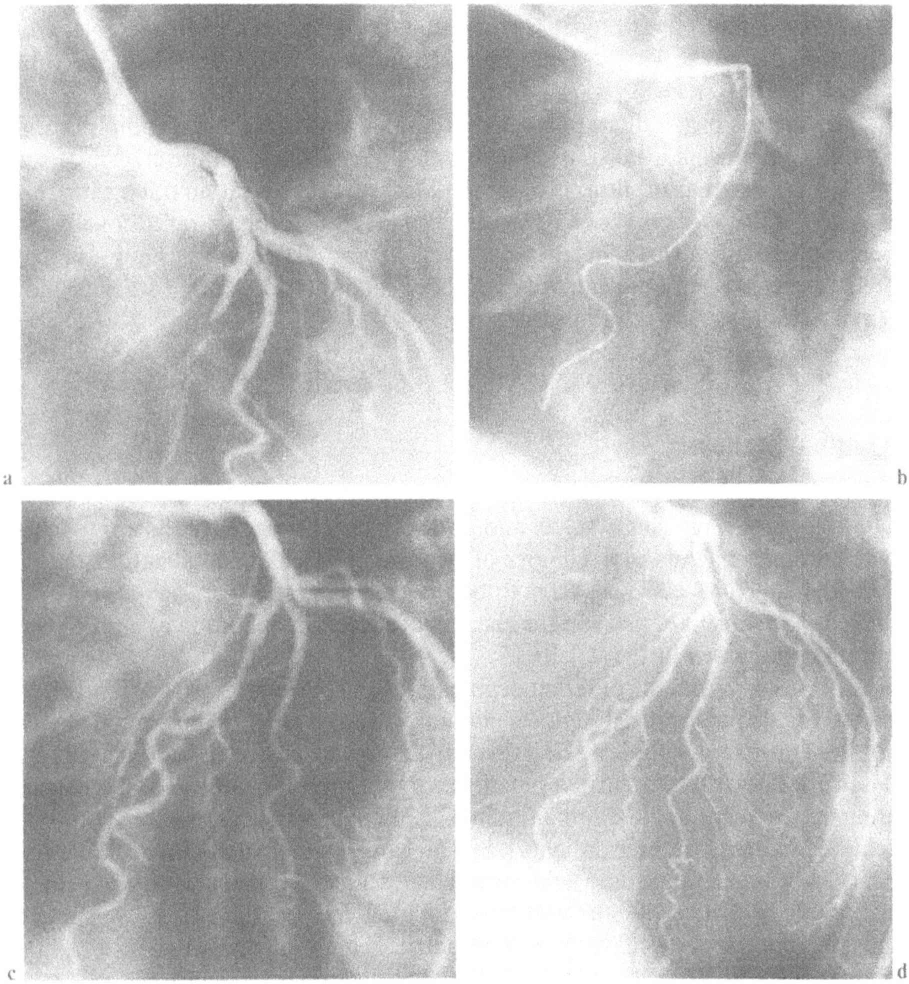

Fig. 16. a Total occlusion of LAD (LAO, cranial projection). The site of occlusion is clearly visible and the course of the vessel can be anticipated from the faint opacification distal to the occlusion. **b** Wire in LAD. **c** Successful recanalization of LAD with residual stenosis and border irregularities (probably representing intimal tear). **d** Control angiography at 6-month followup shows further improvement of LAD patency

Certain precautions must be taken when dilatation of a completely occluded artery is planned, since ischemic complications are not precluded in this situation (see also Chap. 5, p. 54). Usually, the viable myocardium in the territory of the occluded vessel is perfused by ipsi- or contralateral collaterals. Care must be taken not to jeopardize the collateral circulation by the attempt at dilatation. The course of the distal vessel must be known from a recent angiogram or from visualization by collateral filling. A funnel-like "nub" of the coronary artery at the site of occlusion helps determine the proper direction for the dilating catheter and makes attempts at recanalization safer. Figure 16 shows an example of successful

PTCA recanalization of a totally occluded LAD. For such recanalization attempts we commonly use over-the-wire dilatation systems with steerable wires that are not too soft (e.g., Schneider-Medintag or USCI 0.0014-in. steerable wire).

The success of the dilatation attempt also depends on the duration of occlusion. In more recent occlusions of less than 4 weeks' duration the chance of success is high, whereas occlusions of more than 2 months' duration often cannot be recanalized. The feasibility of PTCA in chronic total coronary occlusions is particularly relevant for patients on the waiting list for PTCA who sustain total coronary occlusion without evidence of myocardial infarction, in that some of them remain candidates for angioplasty.

Multiple Stenoses

Multiple stenoses in single-vessel and multiple-vessel disease can be approached with coronary angioplasty. The risk of a coronary vascular complication and the hemodynamic consequences have to be assessed separately for each lesion to be dilated. Assessment of risk and the chances of success in dilatation of multiple stenoses are discussed further Chap. 15.

Localized disease in different segments of one coronary artery (tandem lesions) (Fig. 17) or localized stenoses in multiple vessels (Fig. 18) may often be suitable for coronary angioplasty. However, with more extensive disease diffusely stenosed arteries with complicated stenotic morphology and a damaged left ventricle are more frequent angiographic findings. Complete revascularization cannot be achieved in many of these patients [28]. If it can be anticipated that multiple coronary bypass grafting would achieve a higher degree of revascularization with an acceptable operative risk the patient should undergo surgery. In a few patients only, incomplete revascularization and partial relief of the ischemic insult to the myocardium by dilatation of the most critical stenosis may be justified.

For additional considerations concerning complex PTCA see Chap. 15.

Protective Role of Coronary Collaterals

Coronary collaterals are interconnecting anastomotic vessels that link segments of the same artery (intracoronary collaterals) and segments of different arteries (intercoronary collaterals). Angiographically, these arterial communications become visible when their diameter exceeds 100 μm. With normal or only mildly obstructed coronary circulation these interconnecting anastomoses carry minimal flow and are too small for angiographic visualization. When significant coronary obstruction occurs the distal coronary pressure usually falls, thus inducing a transanastomotic pressure gradient. This transanastomotic pressure gradient leads to increased blood flow through the arterial anastomosis into the territory

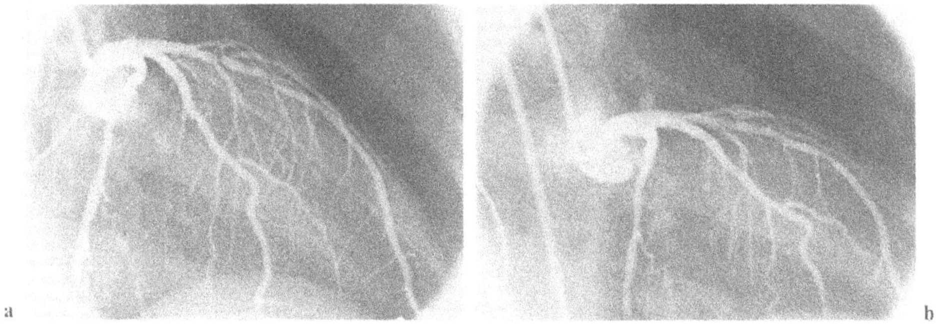

Fig. 17 a, b. Tandem stenoses in LAD (RAO projection) before and after PTCA

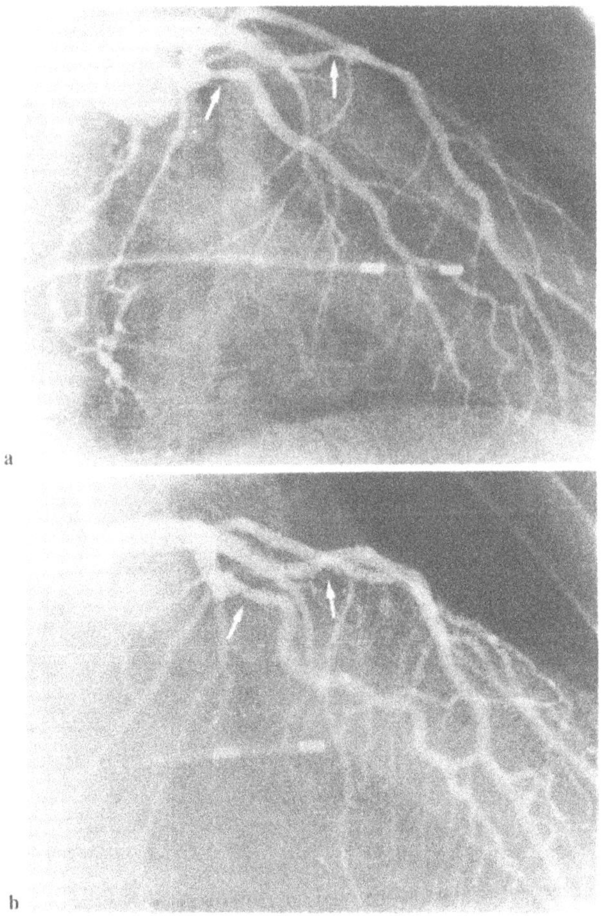

Fig. 18. Localized stenoses in LAD and proximal left circumflex artery (*arrows*) before (**a**) and after (**b**) PTCA

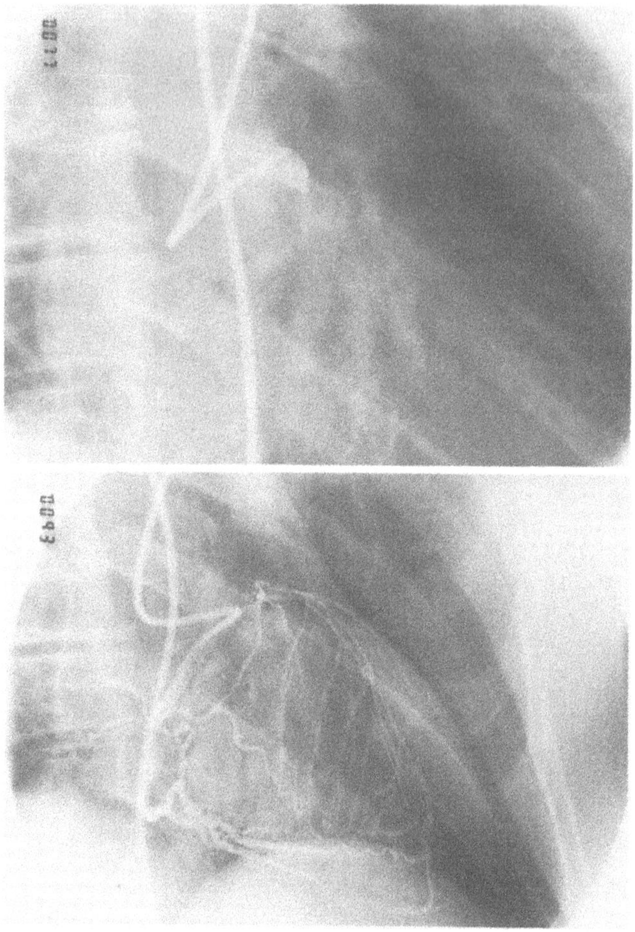

a

b

Fig. 19. Injection of the left MCA (**a**) revealing total occlusion of the left main stem (42-year-old male patient with stable angina pectoris) and of the RCA, (**b**) showing collateral filling of the LAD and the left circumflex system. The left ventricular ejection fraction was normal

of the obstructed artery. With increasing flow, these interconnecting vessels progressively dilate and become angiographically visible coronary collaterals [29].

Thus, development of angiographically demonstrable coronary collateral circulation usually represents an adaptation to obstructive coronary artery disease. The growth of these collateral vessels seems to depend on the duration of the transanastomotic pressure gradient. In patients with acute myocardial infarction and a history of angina pectoris, angiographically visible coronary collaterals were more frequent than in infarct patients without any history of angina pectoris [30]. The extent to which coronary collateral circulation can preserve myocardial tissue is variable and depends on the flow capacity of the collaterals and the amount of myocardium they serve. Figure 19 shows the coronary angiogram of a 45-year-old man with long-standing stable angina pectoris. The left main stem was totally occluded and left ventricular function was normal owing to a well-developed collateral circulation from the right coronary artery.

Coronary blood flow through collateral vessels is frequently sufficient at resting conditions but cannot meet increased demands [31, 32]. Therefore, most of the patients with viable myocardium supplied by collateral flow have more or less marked signs of exercise-induced myocardial ischemia. If collateral circulation originates from a nondiseased vessel the prognosis is better than that of ischemia due to a high-grade coronary lesion with imminent progression to total coronary occlusion.

Clinical studies suggest that patients with developed collateral vessels have smaller infarcts and lower infarct mortality [33–35]. Following acute occlusion of a coronary artery, blood flow into the infarct area by collateral circulation may persist, and even if myocardial infarction is not avoided the size of the infarct may be kept small. Also, residual flow into the postocclusion territory may be improved by means of drugs (e.g., nitrates) or by mechanical means (intra-aortic balloon pump).

Similarly, patients with effective collateral circulation are less likely to suffer severe left ventricular damage in the case of total vessel occlusion during PTCA and may not need emergency coronary bypass surgery. When coronary collaterals are visible on the pre-PTCA diagnostic angiogram there is a tendency to approach the procedure in a more relaxed attitude. However, experience has taught us that angiographically well-developed collaterals do not necessarily guard against severe myocardial ischemia or myocardial infarction in the case of acute iatrogenic vessel occlusion [36] (Fig. 20c). Again, angiographic visualization of coronary collaterals depends (a) on the existence of interconnecting anstomotic vessels and (b) on the balance of the distal perfusion pressures in the interconnecting arteries. Coronary angiography only demonstrates collaterals that are in operation. Potentially functional (recruitable) collaterals are not visualized angiographically.

This can easily be demonstrated by the angiographic disappearance of coronary collateral flow after successful PTCA, indicating a significant increase of antegrade flow in the dilated artery (Fig. 20).

Collateral function can be assessed during coronary angioplasty by measuring distal coronary pressure via the balloon catheter during balloon inflation (distal occlusion pressure or coronary wedge pressure) [37, 38]. These pressure measurements have to be made at low balloon inflation pressures of 1–2 atm to avoid compressing the pressure lumen of the balloon and creating an artefact. Correlation of distal occlusion pressures with angiographic documentation of collateral flow during balloon occlusion of the vessel to be treated by PTCA indicates that distal occlusion pressures of more than 30 mmHg can be considered suggestive of functional collaterals [37]. It has also been shown during coronary angioplasty that the peripheral coronary artery pressure in totally occluded arteries is significantly higher than in arteries with less significant obstruction [39]. These results correspond to intraoperative measurements of distal coronary pressure, which was found to be around 20% of aortic pressure with normal coronary circulation and up to 40% of aortic pressure in patients with significant coronary artery disease [40]. The prediction of recruitable collaterals on the basis of the coronary

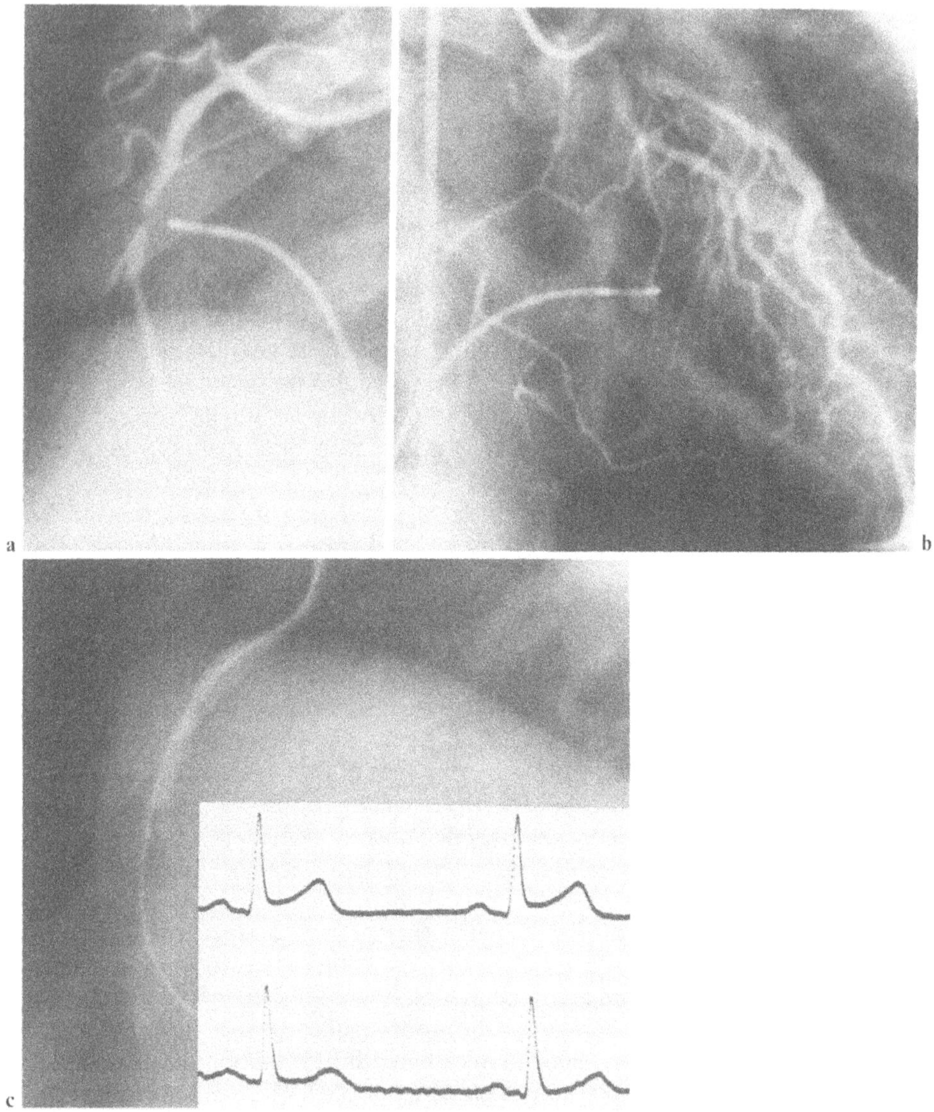

Fig. 20. a The pre-PTCA angiogram of the RCA shows subtotal occlusion in the middle segment. **b** Injection into the left coronary artery allows visualization of well-developed collateral vessels to the territory of the RCA. **c** Balloon dilatation of RCA stenosis. During balloon inflation the patient developed angina pectoris associated with ST elevation (*upper tracing*). Normalization of the ECG (*lower tracing*) after balloon deflation. **d** Successful PTCA result. **e** After successful PTCA of the RCA stenosis injection of the left coronary artery is no longer followed by visualization of collateral vessels

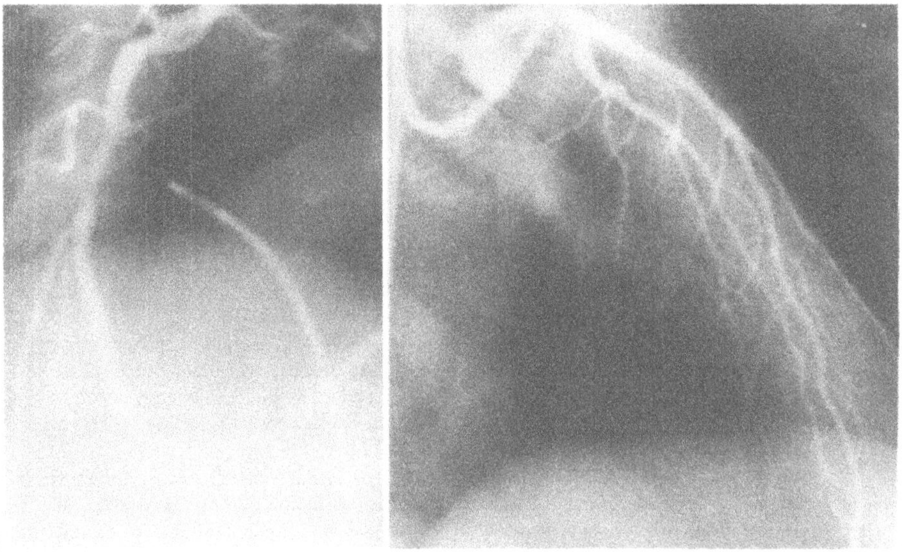

Fig. 20d, e

wedge pressure during coronary angioplasty may be of practical value for patient management should total occlusion of the PTCA vessel occur immediately or some time after the procedure.

The significance of coronary collaterals becomes reversed when they originate from the PTCA vessel and supply a substantial amount of viable myocardium. The total amount of myocardium at risk and the potential hemodynamic insult to the left ventricle in the case of a complication may then be enormous. These are high-risk situations that must be understood by the physician and the patient. If angioplasty still seems the best therapeutic choice, then it is sometimes worthwhile to attempt recanalization of the vessel receiving collateral flow first, to provide for potential reverse collateral flow in case of acute or late coronary events.

References

1. Meier B, Gruentzig AR, King SB, Douglas JS, Hollman J, Ischinger T, Aueron F, Galan K (1984) Risk of sidebranch occlusion during coronary angioplasty. Am J Cardiol 53:10
2. Zack PM, Ischinger T (1985) Late progression of an asymptomatic intimal tear to occlusive coronary artery dissection following angioplasty. Cathet Cardiovasc Diagn 11:41
3. Ischinger T, Gruentzig AR, Meier B, Galan K (1985) Coronary dissection and total coronary occlusion with percutaneous transluminal coronary angiplasty (PTCA): significance of initial angiographic morphology of coronary stenoses. Circulation (in press)
4. Dorros G, Cowley JM, Simpson J, Bentivoglio LG, Block PC, Bourassa M, Detre K, Gosselin AJ, Gruentzig AR, Kelsey SF, Kent KM, Mock MB, Mulhin SM, Myler RK, Passamani ER (1983) Percutaneous transluminal coronary angioplasty: report of complications from the NHLBI PTCA Registry. Circulation 67:723–730

5. Kent KM, Bentivoglio LG, Block PC, Cowley MJ, Dorros G, Gosselin AJ, Gruentzig AR, Myler RK, Simpson J, Stertzer SH, Williams DO, Fisher L, Gillespie MJ, Detre K, Kelsey S, Mullin SM, Mock MB (1982) Percutaneous transluminal coronary angioplasty. Report from the Registry of the NHLBI. Am J Cardiol 49:2011
6. Cowley MJ, Vetrovec GW, Wolfgang TC (1981) Efficacy of percutaneous transluminal coronary angioplasty: technique, patient selection, salutary results, limitations and complications. Am Heart J 101:272
7. Meier B, Gruentzig AR, Hollman J, Ischinger T, Bradford JM (1983) Does length or eccentricity of coronary stenoses influence the outcome of transluminal dilatation. Circulation 67:497
8. Ischinger T, Gruentzig AR, Hollman J, King SB, Douglas JS, Meier B, Bradford J, Tankersley R (1983) Should coronary arteries with less than 60% diameter stenosis be treated by angioplasty? Circulation 68:148
9. Cowley MJ, Dorros G, Kelsey SF, Raden MV, Detre KM (1984) Acute coronary events associated with percutaneous transluminal coronary angioplasty. Am J Cardiol 53:12 C
10. Cowley MJ, Dorros G, Kelsey SF, Raden MV, Detre KM (1984) Emergency coronary bypass surgery after coronary angioplasty: The NHLBI Percutaneous Transluminal Coronary Angioplasty Registry experience. Am J Cardiol 53:22 C
11. Dorros G, Cowley MJ, Janke L, Kelsey SF, Mullin SM, Raden MV (1984) In-hospital mortality rate in the NHLBI PTCA Registry. Am J Cardiol 53:17 C
12. Roberts WC (1972) Coronary arteries in fatal acute myocardial infarction. Circulation 45:215
13. Levin DC, Fallon JT (1982) Significance of the angiographic morphology of localized coronary stenoses: histopathologic correlations. Circulation 66:316
14. Friedman M (1965) The coronary canalized thrombus. Provenance, structure, function and relationship to death due to coronary artery disease. Br J Exp Pathol 80:256
15. Ridolfi RL, Hutchings GM (1977) Relationship between coronary artery lesions and myocardial infarcts: ulceration of atherosclerotic plaques precipitating coronary thrombosis. Am Heart J 93:468
16. Hall DP, Gruentzig AR (1984) Influence of lesion length on initial success and recurrence rates in coronary angioplasty. Circulation 70:(II)176 (abstract)
17. Hill JA, Margolis JR, Feldman RL, Conti CR, Pepine CJ (1983) Coronary arterial aneurysm formation after balloon angioplasty. Am J Cardiol 52:261
18. Bentivoglio LG, Leo LR, Wolf NM, Meister SG (1983) Frequency and importance of unprovoked coronary spasm in patients with angina pectoris undergoing percutaneous transluminal coronary angioplasty. Am J Cardiol 51:1067
19. Gensini GG (1975) Coronary arteriography. Futura, Mount Visco, pp 240–326
20. Gould KL, Lipscomb K (1974) Effects of coronary stenoses on coronary flow reserve and resistance. Am J Cardiol 34:48
21. Wüsten B (1979) Biophysics of coronary artery narrowing. In: Schaper W (ed) The pathophysiology of myocardial perfusion. Elsevier/North Holland Biomedical, Amsterdam, p 285
22. Feldman RL, Nichols WW, Pepine CJ, Conti CR (1978) Hemodynamic significance of the length of a coronary arterial narrowing. Am J Cardiol 41:865
23. Bruschke AVG, Wijers TS, Kolsters W, Landmann J (1981) The anatomic evolution of coronary artery disease demonstrated by coronary angiography in 256 non-operated patients. Circulation 63:527
24. Proudfit NL, Bruschke ABG, Sones FM (1978) Natural history of obstructive coronary artery disease: ten year study of 601 non-surgical cases. Prog Cardiovasc Dis 21:53
25. Ischinger T, Gruentzig AR, Meier B (1983) Perkutane transluminale Koronarangioplastie (PTCA): Ursachen und Häufigkeit von Notfalloperationen. Z Kardiol 72:(II)–66 (abstract)
26. Savage R, Hollman J, Gruentzig AR, King SB, Douglas JS, Tankersley R (1982) Can percutaneous transluminal coronary angioplasty be performed in patients with total occlusions? Circulation 66:330
27. Holmes DR, Vlietstra RE, Reeder GS, Breshnahan JF, Smith HC, Bove AA, Schaff HV (1984) Angioplasty in total coronary artery occlusion. J Am Coll Cardiol 3:845

28. Vandormael MG, Chaitman BR, Ischinger T, Aker UT, Harper M, Hernandez J, Deligonul U, Kennedy HL (1985) Immediate and short term benefit of multilesion coronary angioplasty: influence of degree of revascularization. J Am Coll Cardiol (in press)
29. Newman PE (1981) The coronary collateral circulation: determinants and functional significance in ischemic heart disease. Am Heart J 102:431
30. Karsch KR, Blanke H, Schlueter M, Rentrop P (1981) Relationship between collaterals and history of angina pectoris in acute myocardial infarction. Circulation 64:(IV)107
31. Goldberg HL, Goldstein J, Borer JS, Moses JW, Collins MB (1984) Functional importance of coronary collarteral vessels. Am J Cardiol 53:694
32. Flameng W, Schwarz F, Hehrlein FN (1978) Intraoperative evaluation of the functional significance of coronary collateral vessels in patients with coronary artery disease. Am J Cardiol 42:187
33. Helfant RH, Vikonas PS, Gorlin R (1971) Functional importance of human coronary collateral circulation. N Engl J Med 284:1277
34. Schwarz F, Schaper J, Becker V, Kübler W, Flameng W (1982) Coronary collateral vessels: their significance for left ventricular histologic structure. Am J Cardiol 49:291
35. Schwarz F, Schuler G, Hofmann M, Kübler W (1983) Recruitment of collaterals following acute coronary occlusion reduces infarct size in man. J Am Coll Cardiol 1:591
36. Kutcher MA, Gruentzig AR, Turina M, Craver JM, Jones EL, Douglas JS, King SB (1982) Can emergency bypass surgery following acute failure of coronary angioplasty prevent myocardial infarction? Am J Cardiol 49:956
37. Meier B, Luethey P (1984) Coronary wedge pressure as predictor of recruitable collateral arteries. Circulation 70:(II)266
38. Ischinger T, Gruentzig AR, Hollman J (1983) Reproducibility and localization of cardiac pain with balloon inflation during coronary angioplasty (PTCA). Circulation 68:(III)410 (abstract)
39. Dervan JP, Baim DS, Cherviles J, Grossmann W (1983) Transluminal angioplasty of occluded coronary arteries. Use of a movable guidewire system. Circulation 68:776
40. Oldham HN, Rembert JC, Greenfield JC, Wechsler AD, Sabiston DC (1978) Intraoperative relationship between aorto-coronary bypass graft blood flow, peripheral coronary artery pressure and reactive hyperemia. In: Maseri A, Klasen GA, Lesch M (eds) Primary and secondary angina pectoris. Grune and Stratton, New York, pp 370–373

Chapter 5. Indications and Contraindications for Coronary Angioplasty

THOMAS ISCHINGER

General Considerations

The selection of adequate therapy for patients with coronary artery disease after coronary arteriography is based on the patient's symptomatic status and objective evidence of myocardial ischemia, the angiographic anatomy of the coronary arteries, and the status of the left ventricle. The therapeutic goals are the relief of angina pectoris and the extension of long-term survival. Medical therapy, which is directed primarily at the reduction of myocardial workload, is considered effective if it provides adequate relief of angina pectoris with respect to the patient's individual needs and expectations, with no unacceptable side effects. If medical therapy remains ineffective, myocardial revascularization may achieve symptomatic relief by directly increasing blood flow to the ischemic myocardium. The degree of angina pectoris or limitation of physical activity that is considered unacceptable by a patient varies greatly between individuals. The willingness of patients and physicians to accept these limitations varies with the prospects offered by alternate therapies.

Both coronary bypass surgery and coronary angioplasty have been shown to reduce angina pectoris drastically in symptomatic patients, by increasing myocardial perfusion [1–5]. Coronary bypass surgery has been demonstrated to improve long-term prognosis, e.g., avoid coronary events and prolong life, in subsets of patients with severe coronary artery disease [6–12]. In patients with single-vessel disease extension of survival by surgical intervention has been difficult to demonstrate. There has been no statistical evidence as yet that coronary angioplasty prolongs life. However, the number of vessels involved and the degree of damage to the left ventricle do not sufficiently define the risk of long-term complications. Patients with single-vessel disease are not a homogeneous group of patients with a favorable prognosis. The need for revascularization has to be judged individually on the basis of the clinical course of the patient, the amount of myocardium in jeopardy, and the angiographic morphology of the coronary circulation. A severe proximal stenosis in a left anterior descending artery that supplies a large area of viable myocardium may be a greater threat to the patient that so-called triple-vessel disease if this involves minor branches, more distal coronary segments, or totally occluded vessels. Thus, for a patient with single-vessel disease and demonstrable ischemia owing to a lesion of the proximal left anterior descending artery, we may recommend revascularization even if only mild symptoms or none at all are present.

On the other hand, the presence of coronary stenoses revealed by angiography does not constitute an indication for revascularization. Before any revascularization procedure is considered the correlation of symptoms and myocardial ischemia with the coronary obstruction(s) visualized on the arteriogram has to be determined. This may be obvious in patients with typical angina pectoris and severe single-vessel stenosis. In patients with less severe obstructions (<70% diameter reduction), mild symptoms, or atypical chest pains, ischemia must be demonstrated before revascularization can be considered to be indicated [13, 14]. Various noninvasive exercise tests are helpful in this regard. It is current practice in coronary surgery to bypass mild lesions along with the critical stenoses, while dilatation of hemodynamically insignificant lesions during a complex angioplasty procedure is controversial, because restenoses more severe than the original lesion may occur [14, 15]. Ideally, in patients with multivessel disease demonstration of ischemia in the different areas of the obstructed arteries should be attempted before complex coronary angioplasty is undertaken, to guide the dilatation strategy.

PTCA or Bypass Surgery?

The decision for PTCA or coronary bypass surgery depends on the limitations of the revascularization procedures, the chances to achieve the therapeutic objectives, and the estimated safety of each for the patient.

One limitation of *coronary bypass surgery* is the condition of the distal coronary vessel. If nonbypassable distal stenoses are present, if the disease is diffuse, or if the vessel is too small for effective anastomosis of bypass grafts to be possible, then surgery should not be recommended. In rare instances coronary arteries may not be surgically accessible [16]. Obviously these questions have to be discussed with the cardiovascular surgeon.

The purpose of both coronary bypass surgery and PTCA is complete myocardial revascularization. In most of the patients with severe multivessel disease, it is necessary to revascularize substantial amounts of myocardium for revascularization to be effective. Patients should not undergo surgical revascularization if consequent significant residual myocardial ischemia can be anticipated.

Another limiting factor of coronary bypass surgery is the availability of appropriate conduits as bypass grafts. This is usually no problem with first operations, but it might be more difficult to find adequate vein grafts for repeat operations. However, in most cases the problem can be solved by the surgeon. The increasing use of internal mammary arteries may also be helpful in this respect.

Intraoperative angioplasty or coronary endarterectomy are performed by some surgeons to deal with the problem of diffuse and distal disease, but multiple grafting remains the preferred technique in these cases.

Left ventricular function is a strong predictor of survival after surgical revascularization [17]. If the left ventricle is so severely impaired as to preclude survival of the operation the patient should not be subjected to coronary bypass surgery. Patients with ejection fractions less than 20%–25% are commonly not considered good candidates for surgery. However, if these patients have severe symptoms and have bypassable vessels their condition may be improved by revascularization of a substantial amount of ischemic myocardium. It is obvious that most of these patients are also poor candidates for coronary angioplasty. If the severely impaired ventricle suffers further damage from complications of PTCA the chances of sustaining circulation until emergency surgery and bringing the patient through the operation are extremely low.

Other noncardiac conditions, primarily advanced pulmonary disease, but also renal insufficiency [18], associated vascular lesions, or wasting diseases may constitute a high operative risk or make the patient inoperable. Associated vascular lesions that can potentially cause severe perioperative insults, such as symptomatic carotid artery disease, should probably be managed before bypass surgery, if the cardiac status allows. In other patients coronary bypass surgery needs to be performed first before surgical treatment of associated operable conditions can be considered.

In elderly patients (70 years and older) and patients with prior bypass surgery, operative mortality has been shown to be higher [17]. These patients need not necessarily be denied the benefits of surgical revascularization, but the indications should be applied more stringently.

A potential decrease in long-term survival owing to systemic or neoplastic diseases must be considered in the selection of patients for myocardial revascularization. Severe permanent physical limitations may also reduce the symptomatic benefit these patient would have from revascularization of ischemic myocardium. Obviously, the palliative potential of a less invasive procedure like PTCA is attractive in such patients. But again, if PTCA is preferred over surgical revascularization because the patient has a high operative risk, it must be clearly understood that the operative mortality will be even higher if emergency surgery should become necessary [17].

The main limitation of *coronary angioplasty* is the poor predictability of the reaction of the coronary lesion to balloon dilatation. Coronary dissection or total coronary occlusion are inherent risks in mechanical dilatation of stenotic areas, and the most frequent complications.

A complicated morphology of stenosis seen on angiography (irregular lumen, intraluminal lucencies, etc.) and stenosis location in a vessel curve seem to be associated with an increased risk of vessel dissection [19] or occlusion. The technique may also be less suitable for diffusely diseased coronary arteries, stenoses at major bifurcations, or very tortuous arteries.

In chronic total coronary occlusion angioplasty may technically be feasible in a large percentage (>70%) [20–22] of selected patients, but the early reocclusion rate is reported to be relatively high (>40%) [21, 22]. Attempted recanalization of a totally occluded vessel does not preclude myocardial ischemic complications.

Particularly within the left coronary tree, manipulation with the dilatation system carries a potential risk of iatrogenic obstruction or injury of noninvolved vessels or of the left main system. Therefore, the decision to attempt recanalization of a chronic occlusion in a patient with single-vessel disease must be dictated by the evidence of myocardial ischemia. There are no data as yet to determine the (long-term) benefit of recanalization of occluded vessels that would normally supply infarcted myocardium and whose occlusion is producing insignificant or no ischemia.

In some patients with multiple-vessel disease, however, angioplasty for totally occluded arteries may be part of the dilatation strategy of a complex PTCA procedure.

The ability to reach and cross the coronary stenosis has been markedly enhanced by the steerable dilatation systems, but it is still the major technical limitation of the procedure.

In patients with extensive multiple-vessel disease PTCA may often not achieve the same degree of revascularization as coronary bypass surgery, in which case it will have less chance of improving symptoms and prognosis [23, 24]. If surgery appears superior in achieving the therapeutic goals, angioplasty should not be chosen.

Vessel patency after PTCA is another limiting factor of the procedure. While early patency rates lie between 80% and 90% after coronary bypass surgery, they are lower after coronary angioplasty (<80%). Current data on the development of restenosis, however, do not identify a subset of patients with vessel patency after PTCA so poor as to preclude coronary angioplasty.

The primary limitation to selection for coronary angioplasty is undoubtedly based on the assessment of the degree of risk to the patient if total occlusion of the vessel being treated should occur during the procedure. This consideration may be influenced further by the availability and promptness of surgical support and the experience of the surgical team.

Chances of Success and Patient Safety

With some exceptions, the prospective outcome of coronary angioplasty is usually assessed after a patient has been found to be eligible for coronary bypass surgery. Before the selection of angioplasty for revascularization three important questions should be asked:

1. To what extent can the ischemic myocardium be revascularized by coronary angioplasty as against coronary bypass surgery?
2. What is the risk that the coronary lesion(s) will not respond adequately to mechanical dilatation (local risk of complication)?
3. What are the clinical risks for the patient (myocardial infarction and death) should total occlusion of the vessel occur during the procedure?

In those patients who have discrete accessible lesions with a low potential for local complications in all vessels that otherwise would receive bypass grafts, it can be anticipated that the result of angioplasty will be equivalent to that of coronary bypass surgery. These will be primarily patients with single-vessel disease or localized lesions in two vessels. If an experienced operator is available angioplasty should be recommended to these patients. On the basis of these criteria, patients with triple-vessel coronary disease may also be candidates for angioplasty, but presence of diffused disease and complicated stenoses often reduce the chance of complete revascularization by angioplasty in these patients.

Multivessel disease is also frequently associated with chronic total occlusions and non-bypassable poor distal vessels. With more extensive disease anatomically incomplete revascularization that results in satisfactory palliation [23–25, 32] may have to be accepted more frequently using either procedure – coronary bypass surgery or PTCA.

In selected patients with a low risk of complications and well-suited lesions for PTCA, dilatation of only the "critical" stenosis(es) in the setting of multivessel disease can be an expeditious and effective therapy giving satisfactory palliative results [23, 24, 32].

While the occurrence of coronary dissection or total coronary occlusion due to PTCA cannot be safely predicted, the clinical consequences of total occlusion can be assessed on the basis of the diagnostic coronary angiogram. The main question that needs to be examined is: What will be the residual amount of functional myocardium should acute occlusion of the PTCA vessel occur.

The amount of myocardium at risk is largely determined by the location of the coronary stenosis, with more proximal lesions in vessels with a large distribution area affecting a much higher proportion of the myocardium than distal lesions in less significant vessels [26]. An acute occlusion of the proximal left anterior descending artery may lead to an extensive myocardial infarction involving up to 50% of the myocardium [27]. If the ventricle has been previously damaged in an area unrelated to the distribution of the vessel to be treated by PTCA, then the combination of the previous insult and the acute infarction due to PTCA will result in massive damage to the left ventricle. Angioplasty in the presence of a totally occluded large coronary artery contralateral to the vessel treated by PTCA carries an increased risk of myocardial infarction and death [28]. It can be anticipated that if 50% of the left ventricular myocardium is affected this may lead to severe hemodynamic impairment and reduce the chances of sustaining the patient's circulation through bypass surgery.

The consequences can be similar if the vessel considered for PTCA supplies collateral blood flow to viable myocardium in the distribution area of a chronically occluded coronary vessel. The amount of myocardium that can become acutely ischemic may be extensive. Therefore, recanalization of subtotally or totally occluded vessels that are collateralized from the vessel to be dilated should be attempted first in patients with multiple-vessel disease, with the object of creating reverse collateral flow. The decision as to whether or not to proceed with PTCA may depend on the hemodynamic and angiographic success of this recanalization attempt. Patients for whom coronary angioplasty genuinely would be the first choice of therapy accept this approach.

Coronary angioplasty can be performed more safely in selected patients with double- or triple-vessel disease if it is done stepwise and the result of each dilatation taken account of to minimize the risk of acute obstruction of more than one coronary vessel at the same time and to avoid compromising the blood supply to extensive areas of myocardium. This strategy usually requires that dilatation of the stenosis presenting the most significant threat to perfusion of the left ventricular myocardium (critical stenosis) be attempted first.

Contraindications

Contraindications related to the angiographic anatomy of the coronary arteries and to technical limitations have become rare as a result of the improved catheter technology. Most of the complicated and distal coronary lesions are now accessible. In patients with multiple-vessel disease and lesions that are well suited to coronary angioplasty, a high chance of therapeutic success can be predicted. If angioplasty would result in a lesser degree of revascularization of ischemic myocardium than bypass surgery then coronary angioplasty should not be chosen. A low chance of success for coronary angioplasty represents a relative contraindication. Rare exceptions may be made for patients with high surgical risk.

More importance attaches to contraindications based on the patients' safety. A high risk of occlusive dissection, as judged by the location and angiographic morphology of the coronary lesion [19], coupled with the anticipation of severe hemodynamic insult to the patient precludes coronary angioplasty.

Dilatations in arteries that serve a critical amount of myocardium, such as the left main stem or "last supply vessels," carry an increased risk of massive myocardial infarction and death should total occlusion occur as an immediate or late sequela of the procedure. I therefore consider left main coronary artery disease a relative contraindication for PTCA, although these lesions often appear technically suitable for dilatation. Closure of the left main coronary artery almost invariably leads to severe myocardial damage and collapse of left ventricular function, and is associated with markedly increased mortality even if emergency bypass surgery is immediately possible.

However, patients with high-risk situations may still be selected for coronary angioplasty if the lesion is technically ideally suited and if a high operative risk makes coronary surgery a poor first choice.

Expanded Indications for Coronary Angioplasty

Originally PTCA was described as a technique for revascularization in symptomatic patients with discrete, proximal, subtotal single-vessel stenosis who otherwise would undergo coronary bypass surgery. Therefore, suitability of the potential PTCA patient for coronary surgery – with respect to clinical indication, status of the coronary arteries and operative risk – was considered a prerequisite. However, in a patient whose coronary and symptomatic status does not constitute a clear indication for revascularization according to the current scientific evidence (see Chapter 3), the less invasive technique of coronary angioplasty may be indicated as a supplement or an alternative to medical treatment rather than an alternative to coronary bypass surgery. These considerations apply more often to patients with ideally suitable single-vessel stenoses. The anticipation of a high chance of palliation with a low risk of complications would make PTCA an attractive prospect in these patients. Symptomatic patients with single-vessel disease and stenosis of suitable morphology are ideal candidates for coronary angioplasty. In these patients single stenosis dilatation

Table 1. Angiographic and clinical indications for PTCA

Ideal indications	Expanded indications
Single, concentric, noncalcified, subtotal lesion	Multiple discrete lesions in a single vessel Multiple discrete lesions in multiple vessels
Proximal location	Distal location Complicated lesions Chronic total occlusions
Stable angina	Unstable angina Acute MI Prior CABGS
Proven myocardial ischemia	Proven myocardial ischemia
Candidate for CABGS	Candidate for CABGS

MI, myocardial infarction; CABGS, coronary artery bypass graft surgery

may bring about quick and safe correction of the myocardial ischemia throughout the area affected. Early and late results can be reliably assessed by noninvasive means. Suitable lesions for coronary angioplasty are more frequently found in patients with single-vessel disease, who usually have a shorter history of angina and less severely damaged ventricles than other patients with significant disease [29].

Patient selection is now based essentially on the same criteria as during earlier experience, but has become more permissive. The current potential of coronary angioplasty allows various clinical and angiographic patient subsets to be treated [30] (Table 1). It is estimated that approximately 25%–30% of patients with symptomatic coronary artery disease can now be considered for PTCA [31].

Multiple dilatations (complex PTCA) have been performed with increasing frequency in patients with more extensive coronary artery disease and make up about one-third of the procedures we have performed [32–34]. In carefully selected patients the rates of primary success and complications are comparable to those achieved with PTCA in patients with single stenosis. However, further study of the long-term value of complex PTCA is required.

The young patient (<40 years old) who has coronary lesions suitable for angioplasty deserves special consideration. Since coronary atherosclerosis is a progressive disease, many of the younger patients will eventually develop more extensive coronary disease. Even if coronary angioplasty cannot make bypass surgery completely unnecessary in some of these patients, it may delay the necessity for it until more definite surgical revascularization can be performed later in their lives, when there is a lower likelihood of a second operation [6]. Second coronary operations are associated with a higher risk of complications than are first operations [35].

Angioplasty may be a valuable alternative to reoperation in patients with previous coronary bypass surgery who have recurrent angina due to graft closure or disease progression in the native circulation. Experienced operators achieve success and complication rates similar to those obtained overall with angioplasty. However, recurrence seems to be more frequent after dilatation of an obstruction in the midvein graft or at the proximal (aorta-to-graft) anastomosis. Also, in the case of older vein grafts atherosclerotic lesions may be very friable and should therefore be approached with caution.

Only recently has the application of PTCA been extended to the treatment of unstable angina and acute myocardial infarction, sometimes in combination with systemic or intracoronary thrombolysis (see Chap. 17).

Growing skill, improved results, and refinement of the technique allow more liberal selection of patients for PTCA, but must not lead to its noncritical use. Many functionally insignificant lesions could easily be mechanically dilated in the confident expectation of preventing more advanced disease. However, this preventive concept may be jeopardized or even reversed by the recurrence of stenoses which are more severe than the original lesions [14]. In this event, acceleration of the disease process will be the final result rather than prevention. Therefore, both ends of the current spectrum of indications need critical consideration for appropriate patient selection and good results to be maintained.

References

1. Rahimtoola SH (1982) Coronary bypass surgery for chronic angina: a perspective. Circulation 65:225
2. Marco JD (1980) Myocardial perfusion following bypass surgery. In: Hurst JW (ed) Update II: the heart. McGraw-Hill, New York, p 13
3. King SB, Hurst JW (1980) The relief of angina pectoris by coronary bypass surgery. In: Hurst JW (ed) Update II: the heart. McGraw-Hill, New York, p 71
4. Hirzel HO, Nuesch K, Gruentzig AR, Luetolf M (1981) Short and long term chances in myocardial perfusion after PTCA assessed by thallium 201 exercise scintigraphy. Circulation 63:1001
5. Meier B, Gruentzig AR, Siegenthaler WE, Schlumpf M (1983) Long term exercise performance after PTCA and coronary artery bypass grafting. Circulation 68:797
6. Loop FD, Sheldon WC, Lytle BW, Cosgrove DM, Proudfit WL (1981) The efficacy of coronary artery surgery. Am Heart J 101:86–96
7. European Coronary Surgery Study Group (1982) Long-term results of prospective randomized study of coronary artery bypass surgery in stable angina pectoris. Lancet II:1173
8. CASS Principal Investigators and their Associates (1983) Coronary artery surgery study: a randomized trial of coronary bypass surgery: survival data. Circulation 68:939
9. Hurst JW, King SB (1980) The prolongation of life by coronary bypass surgery: the Emory University Hospital experience. In: Hurst JW (ed) Update II: the heart. McGraw-Hill, New York, p 141
10. Hurst JW, King SB, Logue RB, Hatcher CR (1978) Value of coronary bypass surgery. Am Heart J 42:308
11. CASS principal investigators and their associates (1984) Myocardial infarction and mortality in the Coronary Artery Surgery Study (CASS) randomized trial. N Engl J Med 310:75
12. Mock M, Rinquist I, Fisher L, Davis KB, Chaitman BR (1982) Survival of medically treated patients in the CASS registry. Circulation 66:562
13. Kent KM, Rosing DR, Ewels CJ, Lipson L, Bonow R, Epstein SE (1982) Prognosis of asymptomatic or mildly symptomatic patients with coronary artery disease. Am J Cardiol 49:1823
14. Ischinger T, Gruentzig AR, Hollman J, King SB, Douglas JS, Meier B (1983) Should coronary arteries with less than 60% diameter stenosis be treated by angioplasty? Circulation 68:148
15. Cosgrove DM, Loop FD, Saunders CL, Lytle BW, Kramer JR (1981) Should coronary arteries with less than fifty percent stenosis be bypassed? J Thorac Cardiovasc Surg 82:520

16. Comazzi JL, Jang GC, Marsa RJ, Willis WH (1983) Percutaneous transluminal angioplasty of a large septal artery. Cathet Cardiovasc Diagn 9:181
17. Kennedy JW, Kaiser GC, Fisher LO, Fritz JK, Myers W, Mudd JG, Ryan TJ (1983) Clinical and angiographic predictors of operative mortality from the collaborative study in coronary artery surgery (CASS). Circulation 63:793
18. Kober G, Vollbracht G, Giesecke R, Grützmacher P, Fassbinder W, Kaltenbach M (1985) Transluminale koronare Angioplastie bei Patienten mit chronischer Niereninsuffizienz. Dtsch Med Wochenschr 4:129
19. Ischinger T, Gruentzig AR, Meier B, Galan K (1985) Coronary dissection and total coronary occlusion associated with percutaneous transluminal coronary angioplasty (PTCA): Significance of initial angiographic morphology of coronary stenoses. Circulation (in press)
20. Holmes DR, Vlietstra RE, Reeder GS, Breshnahan JF, Smith HC, Bore AA, Schaff H (1984) Angioplasty in total coronary artery occlusion. J Am Coll Cardiol 3:845
21. Vetrovec G, Cowley M, Wolfgang T (1984) Nonemergent PTCA for total coronary occlusion: immediate and late results. Circulation 70(II):146
22. Libow MA, Leimgruber PP, Roubin GS, Gruentzig AR (1985) Restenosis after angioplasty (PTCA) in chronic total coronary artery occlusion (abstract). J Am Coll Cardiol 5:445
23. Vandormael M, Chaitman BR, Ischinger T, Aker UT, Harper M, Hernandez J, Deligonul U, Kennedy HL (1985) Immediate and short term benefit of multi-lesion coronary angioplasty. Influence of degree of revascularization. J Am Coll Cardiol (in press)
24. Ischinger T, Russ T, Zack P, Aker U, Kennedy H (1984) Complex coronary angioplasty: angiographic and functional results. Eur Heart J 5(I):57
25. Williams DC, Kurzrok S, Riley R, Singh A, Most A (1983) Partial revascularization by single vessel coronary angioplasty: efficacious therapy of multivessel coronary artery disease. J Am Coll Cardiol 1:655
26. Schuster EH, Griffith LS, Bulkley BH (1981) Preponderance of acute left anterior descending coronary arterial lesion in fatal myocardial infarction: a clinical-pathologic study. Am J Cardiol 47:1189
27. De Pace NL, Iskandrian AS, Nadell R, Colby, Hakki AH (1983) Variation in the size of jeopardized myocardium in patients with isolated left anterior descending coronary artery disease. Circulation 67:988
28. Roubin GS, Leimgruber PP, Douglas JS, King SB, Gruentzig AR (1985) Angioplasty in multivessel coronary artery disease: patient selection and dilatation strategy (abstract). J Am Coll Cardiol 5:445
29. Hamby RJ, Katz S (1980) Percutaneous transluminal coronary angioplasty: its potential impact on surgery for coronary artery disease. Am J Cardiol 45:1161
30. Ischinger T, Aker U, Kennedy H (1984) Percutaneous transluminal coronary angioplasty (PTCA): current status and indications. Cardiovasc Rev Rep 5:782
31. Ischinger T, Harper J, Zack P, Russ T, Aker U, Kennedy H (1984) Expanded indications for coronary angioplasty: impact on coronary bypass surgery. Eur Heart J 5(I):57
32. Ischinger T, Russ T, Zack P, Aker U, Kennedy H (1984) Perkutane transluminale Koronarangioplastie (PTCA). Effektive Behandlung von Mehrgefäßerkrankungen. Z Kardiol 73(I):34
33. Dorros G, Singh S, Janke L (1984) Coronary angioplasty in multivessel coronary artery disease. Circulation 70(II):107
34. Hartzler GO, Rutherford BD, McConahay DR, McCallister BH (1982) Simultaneous multiple lesion coronary angioplasty – a preferred therapy for patients with multiple vessel disease. Circulation 66(II):5
35. Loop FD, Cosgrove DM, Kramer JR, Lytle BW, Taylor PC, Golding CR, Groves LK (1981) Late clinical and arteriographic results in 500 coronary artery reoperations. J Thorac Cardiovasc Surg 81:675

Chapter 6. The Cardiac Catheterization Laboratory for Coronary Angioplasty

UMIT T. AKER and THOMAS ISCHINGER

Introduction

Optimal performance of percutaneous transluminal coronary angioplasty (PTCA) requires radiological equipment capable of meeting the special demands of this interventional procedure. These demands, which influence equipment selection, may be summarized as follows:

1. Satisfactory visualization of the coronary arterial tree on a live TV fluoroscopic screen by means of small-volume contrast material delivered at a low flow rate through coaxial catheter systems: necessary for safe manipulation of guidewire and balloon catheter to reach and cross the lesion, especially in tortuous arteries with superposition and in large subjects.
2. Playback of video tape recording of coronary arteriograms, forward and reverse, at 30 frames/s, in slow motion and in freeze-frame, with fidelity approaching cine film quality: necessary for evaluation of coronary pathology in emergency situations and for assessment of the adequacy of dilatation, especially as dilated lesions may have more complex anatomical features.
3. Display of high-quality stationary TV images: necessary for displaying guide shots for route mapping.
4. Facility allowing rapid projection changes, including cranial and caudal views: to assist in directing the guidewire into the desired branches, to ensure correct placement of guidewires and dilatation catheters across the lesion, and to provide optimal visualization of the lesion before and after PTCA.
5. Cine films of highest possible quality, showing fine angiographic details of coronary anatomy: angiographic selection criteria for PTCA require detailed morphology of the lesions; accurate quantitation of the results of PTCA also requires high-quality cine films.

These demands necessitate radiological equipment that is usually not incorporated into the design of routine coronary angiography laboratories. This is particularly true for high-definition TV fluoroscopic imaging and playback equipment and for the desirability of bi-plane systems.

In this chapter, components of cine imaging and video systems will be reviewed with reference to the requirements of a laboratory dedicated to interventional cardiology. A summary of guidelines for selection and configuration of the equipment will be presented. It should be pointed out that the recommendations are for an optimal facility, and not minimum necessary recources for the practice of interventional cardiology.

Description of the basic concepts of x-ray generation, image intensification, cine angiography, and television image display is outside the scope of this review.

The reader can find this information in previously published texts [1, 2]. Optimal resources for diagnostic cardiac catheterization laboratory have already been specified elsewhere [3].

Staffing and space requirements will be considered only for the interventional procedure room. Shared facilities in the catheterization laboratory, such as film processing and review, storage, etc., will be addressed only briefly, since it is assumed that a room devoted exclusively to interventional procedures will be an integral part of an established laboratory. Of course, such a room may also function as a general cardiac angiographic laboratory in institutions whose caseload justifies only one angiographic suite.

x-Ray Equipment

Generators

In the planning of an angiographic laboratory one of the most important decisions is the selection of the x-ray generator, which includes a high tension transformer and control unit. For all practical purposes, the generator will largely determine the performance characteristics of the system.

Some manufacturers propose only one type of generator for vascular applications, while others offer choices of different types and ratings. To take advantage of newer x-ray tubes with higher loadability, generators with high outputs are recommended for PTCA laboratories. Longer source input distance (SID) of "C" or "U" arms or parallelogram type devices and compound projections with steep cranial and caudal angulation require high-output generators for optimal x-ray exposure factors. Transformer design, rectifiers, and contacting method will influence the actual power output of the generators. Both constant-potential generators (up to 200 kW rating) and 12-pulse generators (up to 125 kW) are suitable. This power rating is not excessive in relation to cine angiographic requirements in the PTCA laboratory. For example, in a large adult, a cine exposure in the left anterior oblique projection with a 30° cranial angulation (proposed Society of Cardiac Angiography Terminology [4]) and cine pulse width of 5 ms may necessitate a tube current of 500 mA to keep kilovolt peaking at 90 or below. A current output capacity 1.5–2 times the cine pulse output is recommended to minimize voltage fluctuations [3]. Therefore, a 1000-mA rating at 100 kV is not excessive for PTCA installations. Constant potential generators can supply cine output current over 600 mA if not limited by x-ray tube loading. For tube currents of over 600 mA they are superior to 12-pulse SCR generators.

Furthermore, constant-potential generators include circuitry for secondary cine pulsing and automatic brightness control, obviating the need for a separate cine pulse unit and the expense this would involve. They also offer automatic, sophisticated computerized brightness control in both fluoroscopy and cine mode. This is important for C or U arm stands, because the variable projections demand fast and automatic variation of exposure factors. One manufacturer with grid control x-ray tubes offers bi-plane pulsed fluoroscopy, which is intriguing in PTCA applications.

In PTCA applications, some manufacturers are incorporating modules to the generator control desk to change fluoroscopy dose level. Half the normal dose level during guiding catheter placement can be used to reduce radiation. Two or four times the normal fluoroscopy dose or 30% of the cine dose can be utilized to improve fluoroscopic image quality, for example while negotiating a complex lesion or during control shots to evaluate the status of the lesion.

It is desirable to have the exposure factors displayed at the control desk during or at the end of each run. A useful optional extra is a display of the cine and fluoroscopy factors on the procedure room TV monitor for the operator's review. Constant-potential generators available on the market have pushbutton program selection as well as manual override of the exposure factors.

The same high-tension transformer and control desk are used in bi-plane systems based on constant potential generators. Only one additional tetrode or triode tank and control cabinets are necessary for lateral plane. On the other hand, two transformers, two control desks, and two cine pulsing units are necessary for bi-plane systems using 12-pulse generators. Therefore, price differences between constant-potential and 12-pulse generators are minimized in bi-plane laboratories. Space requirements for rack and cabinets are also smaller with constant-potential generators in bi-plane installations. Both type of generators have a modular design, which allows the user to select only modules necessary for cine operation, avoiding extra cost.

In practice, generators offered by major manufacturers are adequate for satisfactory cine quality and fluoroscopic images when other components of the system are optimized. Constant-potential generators offer some advantages, as outlined above, and may be preferable in bi-plane PTCA installations.

x-Ray Tubes

The demands made by PTCA require an x-ray tube with high loadability, large heat storage capacity of the anode, rapid heat dissipation, favorable focal spot geometry with Gaussian distribution, and reduced extrafocal radiation.

During fluoroscopy, use of a small nominal focal spot is desirable, since it will contribute to better resolution of the TV image and video recording.

C and U arms or parallelograms in common use today have larger source input distance requiring higher x-ray factors than older Craddle or Cardio-diagnost systems. All major manufacturers will supply high-speed (9000 rpm or greater) rotating anode x-ray tubes. The anode disks are compound rhenium-alloyed tungsten with molybdenum, blackened on the back, or have graphite heat sink. The anode diameter should be 100 mm or larger. The anode angle of these tubes is usually 12°, providing a higher tube rating. They come with a small focal spot of 0.6 mm and a large focal spot of 0.9, 1.0, or 1.2 mm, with corresponding ratings of 35–40 kW for the small focal spot and 70–100 kW for the large focal spot. The anode heat storage capacity of these tubes is around 300 kJ (400000 units); heat dissipation is 280–300 W with forced air cooling, obviating the need for liquid cooling, which is cumbersome for rotational systems. These tubes will have adequate field coverage for 9-in. bi-modal or tri-modal image intensifiers supplied

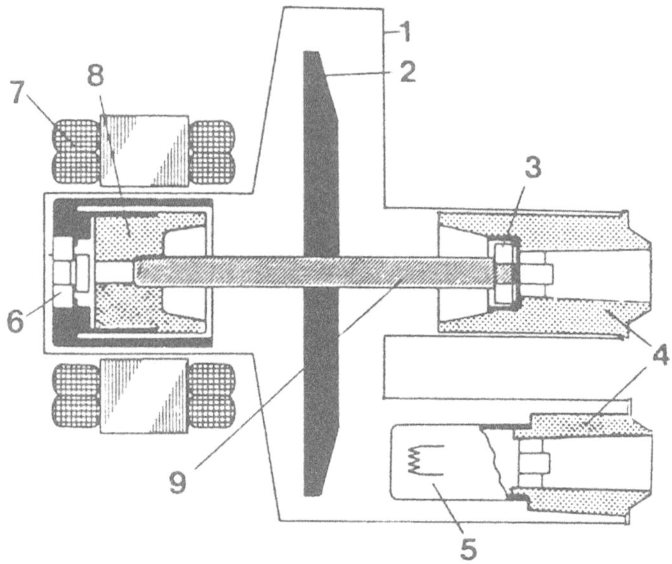

Fig. 1. Ceramic x-ray tube. See text for details. *1,* whole-metal casing; *2,* anode disk; *3/6,* ball bearings; *4/8,* ceramic insulators; *5,* cathode with filament; *7,* stator windings; *9,* anode shaft. (Courtesy of Philips, Gloeilampenfabrieken, Medical Systems Division, Eindhoven, The Netherlands)

with C or L-U arms or parallelograms. An x-ray tube with a 6° or 7° anode angle may be used with 6-in. image intensifiers, directing the anode heel toward the left side of the chest; at 9-in. mode the heel effect may be observed at the periphery depending on SID. One such tube has a 0.3- to 0.6-mm focal spot with 20- to 50-kW ratings and is quite satisfactory for the Cardio-diagnost table. Grid-controlled tubes with low anode heat capacity may require cooling-off periods during long procedures.

A newly introduced x-ray tube has a novel design, the anode disk being supported on a shaft with bearings at both ends. It has a metal envelope with ceramic insulators (Fig. 1). The anode is large, 120 mm, with a heat capacity of 600 kJ (810000 heat units). It is supplied with superimposed 0.2–0.7, 0.5–0.8, and 0.6–1.3 mm focal spot combinations. The power rating of the anode is 20 kW for a 0.2-mm and 85 kW for a 0.7-mm focal spot (corresponding ratings for the cold anode, 24 kW and 103 kW, respectively.) In PTCA installations, a 0.2-mm focal spot enhances fluoroscopic TV resolution, yet a 0.7-mm focal spot provides a high enough rating for cine runs. Because of the small focal spot size and the metal envelope with its beryllium window, off-focus radiation is low. The heat dissipation of the tube housing, with circulating oil and heat exchanger, is 1000 W. Its price is more than three times that of the conventional tubes, but a significantly longer tube life is expected.

An anode heat computer is recommended in PTCA installations where fluoroscopic times longer than are required for diagnostic coronary angiography are combined with multiple cine runs.

In summary, PTCA installations should have x-ray tubes with large, compound anodes rotating, at high speed, with high heat storage capacity (at least 400 000 heat units or 300 kJ), small anode angles (12° or less), and focal spots of 0.6 mm and 0.9–1.2 mm. Small focal spots of 0.2 or 0.3 mm will provide better fluoroscopic image resolution. A new ceramic x-ray tube offers the combination of small focal spots with higher rating.

In systems with short SIDs x-ray tubes with lower ratings but smaller focal spots can be used. At least a pinhole camera picture of the effective focal spot should be provided with the tube, so that focal spot size, shape, and energy distribution can be evaluated before its acceptance. In many x-ray tubes, energy distribution of the focal spot is the edgeband type, which is the least desirable form, and it may be twice the size of one with homogeneous distribution under cineangiographic loading conditions [5]. Small focal spots (0.2–0.3 mm) with the best resolving power have a Gaussian energy distribution (peaked toward the center). Homogeneous distribution is satisfactory in larger focal spot sizes. The resolving power of the x-ray tube focal spot can be measured by a star test pattern.

Image Intensifiers

In the past, single-mode, small (15–17 cm) image intensifiers with cesium iodide input screens were recommended for the laboratories used primarily for the study of coronary artery disease [2, 3]. This recommendation was based on their better resolution, higher gain, and lower voltage requirements compared with large dual- or triple-mode intensifiers used in 15- or 17-cm field size mode for coronary angiography. In recent years, equipment support systems of the C or U arm types, providing rapid positioning for cranial or caudal angulations, have become popular in coronary angiography laboratories, because of the importance of angulated views in imaging of the coronary arterial tree [6, 7]. Support systems of this type should be equipped with large, multi-mode image intensifiers. As will be discussed in a later section, bi-plane systems are desirable in a procedure room used exclusively for interventional cardiology. Equipment support systems in bi-plane configurations capable of compound angular views are exclusively supplied with 23- or 25-cm multi-mode image intensifiers by every major manufacturer. The image quality of the new generation of multi-mode intensifiers is comparable to or better than that of older 15- to 17-cm, single-mode models.

The first major advance in the image tube technology was the introduction of cesium-iodide input phosphor. Thin glass or metal input windows, improved electron optics, decreased light reflection in the output phosphor, improved fiber optics, and other technical improvements have also contributed to the better performance of today's image intensifiers. Different features of input phosphor have conflicting implications for image tube design. Increasing the thickness of input phosphor will increase the absorption of the x-rays (detection efficiency) and decrease the quantum mottle of the image for a given dose. On the other hand, increased thickness of the input phosphor promotes lateral light scatter in the layer, and will cause a decrease in spatial resolution. A compromise has to be accepted between these parameters of intensifier design. Modern cesium-iodide input phosphors have considerably less light scatter, owing to columnar separation of crystals; they offer the advantage of improved resolution. For image intensifiers with large input fields thicker glass is required, which acts as a scatter medium.

Metallic input windows with low absorption, such as titanium or aluminum, in new large intensifiers also reduce x-ray scatter and improve the resolution-to-contrast ratio. Improvements in electron optics and image tube construction have reduced scattering within the intensifier.

Gray glass at the output phosphor decreases halation caused by reflected fluorescent light. Fiber optic coupling at the output phosphor is used for the same purpose. The result of these improvements combined has been a significant reduction of veiling glare in images.

An increased detective quantum efficiency and conversion factor permit lowering of the radiation dose per frame, thus decreasing radiation exposure to the patient and personnel. Furthermore, reduced radiation per frame allows cine exposures with lower kilovolt peaking, improving patient x-ray contrast. In modern image intensifiers, 12- to 15-μrad/frame are generally adequate for field sizes of 23–25 cm, and 22- to 25-μrad/frame for field sizes of 14–17 cm. Ultimately, the angiographer must decide at what dose level quantum mottle appears to be least pronounced in clinical studies. Increasing dose levels to achieve a further minor reduction in quantum noise will drive up kilovolt peaking and will result in loss of x-ray contrast, besides increasing the radiation doses to the patient and personnel. In PTCA applications with longer fluoroscopic times and additional cine runs, exposure of the operator to x-irradiation becomes an important consideration in selection of the optimum radiation dose level per frame.

Two measurements are proposed for evaluation of an image intensifier: detective quantum efficiency (DQE) and modulation transfer function (MTF) [8–11]. It is not possible to measure these at the site where the equipment is installed, but they should be supplied by the manufacturer for the model of image intensifier offered. Conversion factor, contrast ratio, and resolution figures should also be provided. Good-quality multiple-mode intensifiers of newer designs will have a contrast ratio over 16:1, and not infrequently 18:1 or 20:1. The conversion factor for 23- to 35-cm fields should be at least 100 cd/m^2/mR/s. For a titanium input tube, factors as high as 220 cd/m^2/mR/s have been quoted. For 14- to 17-cm fields it should be over 50 cd/m^2/mR/s. Limiting resolution should be 2.5–3.0 lp/mm on film for large fields and 3.5–4 lp/mm for small fields. Contrast ratio and limiting resolution can easily be measured at the installation site. Perhaps the best index of image intensifier performance is the clinical image quality on cine films when frame dose rate, calibration, and film processing are optimized. High gain and resolution do not necessarily ensure good image quality.

In dual mode intensifiers, field sizes vary from 25–23 to 17–14 cm, making a smaller field with some degree of overframing optimal for coronary angiography. In triple-mode intensifiers, additional electron optical magnification to a field size of 12 cm is available. This smaller field provides improved resolution in the TV image, and it may be useful in PTCA when complicated lesions have to be crossed or branches with a difficult anatomy have to be crossed.

In summary, new PTCA installations will be offered with large multiple-mode image intensifiers as component parts of the C or U arms designed for compound angulations and bi-plane systems. However, in these larger intensifiers resolution and contrast ratio, DQE, and MTF are at least as good as, and often better than in smaller, single-mode intensifiers. They offer the additional advantage of electron optic magnification for different field sizes. Increased voltage requirements for smaller fields of multi-mode intensifiers do not constitute a problem in new installations, because of the availability of generators with high power ratings and x-ray tubes with high loadability. The individual user should request and obtain image tube specifications, and they should be within the above-mentioned ranges for high-quality image tubes. Input dose behind the grid, contrast ratio, and resolution limit should be measured at the installation site before acceptance and should correspond to the quoted specifications.

Cine Pulse Systems and Automatic Brightness Control

In all modern cine systems, x-ray output is intermittent and synchronized with the cine camera to allow exposures only when the camera shutter is open. Pulsing of the x-ray output is obviously necessary to avoid pointless extra radiation to the patient while the camera shutter is closed. Pulsed radiation is also the means by which exposure time is set for each cine frame. Motion blurring during cine runs is eliminated by x-ray pulses of short duration. The camera shutter, in addition to generating the synchronization signal, helps to prevent afterglow of the output phosphor reaching the next frame after cessation of x-ray pulses in high frame rates (60/s or more). The image intensifier is moved over anatomical parts of different densities during panning, and the brightness of the output phosphor would change significantly if x-ray factors were to remain the same. Since the camera lens aperture is fixed in cine systems it becomes necessary to vary x-ray factors during cine runs to maintain a predetermined level of brightness at the output phosphor for proper exposure of cine film. Duration of exposure, voltage (kVp) and tube current (mA) are the x-ray factors which determine the degree of film blackening. All three factors are used singly or more often the combination for automatic brightness control.

Most modern cineangiography equipment provides cine pulsing by switching x-ray output off and on at the high-tension side of the generator (secondary switching).

In systems based on 12-pulse generators, secondary switching is accomplished by one of two methods: (a) Tetrodes or triodes at the high-tension side of the generator are used to turn the x-ray off and on; (b) current flow is pulsed through a grid control x-ray tube while the high tension stays on.

For the automatic brightness control a photomultiplier reads the brightness level of the output phosphor. Its signal is compared with a preadjusted calibration signal for correct film density. The difference is fed to the voltage regulator of the generator which drives the kilovolt peak up or down to bring the output phosphor brightness to appropriate levels. The photomultiplier is usually adjusted to read a limited area in the central portion of the image field; therefore, the manner in which centering and panning is carried out will influence film density. In general, the region of interest should be in the central area read by the photomultiplier. Units of this type will usually have pushbutton program selection of cine factors determined according to the kilowatt rating of generator, cine pulse unit, and x-ray tube. For each selection station exposure time (usually 3 or 5 ms for adult coronary work), frame speed, focal spot size, and maximum filming duration are fixed; brightness is maintained by fluctuation of voltage and tube current up to a maximum chosen according to other fixed parameters and power ratings.

The second method of cine pulsing used in systems based on 12-pulse SCR generators is secondary switching through a grid-controlled x-ray tube. In x-ray tubes of this type a negative voltage is applied to a filament grid, completely cutting off the tube current. When the camera shutter is open the bias voltage is lowered and x-ray emission begins. Therefore, intermittent negative grid voltage acts like a switch on the secondary side of the transformer. Automatic brightness control is achieved by varying the duration of exposure (varying pulse width of the x-ray emission) through grid control. Because of the proximity of the cathode filament and focusing cup, the negative voltage necessary for pulsing is not very large. The response time is very fast, and the pulse waveform is square. However, automatic control of brightness by the modulation of exposure time alone is not adequate; therefore, this mode of automatic brightness control is supplemented by voltage override. In practice, an upper limit of pulse width is set depending on the heart rate and motion of the part to be filmed. A lower kilovolt peaking limit is selected with reference to the density of the anatomy to be filmed. Focal spot size is selected by a separate control. A test button at the control desk and a test position at the operator's foot switch are provided. Exposure factors, except tube current are computed and displayed by the microprocessor during a test run at half the cine doses for patient transparency measurement. During actual cine runs, if adequate brightness is not attained at the maximum pulse width selected the selected kilovolt peak value is overridden by the computer until the maximal kilovolt peak is reached. At this point, if brightness is still inadequate, pulse width increases above the preselected upper value up to a maximum of 10 ms. When subject density diminishes, exposure factors are decreased in reverse sequence. If the preselected low limit voltage value is too high for the patient the pulse width may decrease to very short exposure times and the mA per frame may be less than optimal. Although response time of pulse width modulation is almost instantaneous, the voltage is changed through carbon rollers with a slower response time, as described above. When a large voltage adjustment is needed the initial part of the run may not be properly exposed. However, in practice this has been a rare occurrence with new microprocessor-based generators. Technician and/or operator interaction will enhance the performance of the system. Exposure factors, focal spot size, percentage of remaining heat units, and run time, along with an exposure indicator, can be displayed on the operator's TV monitor as an option to facilitate this interaction. A lock-in feature is provided as in other systems. One advantage of this system is pulsed fluoroscopy, which is discussed below.

The cine pulse unit is an integral part of any constant-potential generator. Consequently, the choice of cine pulse system and the means of automatic brightness control will depend on the type of constant-potential generator selected.

These generators have secondary switching by way of tetrodes or triodes. Analog computers and microprocessors control the exposure factors for automatic brightness control. Their response time for voltage modulation is extremely fast with power tetrodes or triodes, around 1 kV/μs. Single-frame photo-timing is possible. They can provide very high tube current values if not limited by x-ray tube rating. They also measure patient transparency before the start of the cine run, and the computer determines the optimal exposure factors.

There are two methods of evaluating patient transparency: (a) automatic use of test shots immediately before the cine run at very low dose levels; and (b) during fluoroscopy.

For bi-plane operation, each of the above-described cine pulse units fires alternately on two planes, 180° out of phase to prevent fogging. In addition, alternate blanking of image intensifiers is useful to prevent recording of scatter radiation.

In a PTCA installation, automatic dose rate control during fluoroscopy should be provided.

In constant-potential generators, voltage and tube current vary co-directionally for automatic brightness control. Fluoroscopy is not pulsed. The dose rate can be set by a programmable fluoroscopic voltage and tube current ranges. The operator should decide on the adequacy of the dose level. Entry doses up to 10 R/min at 110 kV can be provided.

In PTCA applications the variable dose rate is useful to improve image quality of the TV monitor, for example when crossing a stenosis or for evaluation of the dilatation without going to cine dose levels. Higher fluoroscopy dose levels are used for video tape recording for immediate review.

In summary, automatic brightness control and cine pulse units supplied with constant potential generators and the grid-controlled system are suitable for PTCA applications. The power rating of the pulsing units should be at least 50–60 kW. In a grid-controlled system, the high demands placed on the x-ray tube may require frequent replacement of this relatively expansive component. The system also requires closer operator interaction for optimum performance. Constant potential generators require almost no interaction for exposure and automatic brightness control and have generally higher ratings. Fluoroscopic dose rate control with variable dose level is a desirable option in PTCA applications.

Video Systems, Video Tape Recorders, Video Disk Recorders

High-fidelity video imaging and playback capability are essential for the safe and optimal practice of PTCA. In fact, the quality of a fluoroscopic TV image, perhaps more than any of its other features, influences the selection of a system for a laboratory dedicated primarily to interventional cardiology. Of course, performance characteristics of image intensifier, x-ray tube, and optics will affect the quality of the TV image; however, to utilize the superior capabilities of the other imaging components, the TV chain and playback instruments must be capable of providing images with definition approaching that of cine film.

Management decisions may have to be made much more frequently in the course of coronary angioplasty than in routine diagnostic coronary angiography.

The operator has to rely on review of the TV images for such decisions. Evaluation of the angiographic adequacy of the dilatation will also require a high-fidelity playback facility in the laboratory. The need for an optimal live TV image for safe manipulation of the guidewires and dilatation catheters is obvious.

All TV cameras for cardiac catheterization laboratories are supplied with a Vidicon-type pick-up tube or one of its modifications, such as Plumbicon or Chalnicon. These newer tubes have unity brightness response and higher light sensitivity. A recently introduced Plumbicon pick-up tube has a 2-in. target area (Frogshead) with the potential for increased resolution. Vidicon pick-up tubes have inherently long lag, leading to blurring of rapidly moving structures. The lag should not be more than 10% of the peak video signal measured after the termination of x-ray exposure. Frogshead Plumbicon or Vidicon tubes used in high-resolution systems have a slightly higher lag, which results in averaging of the quantum mottle detected by these systems and leads to more acceptable viewing conditions; however, if excessive it will lead to motion blurring. The dynamic range (ratio of logarithm of maximum to minimum brightness) of a good Plumbicon is approximately 1000. The signal:noise ratio may be from 500 : 1 to over 1000 : 1. For automatic fluoroscopic dose control some units use the signal from the photomultiplier or the silicone reading cell, measuring the brightness of output phosphor as in cine mode. To prevent blooming, the average brightness is sensed within the measuring field at the output phosphor. The size of measuring field can be varied for this purpose, to include areas of varying density to help the brightness averaging. More modern units read video signals for brightness control. Similarly, averaging of video signal is used to decrease blooming.

Use of the peak video signal for automatic dose rate control would increase blooming. In some units the peak signal is clipped to avoid blooming. For image stabilization, automatic dose control and automatic gain control are coordinated in some TV systems. Circular blanking is provided by some manufacturers to improve the contrast. TV camera lens automatic aperture control is used to adjust the amount of the light reaching the TV pick-up tube. A manual iris diaphragm is recommended for optimal light levels during fluoroscopy and panning [12]; however, many operators may find manual adjustments cumbersome, especially when expert technical assistance is not available. In view of the varying mode of image stabilization and brightness control the designer of the procedure room should clarify these points with the manufacturers. A visit to a laboratory where the system under consideration is operational is quite helpful.

There is controversy about the relative merits of standard 525/625 (60/50 Hz line frequency) and high line rate, high bandwidth TV systems. In theory, high line rates should increase the vertical resolution. To keep vertical and horizontal resolutions equal, the bandwidth should also be increased. At 525 vertical lines, a bandwidth of 4.5 or 5 MHz is required to achieve a horizontal resolution equal to the vertical resolution. The increase in bandwidth to maintain equal horizontal and vertical resolution is related to the square of the increase in the vertical line rate; hence, at 1023 vertical line rate, a 20- or 25-MHz bandwidth is needed. It is generally stated that this increase in resolution is actually detrimental for television view, since x-ray quantum mottle is more clearly detected and more electronic noise is introduced to the system by higher bandwidths. As mentioned above, blooming can also be distracting if image stabilization and aperture control are not optimized. On the other hand, high-line-rate TV allows the operator to review the TV monitor from a distance of 1.2–1.5 m, with better perception of fine details. Blooming has not been prominent with newer TV chains with better image stabilization. Since high-resolution TV systems can only have a 1 : 1 aspect ratio, a round TV raster is smaller than images of standard TV lines displayed with 4 : 3 aspect ratio filling the entire TV monitor screen. Therefore, it is imperative that high-resolution TV monitors should be provided with booms that can be positioned in close proximity to the catheterization table. Authors have used two different high-resolution systems in PTCA applications, one a switchable system of 525/1049 lines with a Frogshead pick-up tube, and one with 1023 grid control-pulse fluoroscopy, and have found them superior to standard TV monitors for review of live fluoroscopy images.

Resolution power of a TV chain is determined by the number of scan lines covering a given area. Consequently, resolution will increase in a given line rate when a smaller field size is used in multimodal image intensifiers. In high-fidelity systems, resolutions up to 2.8 lp/mm may be obtained in 12-cm image-intensifier fields [12]. Additional geometric magnification may further increase resolution if not limited by focal spot size and penumbra effect. An example of the relationship between image field area, focal spot size, magnification, and resolution limit of TV chain is shown in Fig. 2. X-ray tubes with smaller focal spots will contribute to better fluoroscopic resolution, as mentioned above. A resolution limit of 3.5 lp/mm has been quoted in 5-in. mode at 1 : 1 magnification in one system with a 1049-line TV chain and a 0.2 focal spot of the x-ray tube. Of course, similar resolution cannot be obtained for low-contrast vessels.

Broadcast quality, type C helical, 1-in. reel-to-reel tape recorders are most suitable for playback of TV images in PTCA applications. These recorders have

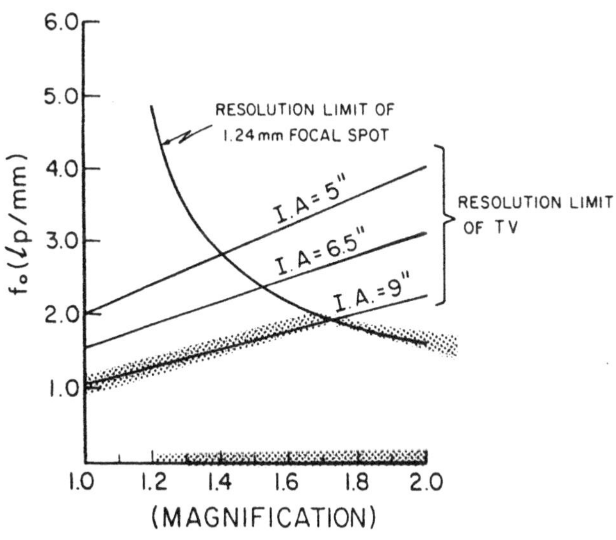

Fig. 2. Effect of focal spot size, image-intensifier input field, and geometric magnification on the resolution limit of TV. (From Kruger, Mistretta, and Riederer 1981, as reprinted in ref. [16])

the capacity for slow motion and freeze frame with no flicker or noise bar in either forward or reverse directions. Some units have digital time-base correction. In the freeze-frame mode, video fields rather than frames are played back, to prevent border motion and jitter. Resolution on playback is slightly lower than with live TV images. These video tape recorders (VTRs) have excellent signal:noise ratios over the range of 39–49 decibels and at a bandwidth of 10 MHz. The quality of playback images is almost equal to cine definition [13]. In bi-plane installations, two tape recorders are necessary. Although expensive, these VTRs will markedly enhance accuracy and speed of image reviewing, and are well worth the initial expense. In contrast, video cassette recorders have significantly lower resolution; search and playback is slower; freeze-frame images cannot be displayed with any acceptable degree of fidelity; and image jitter and horizontal noise bars are common. If the video signal is fed through the operator's live TV monitors to the VTR, slight deterioration of image resolution will occur. For this reason it is best to have the video signal split to VTR and live TV through a distribution amplifier. Tape recorders may be wired to have automatic recording during cine runs, or if desired only VTR recording with higher exposure values as an optional extra with generators and cine pulse units, as discussed above.

Display of guide shots in the procedure room side by side with live images has significant advantages for routeing, accurate dilatation catheter placement, and comparison of lesions before and after dilatation. Display of stationary TV images is best accomplished with video disk recorders (VDRs). One popular line of VDR offers models with disk storage from 500 to 1200 fields, corresponding to real-time recording of 8.3–20 s. Recording and playback can be varied from real time to one field every 3 s or single images forward and reverse. Either one TV field or two interlaced fields, i.e., one TV frame, can be recorded or played back. Any section of the disk can be directly accessed for rapid location of the desired images. Signal:noise ratio is 43 decibels or greater and bandwidth, 6 MHz or 10 MHz. There are VDRs for operation on any available TV line rate. Recording is done during cine injection with a video signal coming through VTR; if desired, a recording can first be made on a VTR and a selected portion of the run can be transferred from the VTR to a VDR. On bi-plane installations it is best to have two separate VDRs and control units. Two VDRs and one control unit can be arranged in bi-plane systems; in this case, every other frame on each VDR will be blank during recording runs, because of alternate firing for x-ray synchronization. With a video switcher, a single control unit and a single VDR can be used in bi-plane installations. However, the best configuration is the one that allows freeze-frame guide shots in both planes on separate TV monitors, side by side with live TV images. This arrangement requires four monitors in the procedure room stacked in a boom, and four small TV monitors for the technician in the control room. A single video field can be displayed in freeze frame from a VTR on the live TV monitor and will stay on every time the fluoroscopy is off. If any recording is made on VTR, the tape has to be wound back to the same field. This mode of display is not only inconvenient, but it also causes undue wear and tear on the recorder.

In summary, high-resolution TV chains with correspondingly high bandwidths are recommended for PTCA application. They should have appropriate image stabilization circuitry. The playback capability should be based on broadcast quality, helical C-type reel-to-reel VTRs with time-base correction. Guide shots can be best played by VDRs and separate TV monitors side by side with live TV monitors for optimal viewing conditions. If finances do not allow incorporation of VDRs into the system images have to be played back on the operator's live TV monitor.

Grids, Collimation, and Semitransparent Diaphragms

Grids are incorporated to the image intensifier housing in front of the input phosphor with the objective of improving image contrast by reduction of scatter radiation. This purpose is achieved by increased radiation to the patient, since the grid also reduces the primary transmission by as much as 50%. A linear, focused grid should be used within the range of its focusing distance. A grid with 8 : 1 ratio and 40 lines/cm is best suited to kilowatt peaking below 90.

The collimator, with at least three pairs of lead shutters, should be used to reduce scatter and limit the primary beam to the exposure field. In the newer support systems, with varying SIDs achieved by changing the image intensifier height, collimation automatically adjusts to the field size. Some manufacturers provide circular collimators or iris type diaphragms.

A semitransparent sickle-shaped diaphragm with gradual tapering toward the edge can be positioned over the cardiac border adjacent to the lung field to minimize density differences.

Optics, Framing, and Camera

Cine optics are part of the system design conceived by the manufacturers. The optional features are the focal length of the camera lens and the type of distributor.

The focal length of the camera lens is selected according to the degree of framing desired. The distributor is chosen according to the number of ports needed. If a spot film camera is added to the system a distributor with three ports will be needed. Our own experience suggests that spot filming is rarely, if ever, used for coronary artery imaging, even in the laboratories where this option has been incorporated into the equipment. Some add-on digital subtraction angiography equipment manufacturers may require a TV camera with gain and signal:noise ratio different than those of the camera used for diagnostic fluoroscopy. The TV cameras of this type have more noise and blooming during diagnostic fluoroscopy. Therefore, in this type of installation a distributor with three ports is necessary to accommodate the additional TV camera for digital angiography.

Some degree of overframing is necessary to avoid wasting image area with resultant unnecessary radiation to the patient [2]. Overframing will also increase magnification and contribute to better resolution on the cine film. In our experience, maximal horizontal overframing is quite satisfactory for coronary work in dual- or triple-mode intensifiers as well as in single-mode 17-cm image tubes. The reader is referred to the report of Inter-Society Commission for a detailed discussion of overframing [3]. The camera lens focal length will vary from 80 to 135 mmHg, depending on the size of output phosphor and the degree of overframing desired. To have the benefit of its best optical characteristics, the camera lens should be fast enough to allow 2 f stops from the maximum aperture. Large lens apertures are no longer necessary in modern systems, because of improvements in image intensifiers. The input dose to the image intensifier should be adjusted to assure minimum acceptable quantum noise, as discussed previously. Relatively slow, fine-grain, large-latitude cine films should be used and developed to an average gradient of 1.2–1.5. Then, the f stop is adjusted to place cardiac density on the characteristic curve of the film to a density of 1.0 or base fog plus 1.0, depending on the type of projector and projection conditions used. In modern systems with the cine films currently available, f stop will fall within the critical resolution of the lens if this procedure is followed. Final adjustment of the appropriate f stop of the camera lens can be then decided, on the basis of the clinical results. Too-small f stops should be avoided, since image contrast and resolution may be decreased owing to diffraction; a too-large f stop may cause vignetting on the image. At the range of f stops generally used, depth of focus is not a critical consideration.

All major manufacturers supply 35-mm Arritechno cameras as the only option with newer equipment support systems. Generally, a film rate of 30 frames/s is satisfactory unless the heart rate is rapid and a fast-moving arterial segment is being filmed, e.g., the AV groove portion of the right coronary artery in the RAO view. Although 60 frames/s will provide better viewing conditions, increased radiation exposure and film cost should be taken into account before routine adoption of high-frame-rate filming in coronary angioplasty.

Angiography Table and Rotational Equipment Support Systems

In all new cardiac catheterization laboratories, the equipment support system is rotational. The older floating tabletop–rotational cradle combination had the advantages of short SIDs and better radiation protection for the operator. In these old systems, angulated views could only be accomplished with improvised add-on devices, such as mechanical coupling of image intensifier and x-ray table by a rod (LED system of GE Co.) or swinging the tabletop on a pivot and ball bearings [14]. Of course, patient discomfort was still a problem on a rotating cradle. Rotational support systems offer the advantages of easily obtained angulated views, which are so important in defining coronary anatomy, and comfort for the supine patient, especially during long procedures. Catheter stability is a definite advantage. Disadvantages of rotational systems are long SIDs and increased radiation exposure to the operator. Since table height and/or U arm height are variable in these systems, the patient entrance distance will vary, with resultant changes in fluoroscopic dose rate and hence in fluoroscopic quality. Fluoroscopic dose rate adjustment in response to varying SID is desirable.

In the AP plane, rotation and angulation are obtained by a U arm with a parallelogram, an L-U arm combination, a C arm with rotation on two axes, or a U arm with fixed SID with a swinging x-ray trolley. In bi-plane systems, lateral

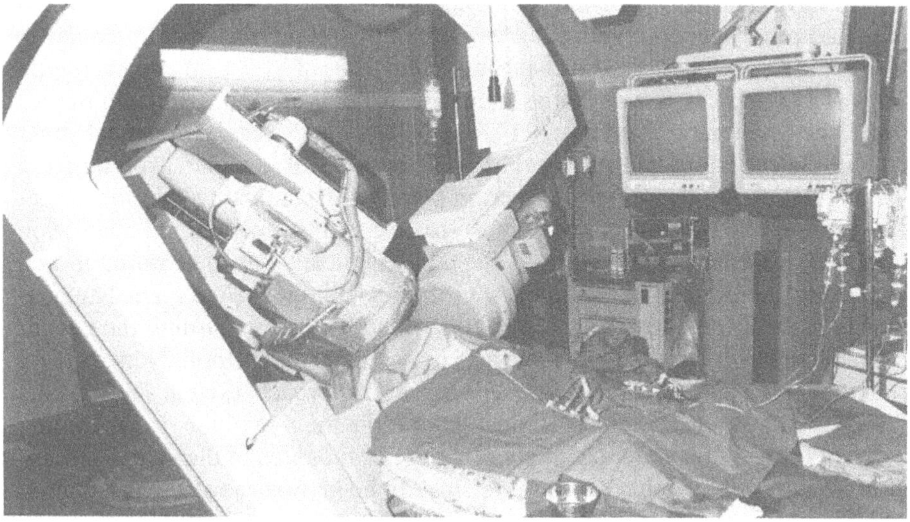

Fig. 3. Bi-plane x-ray system as used by the authors (T. Ischinger, Klinikum Bogenhausen, Munich). U arm, with parallelogram for the AP, and an arc for the lateral plane (Philips Polydiagnost C with L arc)

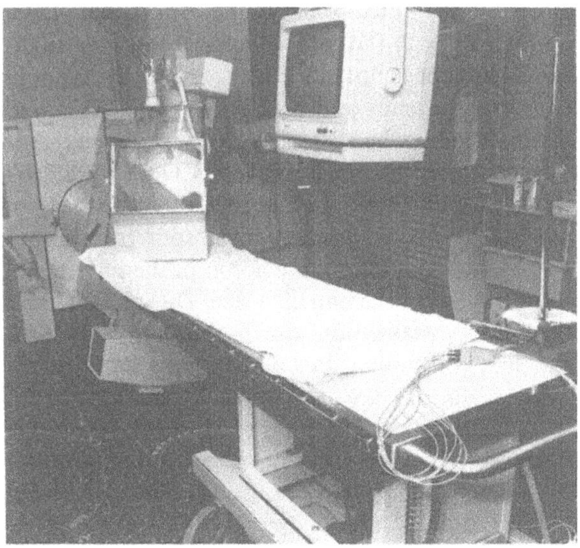

Fig. 4. A single-plane system with mobile U arm for panning and trolley type x-ray table that can be detached for patient transport. (Philips Cardiodiagnost, St. Louis University Hospital)

plane support is provided as follows: For a parallelogram, a lateral C arc (Fig. 3); for an L-U arm, a ceiling-mounted, mechanically coupled x-ray tube and image intensifier with robotic controls for angulation and rotation; second lateral C arm for the C arm systems. For the U arm with fixed SID and swinging x-ray trolley there is no bi-plane provision (Fig. 4). The x-ray systems currently in use in our own unit for interventional procedures are those shown in Figs. 3 and 4.

We have had the opportunity of using parallelogram and L-U devices and have had past experience with C arms. Ease of operation is essentially similar in all three systems. These systems have minimum SIDs of 81–85 cm and maximum SIDs of 113–115 cm. Travel of the image intensifier is around 30 cm. On the AP plane, the rotation range is from $\pm 100°$ to $\pm 90°$ with 45° cranial or caudal angulations. On the lateral plane, generally $-30°$ to $+90°$ RAO lateral rotation and 45° angulation are possible. However, in practice, the cranial angulation is generally limited by the patient's size to 30° to 25°; with steeper cranial angulation the LAO rotation becomes limited. The table frequently has to be raised to well above isocenter, to obtain enough LAO rotation with the desired cranial angulation to prevent the x-ray tube from hitting the table edges. Turning the patient on to the right side on the x-ray table may be necessary and helpful. None of these rotational systems is satisfactory for the brachial approach, even in single plane; for LAO rotation it is necesary almost to straddle the x-ray tube. Furthermore, controls for rotation and table panning cannot be mounted to the operator's left: custom-built rails or other support systems can be improvised at the installation site. Of course, with bi-plane systems the brachial approach will be even more difficult, if not practically impossible. Therefore, PTCA through the brachial approach is most comfortably performed with single-plane equipment. On all the bi-plane equipment mentioned above, the lateral plane can be moved outside of operating field. For the brachial approach, the authors have had long and favorable experience with a U arm system with swinging x-ray trolley (Cardiodiagnost table, from Philips). Although rotation is limited to 60° in the orthogonal plane, slight rotation of the patient on the trolley to the side will provide steeper angulation. Because of the short SID, x-ray tube is not in the way. The trolly has only a canvas top, with excellent x-ray transparency and very good patient comfort. With steeper angulations, the table edge may be visible on the x-ray picture. Another advantage of the system, as mentioned above, is its short SID, which allows adequate x-ray factors with a generator and cine pulse of lower kilowatt rating, x-ray tubes with relatively low loadability with small focal spot for sharper fluoroscopic images. Cranial and caudal angulations are accomplished by swinging the tabletop up to 30°–45° depending on the patient's size. During PTCA, if two angulated views are optimal for visualization and evaluation of lesions, swinging the table is somewhat time consuming, but perhaps not significantly more than in other systems when rotations are performed by the motor. Of course, all other systems can be rotated by hand with faster motions. In laboratories where the brachial approach is used frequently or predominantly, if the volume of work justifies more than one angiographic suite, Cardiodiagnost equipment in at least one room would be quite desirable.

In contrast to the brachial approach, bi-plane systems are preferable for angioplasty through the femoral approach. The main advantage of bi-plane systems is the expediency with which fluoroscopy on two planes can be carried out. The operator can choose the most suitable projection and angulation on each plane, corresponding to the guide shots. Then equipment can be practically stationary during the procedure, with fluoroscopy on the one plane or the other as needed. Since degrees of rotation and of angulation are not changed, these projections correspond more closely to the freeze-frame images of the guide shots on

VDR or VTR playback. Procedure, fluoroscopy time, and radiation exposure can be shortened in comparison with single-plane systems, since recentering after each change of projection is eliminated. Rapid fluoroscopic switching in two planes during guidewire manipulation permits better spatial orientation.

Digital readout of both orthogonal rotation and cranial-caudal angulation should be provided for facile and accurate duplication of the same projection used in control (guide) shots for comparison with post-PTCA cineangiograms.

A handle for rotation, angulation, and table movements is very useful in single-plane systems, since it enables the operator to have total control. In bi-plane systems, AP and lateral supports can be locked and rotated simultaneously.

Tables provided with C and U arms or with parallelograms are built on a relatively narrow base which contains panels for connections to signal conditioners of the physiological recorders and footswitch plus auxiliary power outlets. The authors have incorporated suction and oxygen supply lines to the base, freeing the floor space around the table. In some laboratories, a defibrillator is also mounted on the base of the table. One manufacturer also offers a ceiling-mounted table; gas supply lines and cables running to the connecting panels in the base are enclosed in the ceiling suspension and the telescope. Tabletops should be carbon fiber, which has good radiolucency. Longitudinal table travel is limited by the depth of the C or U arm, but generally has adequate coverage of the femoral area. Vertical motion should be adequate for adjusting to the operator's height.

In summary, bi-plane x-ray systems are preferable in interventional laboratories. For the brachial approach, a single-plane configuration or siting of the lateral support system outside the field of action in a bi-plane system will provide better working conditions.

Digital Subtraction Angiography in PTCA

An excellent review of technical aspects of digital subtraction angiography (DSA) has recently been provided by Kruger and Riederer [15]. Diagnostic quality images of coronary arteries can be obtained by pulsed digital DSA [16, 17]. However, the utility of digital subtraction imaging in coronary angiography, and more specifically in PTCA (road mapping [31]), is questionable at the present state of the art. Very good contrast can be obtained in subtracted images of coronary arteries by using injection volumes of 2 cm^3 or less, thus saving 20–50 cm^3 opaque material in the usual four to ten cine runs required for guide and post-PTCA coronary angiograms: this amount would not have any clinical importance in most instances. When diagnostic coronary angiography and PTCA are combined in the same session the saving in opaque media is a useful feature of DSA, especially with regard to economy in left ventricular cineangiographic injections [18]. Although TV and hard-copy images of the digital angiograms would be available for review in a relatively short time, playback of cine runs in a high-definition video system is faster, with equal if not better image quality. In laboratories without high-definition TV chains DSA may provide better image display and post-processing capabilities (edge enhancement, etc.).

In comparison with cineangiography, pulse mode DSA does not offer the advantage of reduction in radiation exposure.

In the future the most useful aspect of DSA in PTCA applications may be lesion quantitation, either by automatic border recognition or by videodensitometric methods. Estimation of coronary flow or relative changes in the flow may also be possible by videodensitometry.

Contrast Injectors

Only a few laboratories have contrast injectors for coronary artery visualization, although their modern versions are perfectly capable of delivering small amounts of contrast material reliably and at the low flow rates required for intracoronary injections. In interventional cardiology injections are usually given by hand, although power injectors may make opaque medium delivery easier. With ACS dilatation catheters, balloon inflation may occur during injection through the guiding catheter with power injectors [19]. This phenomenon is probably due to the milking effect of high pressure in the guide catheter lumen around the balloon channel which surrounds the shaft of the dilatation catheter. We have observed this same phenomenon when using 2-cm^3 hand injectors, which are capable of generating more pressure than 10-cm^3 injectors. Power injection has also been used through the distal part of USCI/Schneider-Medintag balloon catheters [20].

The characteristics of acceptable power injectors have already been defined [3].

Summary and Guidelines for x-Ray Equipment Selection

The principal features of an ideal facility for the optimal performance of PTCA have been outlined in a report of the Executive Committee of National Heart, Lung, Blood Institute PTCA Registry [21]. Particular demands of PTCA on the x-ray equipment have been enumerated in the Introduction to this chapter. The acquisition of optimum x-ray resources is dependent on the level of financing, which in turn is determined on the basis of the total caseload of the laboratory in general and the number of expected PTCAs in particular. High volumes will justify an angiography suite devoted solely to PTCA, which would facilitate the full utilization and amortization of the equipment. If the caseload or the financing does not permit a room exclusively for PTCA, an existing angiography laboratory may be upgraded. The purpose of this summary is to provide guidelines for equipment selection according to the imaging priorities required by PTCA and the level of financing available. The quality of local service from the x-ray equipment supplier should be one of the primary factors in selection.

1. PTCA room with optimal x-ray equipment
   a) A rotational bi-plane equipment support system capable of compound angulations in both planes; carbon fiber top, pedestal base or ceiling-mounted x-ray table.

b) High-resolution multimodal image intensifiers with previously listed specifications.
c) X-ray tubes of high loadability, with previously listed power ratings and focal spots.
d) A constant-potential generator equipped for bi-plane operation. Provision of variable fluoroscopic dose levels. Power ratings of x-ray components should be matched.
e) Bi-plane high-resolution, high-bandwidth, TV chains with options and circuitry providing good image stabilization, uniform resolution, and prevention of blooming.
f) Two broadcast-quality, type C, helical VTRs, preferably with time-base correction for playback of TV or cine images and two VDRs for playback of guide shots or other desired cine runs in freeze-frame.

2. At the next level of funding, a single-plane duplication of the above system; VDR could be omitted and freeze-frame images, displayed from VTR on a second TV monitor in the procedure room or on the single TV monitor provided for the operator.
3. At the next level, the high-resolution TV chain can be substituted by a standard-line-rate, high-fidelity TV system. At the last level of economy, the reel-to-reel videorecorder may be substituted by a high-quality videocassette recorder. It must be emphasized that a videocassette recorder is grossly inferior to broadcast-quality reel-to-reel recorders for PTCA applications.

In upgrading of an existing system, additional investment should be first made for upgrading the TV chain and playback capabilities. The next stage of improvement in a 12-pulse system should be upgrading of the cine pulse unit and the x-ray tube to higher power ratings. It is assumed that the room considered for upgrading will already have a rotational system with cranial and caudal angulation facilities.

Cine Film Processing, Quality Control, Cine Film Viewing, and Lesion Quantification

The cine processor should be of professional quality with good agitation features, no significant variability of film transport speed at a given setting, and very tight temperature control, to not more than ± 0.3 °C [3]. A replenishment system with flow meters is essential; replenishment by flooding is not acceptable. The water supply should be filtered; if the installation is in an older building with iron water pipes the quality of the water supply becomes a problem and special measures are necessary. In hot climates the water temperature may be higher than in the developing tanks during summer months, and a chilling unit has to be incorporated into the water supply line. Small tabletop processors are not adequate for cardiac catheterization laboratories.

For coronary angiography, a film with wide latitude and fine grain is the ideal choice, since the structures to be filmed are basically in shades of gray with small diameters and low x-ray contrast. These films should be developed to an average gradient of approximately 1.2, and not above 1.5. A rather wide toe on the characteristic curve is desirable, since most of the gray shades will be closer to the toe. Accordingly, the cardiac density should be on 1.0 or base fog +1.0, depending on the projectors used. The lens aperture should be set to obtain these values, as mentioned previously. A common misconception among cardiologists is that it is necessary to obtain contrasty cine films which are pleasing to the eye in their black and white appearance. Actually, the information content of these images is inferior to that of cine film with low contrast and wide latitude, which looks somewhat grayer. In modern cine systems with high gain and brightness there is no need for high-contrast and high-speed films. The cost is another factor in selection of cine film in very high volume laboratories.

Quality control in the angiographic laboratories should start with quality control of cine film processing. If this variable is not controlled it is impossible to judge the changes in the x-ray equipment performance. In initial calibration procedures of angiographic equipment, selection of cine film and its proper development to obtain the desirable characteristic curve is one of the essential steps. Not uncommonly, inferior cine film image quality is the result of poorly controlled film processing rather than inadequate x-ray equipment.

A quality control program may appear superfluous in a laboratory when development factors remain constant and high-quality films are regularly produced. Even in these circumstances, an ongoing quality control process assures more uniform and consistent results, probably due to increased awareness and diligence of the personnel. Furthermore, potential problems are easily detected; for example, a systematic change in film contrast near the time of changing the chemicals may indicate that replenishing rates are not adequate, or a sudden change in film quality may be due to malfunctioning of the recirculation pump. If image deterioration occurs without any change in measured processing factors the problem may be attributable to the x-ray equipment.

A cine run using an x-ray phantom at the beginning of each day in each room is a useful safety measure, preventing the occurrence of no x-ray exposure with a fully prepared patient on the catheterization table. The cine film magazine should be cleaned with each reloading. Film gates should be cleaned and sprayed daily with antistatic solutions or with each loading, depending on the cine film used. Fluoroscopic dose rate measurements, half-value layers of the x-ray tubes, limiting resolution and contrast ratio of intensifiers, x-ray calibration factors, alignment of the collimators, shutters, and the system in general should be part of the periodic quality control checks. These measurements can be carried out by a trained inhouse technologist, or they may be part of a preventive maintenance and service contract with the manufacturer of the x-ray equipment. A record of these measurements should be kept for monitoring the changes in image intensifier and x-ray tube performance. Replacement time for image intensifier insets and x-ray tubes can be objectively determined on the basis of serial measurements, avoiding a period of gradual image deterioration until it becomes grossly apparent. Another benefit of quality control with careful monitoring and record keeping is the justification of replacements at the administrative level.

Cine film viewing will require a quality projector and a projection screen. No single model on the market combines all the desirable features of a 35-mm cine projector. Image optics of 35-mm projectors are based on either a rotating prism or the intermittent film advance principle.

With rotating prism optics, film advance is synchronized with rotation of a prism using a mechanical drum which engages the film perforations in the film gate. The film motion is continuous at variable speed; the individual frames are projected on the same optical path by synchronization of film travel speed and degree of rotation of the prism. Individual frames are in complete focus when parallel to the facets of the prism; thus, the higher the number of facets, the better the quality of the projected image. Older models of optics of this type have 12-face prisms and newer ones, 16-face prisms.

In intermittent film advance optics, the individual frames are rapidly pulled into the film gate and projected while stationary through a synchronized rotating shutter, after which the shutter is closed and the next frame is pulled to the gate using a film advance claw or belt. Frame switchover time is short, usually around 10 ms to prevent flicker in slow frame rates. Film playback speed is not continuously variable, as opposed to that with rotating prism optics; different settings at multiples of line frequency or simply high and low speeds are provided in two different models of this type. Theoretically, intermittent film advance projectors should yield sharper images than rotating prism types during review in motion, but single-frame resolution should be equal in both types. Intermittent film advance projectors are noisier than rotating prism types. They may cause more wear and tear on the film and the film loading has to be done more carefully to prevent damage; the downtime may be more than that of the rotating prism projectors.

Options and accessories vary widely between different models and should be chosen by the user according to the specific needs of the laboratory. Film path reversal and image rotation options are useful in a laboratory receiving a large number of referral films from other facilities with different film winding. Side-by-side projection of two films may be selected as a second projector in PTCA laboratories when comparison of the studies before and after PTCA or follow-up examination are made for both research and clinical purposes.

In angiographic evaluation of PTCA results a common practice is computation of stenosis as a percentage by caliper measurements of the most severe narrowing and the adjacent normal segment before any branch take-off in one or two projections; measurements in two perpendicular projections are usually averaged. In some laboratories the most severe stenosis in one plane is recorded. This practice of measurement in stationary single cine frames is contrary to the generally known and frequently stated principle of cine film review in motion. The eye integrates several frames of a motion picture. The physiological image integration smoothes out the quantum mottle in the individual frames; noise is reduced, and information content is improved by image averaging. In fact, the variation in the appearance of a tight lesion from frame to frame is frequently observed in stop motion analysis. Unfortunately, there is no substitute for single-frame analysis for lesion quantification, regardless of whether hand caliper measurements or sophisticated computer technology are used.

The main advantage of electronic calipers is the elimination of manual calculations of the proportion of the luminal diameter occupied by a stenosis or the reduction in cross-sectional area; they save time, but without necessarily improving the accuracy over that obtained with hand-held caliper measurements. There is the advantage of reduced intra- and interobserver variation, although perceived image quality on single frames is inferior to subjective evaluation of film in motion.

Border tracings of the coronary arteries do not take into account irregular intraluminal protrusions of the plaques with varying degrees of contrast. Postangioplasty lesions are highly irregular, and very typically tracing of their outside borders may not yield the actual cross-sectional area due to plaque fracture and unidirectional stretching of the arterial segment; a crescent-type morphology along the line of plaque fracture is quite common, rendering estimation of cross-sectional area from border tracing on two projections very difficult.

A recently proposed computerized lesion quantitation program transfers cineangiographic images to video signal with subsequent videodensitometric analysis [22]. Theoretically, this mode of analysis should not be dependent on geometric configuration. Indeed, good correlations were found between videodensitometric measurement of degree of stenosis plus reduction of cross-sectional area and actual sizes of the lesions in phantoms simulating eccentric stenoses. In a few patient studies there was good correlation between videometric measurements and histological planimetry at post mortem. Analysis by these methods can potentially be performed online in the PTCA laboratory, using DSA imaging if reliable corrections for background density can be made and the pixel density is adequate for discrete, severe stenotic lesions.

Inadequacies of angiographic quantitation in pre-, and especially post-PTCA lesions require assessment of additional indices of myocardial perfusion. Development of a quick and reliable method of coronary flow measurement, possibly a videodensitometric method, will constitute a significant improvement in evaluation of the results of coronary angioplasty.

In assessment of the prognostic significance of coronary lesions, in addition to the vessels involved and the degree of stenosis other factors, such as amount of myocardium in jeopardy and the presence of collateral flow, should be taken into consideration [23, 24]. A computer-based system of coronary scoring for this purpose has been described.

Physiological Recorder, Signal Conditioner, Data Processing

A multi-channel recorder is necessary in the PTCA laboratory, as in any cardiac catheterization room. A photographic recorder with a rapid developer is best. Jet ink or heated stylus recorders are acceptable, provided that at least two pressure channels can be superimposed with the same baseline. The paper cost they entail is less than that for the photographic recorders. In the case of photographic recorders, signal splitting to a monitoring oscilloscope and to the photographic paper with position and gain adjustment by a single control is most practical and convenient for the recording technician. Otherwise, a periscope showing the trace position on the paper should be provided with photographic recorders. This capability is not present in some photographic recorders that are retrofitted to older systems, and the lack of it makes accurate positioning and calibration of the channels very difficult.

A minimum of two pressure preamplifiers should be provided. A further one or two pressure channels is highly desirable, since direct monitoring of arterial pressure may be necessary in critically ill and unstable patients; arterial pressure recorded through the guide catheter with the dilatation catheter in place is highly damped. In patients who require intra-aortic balloon pumping before or during PTCA, balloon inflation and deflation may be best monitored by the pressure curve contour. An additional pressure channel may also be necessary for patients who have had Swan-Ganz catheter monitoring. The pressure transducers should be calibrated against mercury, and equal sensitivity should be ensured. The zero opening level of each transducer should be the same, and at the level of the phlebostatic plane; this is particularly important in PTCA in evaluation of gradient across the stenosis during dilatation. The manifold or the clamps supporting the transducers should be mounted on the angiographic table rather than on a separate stand, since the height of the angiographic table is frequently changed in rotational equipment systems in PTCA laboratories.

A minimum of two ECG channels should be available. In dilatation of left anterior descending and circumflex artery lesions, monitoring of a chest lead by placement of a nonradiopaque electrode is highly useful.

For research purposes, additional signal conditioners may be useful; recorders with easily interchangeable plug-in preamplifiers are best.

Some of the multi-channel recorders are provided with alphanumeric quotation capabilities, which are useful for record keeping. One such recorder also provides an option for continuous display of the mean gradient between guide and balloon catheters.

In addition to a monitoring oscilloscope on the recorder chassis or in the control room, a slave monitor should be provided in the procedure room, located in the same visual field as the TV monitor for comfortable review by the operator.

Although not necessary for the PTCA procedure itself, a reliable and rapid means of determination of cardiac output, for example by thermodilution, should be available, since it is occasionally needed in the management of critically ill patients, for example during thrombolytic therapy or PTCA for acute myocardial infarction. Access to rapid blood gas analysis is also necessary.

Some multi-channel recorders are provided with a separate microprocessor-based computer for on- or offline analysis of the hemodynamic data, report generation, recording of clinical data base, and archiving. Programs for report generation, data base, and archiving can be customized. With microcomputers and multiple terminals networking is possible involving procedure room, projection room for image analysis, and data center for archiving and information retrieval. In large cardiac units the data can be fed into a central computer. The preparation of forms suitable for computer entries of clinical data base, pre- and post-PTCA angiographic findings, hemodynamic data, and follow-up information is extremely useful. A personal computer with adequate disk space may be used for data processing and information management in the laboratory. The same computer with different terminals can also be used for angiographic analysis when provided with lesion quantitation programs and electronic calipers and also for ventricular volume and wall motion analysis. If there is a digital subtraction angiography unit in the room, the computing facilities of this unit will be adequate for ventricular wall motion and volume analysis with the programs commercially available. Probably such units will also have commercially available programs for quantitation of stenosis based on border recognition in the near future. This field of data analysis is in a state of rapid change, and rapid improvements and progression are expected.

The Society of Cardiac Angiography has recently initiated a computerized PTCA Registry providing data retrieval for participating laboratories.

In laboratories with smaller caseloads a separate PTCA log with limited but relevant entries is useful and necessary.

Emergency Equipment

The PTCA room should contain all the necessary equipment and medication for management of all cardiovascular emergencies.

A crash-cart should be in the room, containing drugs (including intracoronary nitrates, calcium, antagonists, streptokinase, and urokinase), intubation equipment and ventilation bags, arterial and venous cannulation equipment, and IV lines and fluids. Its content should be checked daily and replenished as necessary.

A DC defibrillator should be present for use exclusively in the procedure room, as in any cardiac catheterization laboratory. Its actual discharge should be determined according to electrical safety procedures of the hospital, and actual numbers of joules delivered should be recorded for corresponding meter values. Battery-operated, rechargeable, compact models are best. Some of these compact models are equipped with a single-channel, small ECG monitor. These units can be used during the transfer of patients from the PTCA laboratory to the intensive care unit or the operating room. The authors prefer to have a small defibrillator with monitoring oscilloscope for exclusive use in each catheterization room plus a single unit with monitoring facilities for patient transfer. This arrangement saves costs and also allows a defibrillator to be permanently sited at a convenient location in each room. DC defibrillators in the PTCA room should be provided with a synchronization signal for conversion of supraventricular arrhythmias or ventricular tachycardia.

Some angiographers routinely place a temporary pacemaker in the right ventricle before starting PTCA; others rarely see a need for its use. Regardless of whether this is done or not, a temporary pacemaker unit and pacing catheters should always be available in the catheterization room.

An intra-aortic balloon counterpulsation console should be available on demand for emergencies in the PTCA laboratory. When high frequencies of coronary bypass surgery and PTCA justify it, a balloon console may be allocated exclusively to the PTCA laboratory. Percutaneous balloon introduction kits and intra-aortic balloons with central lumen for guidewire introduction and subsequent arterial pressure monitoring are best. In units with smaller caseloads and only limited use of intra-aortic balloon pumping it is a good policy to alert the technician to the possibility that intra-aortic balloon support will be required, particularly in the case of high-risk patients. Depending on the location of the cardiovascular surgical facility and its distance from the PTCA unit, arrangements must be made for surgical standby during transportation of PTCA patients if surgery should become urgently necessary.

Space Requirement and Architectural Considerations for the Interventional Laboratory

The interventional laboratory consists of the procedure, equipment, and control rooms, similar to an optimally designed cardiac catheterization laboratory.

The procedure room houses an x-ray table, a rotational support system with image intensifier and x-ray tube, TV monitors, an oscilloscope, and readout devices. Every effort should be made to keep the floor space free of wires; transducer cables should be connected to the panels in the table base and tunnelled through the floor or pulled over the ceiling to the control room. Power outlets in the base should be used for connection of auxiliary equipment, if necessary. Depending on the space available, some components of x-ray equipment that are not noisy and do not involve excessive heat generation can be located in the procedure room. Indirect lighting provides a more pleasing environment. Tungsten lights with rheostat control will provide the desired level of illumination. Fluorescent lights are undesirable because of the possibility of creating electrical interference. A small surgical light with movable joints can be ceiling mounted; it must be possible to project it to either side of the patient. Connections can be made to a footswitch with an automatic turn-off surgical spot light during fluoroscopy or cine runs. A radiation shield for protection of the operator should be mounted on ceiling tracks for easy positioning. In general, the room should be free of any equipment that is not necessary for performance of the procedure.

The average size of an interventional room should be approximately 8×6 m or 48–50 m^2. Minimum dimensions of 8×5 m will require every measure to free the space in the room. A larger room measuring 9×7 m would allow freer motion of auxiliary equipment, such as respirator and balloon pump, and on rare occasions the use of a circulatory assist device. Different modes of interventional procedures in the future may also tax the floor space in the procedure room; planning for a larger room than is customary at present may be desirable in new facilities.

The equipment room should contain the transformer and the components of x-ray apparatus with high heat generation and noise. If possible, all electronic components should be placed in the equipment room except the generator control desk, which should be in the control room. The equipment room should be located in such a way as to allow short high-tension cables to the procedure room (20 m for 12-pulse generators with cine pulse unit and 12 m for high-tension generators).

The control room should be large enough to house the generator control desk(s), tape deck(s), and controls, VDR(s) control, physiological recorder, TV monitors, and oscilloscope for the technician. The equipment should be arranged in a cockpit configuration to allow the technician access to the x-ray controls and physiological recorder. VTR may be operated by remote control from the desk in the cockpit, or the controls can be incorporated into the generator control desk. VDR controls should also be incorporated into the desk in the cockpit, for access by the same recording and monitoring technician. A good view of the procedure room must be possible from the control room, through leaded glass or lead-impregnated plastic panels. A separate entrance to the procedure and control room is recommended, to limit and separate the traffic to each room. For a bi-plane installation the dimensions of the control room should be at least 4×2.5 m.

Personnel Requirements

1. Monitor and recording technician: The same person can operate the physiological recorder, VTR, and VDRs and monitor the x-ray factors at the cockpit in the control room.
2. A circulating nurse in the procedure room.
3. A scrub nurse at the table for equipment preparation and assistance during the procedure.
4. Some operators may require an additional nurse at the table if the procedure is performed by a single physician; others may elect to work with only one nurse at the table, depending on the system used.

In laboratories with heavy scheduling and frequent, complex PTCAs, a swing shift will be necessary to avoid excessive overtime for the first shift of nurses and technicians.

Depending on the volume of PTCAs, a secretary or data technician assigned to the interventional program is extremely useful for scheduling, data entry, and follow-up information.

The nurse assigned to the holding area of the cardiac catheterization laboratory will generally be able to care for PTCA patients before as well as after the procedure.

Radiation Protection

The reader is referred to standard texts for review of the principles of radiation biology and safety [2, 25, 26]. There is no agreement on the existence of a minimum threshold below which the radiation exposure is safe. Radiation exposure to the personnel should be kept to a minimum. Radiation safety guidelines for cardiac catheterization laboratories have recently been outlined [27]. The maximum acceptable level of radiation has been progressively reduced over the decades. The latest recommendations from the National Council on Radiation Protection and Measurements (NCRP) are 75 rem for hands, 30 rem for forearms, 15 rem for thyroid, and 5 rem for lens and whole body [26]. Angiographers who perform PTCA are probably exposed to more radiation than any other medical practitioners, owing to long fluoroscopy times at somewhat higher dose rates to improve TV images plus cine runs for guide and post-PTCA control angiograms.

The equipment used has inherently more scatter, especially in angulated views, in particular in LAO projection with cranial angulation (Fig. 5). Radiation exposure to the angiographer in rotational systems and its reduction by radiation shields have been described previously [28–30]. Although conclusions reached in these studies can be extrapolated to PTCA practice, no direct measurements of exposure to PTCA practitioners have so far been published. An angiographer who performs 20–30 coronary angioplasties a month, including a number of complex PTCAs plus a moderate number of diagnostic studies, may be exposed to 350–400 rem measured at the neck level outside the thyroid guard when a rotational system with tight collimation but without radiation shield is used (personal observations). All personnel in the procedure room should wear protective coats, with 0.5 mm lead value on the front and 0.25 mm on the other surfaces, and a thyroid guard. Lead eyeglasses with side panels may significantly reduce the exposure of the lens; however, many PTCA angiographers refuse to wear them because they find them uncomfortable and distracting. A ceiling-mounted radiation shield made of leadglass or plastic with flexible leaded rubber bands attached to the bottom significantly reduces the radiation exposure to the operator [28, 29] (see also Fig. 4). These shields are now commercially available through the x-ray manufacturers. We have found some of these radiation shields heavy and cumbersome to use; some are quite light and easy to position. Radiation masks similar to those worn by welders have not become popular among angiographers, since they are cumbersome and distracting during longer procedures.

No personnel not directly involved in the procedure should be in the room. A separate control room should be an essential design feature for any new laboratory. Personnel needed anywhere else than at the operating table should stand as far away as possible from the x-ray source, since the radiation level will fall according to the law of inverse squares.

Radiation exposure of personnel should be carefully monitored and recorded. The badges should be worn at neck level under or outside the lead coat or thyroid guard.

There should be frequent checks of collimation and fluoroscopic dose levels. Optimization of the image chain will help to reduce the exposure levels. The lower fluoroscopic dose rate options offered for PTCA installations should be more frequently utilized during the procedure if available in the laboratory concerned. With the availability of high-fidelity TV chains and playback units, economy in cine runs is possible.

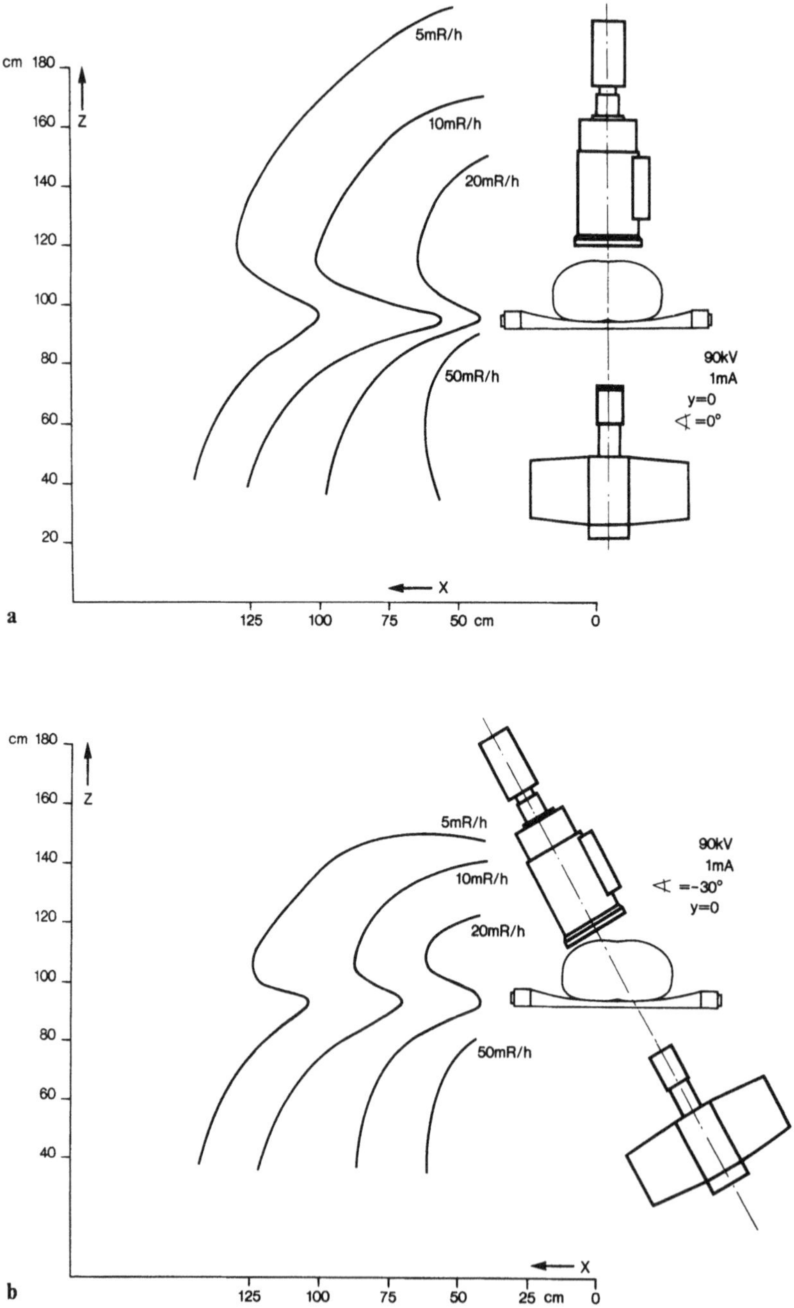

Fig. 5 a–d. Distribution and intensity of scattered radiation around the x-ray table (isoexposure rate curves) with a U arm (Philips Cardiodiagnost) in the vertical and 30° right and left projections at 90 kV and 1 mA [30]. **a–c** Scattered radiation perpendicular to the major axis of the body: **a** vertical projection; **b** 30° right anterior oblique view; **c** 30° left anterior oblique view. There is a marked outward displacement of the curves below the table. This effect is particularly pronounced with the 30° left anterior oblique projection. **d** In the plane parallel to the major axis of the body the isodose curves are practically symmetrical

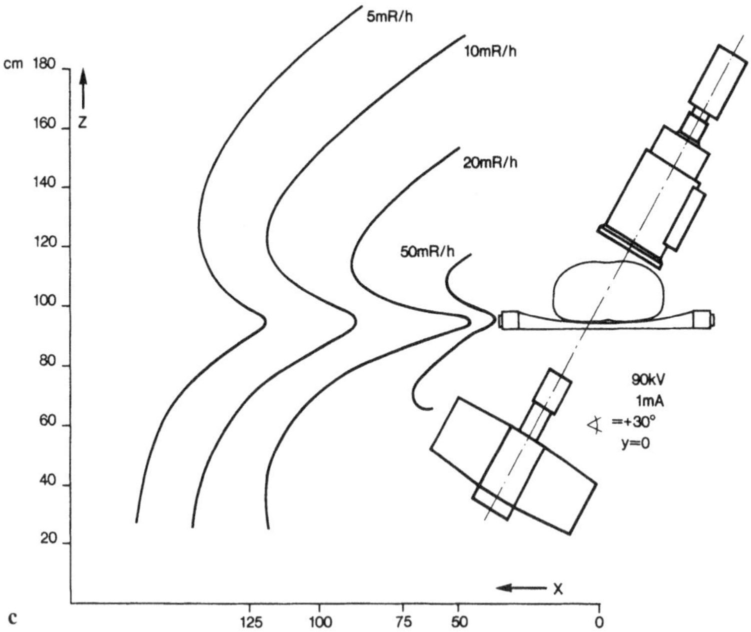
5mR/h
10mR/h
20mR/h
50mR/h
cm 180
160
140
120
100
80
60
40
20
Z
90kV
1mA
∢ =+30°
y=0
X
125
100
75
50
0

c

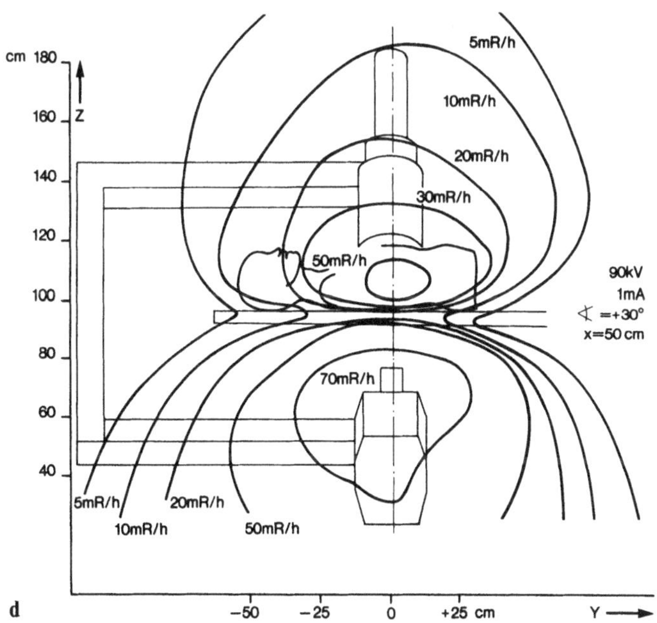
5mR/h
10mR/h
20mR/h
30mR/h
50mR/h
70mR/h
cm 180
160
140
120
100
80
60
40
Z
90kV
1mA
∢ =+30°
x=50 cm
5mR/h
10mR/h
20mR/h
50mR/h
−50
−25
0
+25 cm
Y

d

Shared Facilities in the Cardiac Catheterization Laboratory

The most logical site for the interventional cardiology suite is within the cardiac catheterization laboratory, to allow efficient use of common facilities and close interaction with diagnostic cardiac catheterization activities. It is desirable to site the angiographic suites, the holding area, equipment store, clean supply room, and other procedure-related functions in the same geographic area. Office space and filing cabinets should be located in close proximity, but separated from the patient flow. The reception area and the waiting room for relatives should be located conveniently for easy access from the patient area and administrative section.

Clean Supply Room. Because of the large number of items involved, PTCA equipment should probably be stored in a separate section of the supply room, or alternatively a separate supply room may be provided for PTCA equipment. We have found it practical to stock a small number of each item in close proximity to the PTCA rooms and use a separate storage area for total stock. A system of shelves or organizers is highly useful to allow rapid location of the type of equipment needed urgently during the procedure.

A small separate room with a washbasin, counters, and shelves is useful for cleaning, preparation, and packing of reusable equipment.

In laboratories that do their own gas sterilization a separate room with ethylene oxide venting should be provided.

Holding Area. A holding area, with adequate space and dividing curtains for each stretcher, should be provided. ECG monitoring with telemetry and a multi-channel monitor at the nurse's desk is highly desirable in this area. Wall outlets for oxygen and suction, similar to those in recovery rooms, are practical.

Dark Room and Processing Facilities. Location of the dark room and processing facilities within the angiographic suites has proved very practical for us. If they cannot be located within the same area they should be in close proximity.

Projection and Viewing Facilities. Film viewing and reporting booths and a projection and/or conference room should be sited between the administrative wing and the angiographic suites or can be incorporated into the office area.

A limited amount of recent cardiac catheterization films can be stored in the projection area for easy access. A film file room with movable racks for economy of space should be provided.

Common Room. A lounge for nurses and technicians must be provided in a busy laboratory. It should have facilities such as refrigerator, microwave oven, etc.

Acknowledgement. We thank Dr. H. Mohr, of Philips International B.V., 2000 Hamburg, Federal Republic of Germany, for his critical review of the manuscript and valuable suggestions.

References

1. Ter-Pogossian MM (1967) The physical aspects of diagnostic radiology. Hoeber Medical Division/Harper and Row, New York
2. Christensen EE, Curry TS, Dowdey GE (1978) An introduction to the physics of diagnostic radiology. Lea and Febiger, Philadelphia
3. Inter-Society Commission for Heart Disease Resources (1983) Report. Circulation 68:893 A
4. Paulin S (1981) Terminology for radiographic projections in cardiac angiography. Cathet Cardiovasc Diagn 7:341
5. Milne ENC (1974) Characterizing focal spot performance. Radiology 3:483
6. L'Esperance J, Saltiel J, Bourassa MG (1974) Angulated views in the saggital plane for improved accuracy of cine coronary angiography. AJR 121:738
7. Aldridge HE (1984) A decade or more of cranial and caudal angled projections in coronary arteriography – Another look. Cathet Cardiovasc Diagn 10:539
8. Beekmans AAG et al. (1981) Quality control of image intensifiers. Proceedings of AAPM Meeting on Acceptance Testing, 1–25 October 1981, Chicago
9. Linfoot EH (1964) Fourier methods in optical image evaluation. Pitman, Bath
10. Hay GA (1978) X-Ray imaging. J Phys [E] 11:377
11. Kuhl W, Schrijvers JE (1977) Design aspects of x-ray image intensifiers. Acta Electronica 20:41
12. Gray JG, Woodrow ME, Smith HC, Holmes DR (1984) Technical considerations for cardiac laboratory high definition video systems. Cathet Cardiovasc Diagn 10:73
13. Holmes DP, Smith HC, Gray JE (1984) Clinical evaluation and application of cardiac laboratory high definition video systems. Cathet Cardiovasc Diagn 10:63
14. Mudd JG, Tricamo J (1981) Conversion of a fixed x-ray table for axial views. Cathet Cardiovasc Diagn 7:319
15. Kruger RA, Riederer SJ (1984) Basic concepts of digital subtraction angiography. J. K. Hall, Boston
16. Tobis J, Nalcioglu O, Iseril T, Johnston WD, Roeck W, Castlemane T, Bauer E, Montelli S, Henry WL (1984) Detection and quantitation of coronary artery stenosis from digital subtraction angiograms compared with 35 mm film cineangiograms. Am J Cardiol 54:489
17. Zack PM, Aker UT, Ischinger T, Russ T, Vlahovich GV, Kennedy HL (1984) Angiographic detection of coronary collaterals: a comparison of conventional cine and digital subtraction angiography. Clin Res 32(2):219A
18. Tobis JM, Nalcioglu O, Johnston WD, Siebert A, Roeck W, Iseril T, Elkayam U, Henry WL (1983) Correlation of 10 ml digital subtraction ventriculograms compared with standard cineangiograms. Am Heart J 105:946
19. Van Gelder LM, van der Krieken AM, El Gamal MIA, Bonnier JJRM, Michaels HR (1984) Balloon inflation caused by contrast injection through the guiding catheter. Cathet Cardiovasc Diagn 10:253
20. Sanders M, Shani J, Saviano J, Rivera M (1984) Distal coronary power injection during PTCA. Cathet Cardiovasc Diagn 10:603
21. Williams DO and Members of the Executive Committee of the NHLBI Percutaneous Transluminal Angioplasty Registry (1982) Guidelines for the performance of percutaneous transluminal coronary angioplasty. Circulation 66:693
22. Nickels AB, Gabrielli CFO, Fenoglio JJ, Esser PD (1984) Quantification of relative coronary arterial stenosis by cinevideodensitometric analysis of coronary arteriograms. Circulation 69:512
23. Gensini JJ (1975) Coronary arteriography. Futura, Mt. Kisco, p 488
24. Gensini JJ (1983) A more meaningful scoring system for determining the severity of coronary heart disease. Am J Cardiol 53:606
25. Pizzarello DJ, Witcofski RL (1975) Basic radiation biology. 2. Lea and Febiger, Philadelphia
26. National Council on Radiation Protection and Measurements (1971) Basic radiation protection criteria. NCRP, Washington (Report no. 39)

27. Laboratory Performance Standards Committee, The Society of Cardiac Angiography (1984) Guidelines for radiation protection in the cardiac catheterization laboratory. Cathet Cardiovasc Diagn 10:87
28. Balter S, Sones FM Jr, Brancato R (1978) Radiation exposure to the operator performing cardiac angiography with U-arm systems. Circulation 58:925
29. Gertz EW, Visneski JA, Gould RG, Akin JR (1982) Improved radiation protection for physicians performing cardiac catheterization. Am J Cardiol 50:1283
30. Mohr H, Rentrop P (1977) Strahlenverteilung an einem U-Stativ in der kardiologischen Praxis. Z Kardiol 66:74
31. Tobis J, Johnston W, Montelli S et al. (1985) Digital coronary road mapping as an aid for performing coronary angioplasty. Am J Cardiol 56:237–241

Chapter 7. Angioplasty Equipment and Supplies: Technical Considerations

MICHEL VANDORMAEL, THOMAS ISCHINGER, and ROBERT ROTH

Introduction

Percutaneous transluminal coronary angioplasty (PTCA) is a complex procedure that requires appropriate laboratory facilities and special training of the team who performs it. Although PTCA is performed in the cardiac catheterization laboratory with techniques similar to those used in routine diagnostic cardiac catheterization and coronary angiography, it is far more complex, requiring skills and knowledge beyond those necessary for conventional diagnostic procedures [1].

Several questions that arise when the setup and performance of PTCA are considered: What equipment and instrumentation are necessary? What is an adequate startup inventory? How does this equipment work and how is it set up? This chapter will discuss the equipment and instrumentation necessary for the performance of PTCA. It will provide technical information that will facilitate the performance of PTCA. Great attention to detail is required, as an effective point of technique can make the difference between success and failure in angioplasty. Technical considerations such as setup, use, and care of the angioplasty equipment are a crucial factor in the outcome of PTCA.

This chapter will describe the instrumentation currently used for PTCA at St. Louis University Medical Center and at Munich-Bogenhausen Hospital, Munich, FRG. This is not intended to be an endorsement of any particular device, but a discussion of our experience with the various items of equipment available.

Equipment

PTCA is performed with a coaxial catheter system consisting of two catheters: a guiding catheter and a dilatation or balloon catheter [2–5]. Guide catheters are available in a variety of shapes to provide a means of coronary ostial engagement and to permit passage of the dilatation catheter through the inner lumen into the coronary artery to dilated. A percutaneous introducer sheath is used to facilitate guide and balloon catheter changes. Balloon catheters are available in a number of sizes, with inflated diameters ranging from 2 to 4.2 mm. Selection is based on the severity of the stenosis and on the vessel diameter.

A recent advance in the technique of PTCA has been the development of steerable balloon dilatation catheters [6, 7]. Dilatation catheters are placed in the coronary artery with the help of various thin, flexible guidewires with shapeable tips. The wire is inserted in the central lumen of the balloon catheter and can be maneuvered by the angioplasty operator to negotiate difficult turns, avoid side branches, and engage eccentric lesions. Once the guidewire has been passed across the lesion to be dilated, the dilatation catheter is moved forward over the wire through the stenosis. Several different guidewires are available to optimize the chances of safe placement of the balloon segment across the lesion.

A number of accessories belong to the PTCA system: Y connectors, to allow both pressure measurement and contrast injection; balloon inflation devices; guidewire introducers; and guidewire torque devices. PTCA is facilitated when all the accessories necessary are prepacked and sterilized in a special angioplasty tray.

Dilatation Catheters and Wires

There are now several dilatation catheter systems available for the performance of coronary angioplasty. (See *Appendix* for a list of manufacturers.) Extensive experience has been collected, essentially with two systems, the Schneider-Medintag/USCI and the ACS (Advanced Cardiovascular Systems). The USCI system is somewhat similar to the Schneider-Medintag system. The availability of several systems means that the operator can select a catheter system with characteristics to suit the varying anatomic demands of each PTCA procedure. The approach may then vary depending on lesion severity, morphology, length, location, and accessibility.

Original System

The original angioplasty catheters, introduced by Schneider-Medintag and commercially available also, under license, from USCI, were the G, DG, J, and DJ series (Table 1). These catheters have a double lumen: one central lumen com-

Table 1. Dimensions of the original angioplasty catheters

Catheter type	Balloon diameter (mm)	Balloon length (mm)	Shaft diameter (F/mm)	Shaft length (cm)	Ave deflated profile (in.)
G	3.0	12	4 (1.32)	140	0.053
G	3.0	20	4 (1.32)	140	0.053
G	3.7	20	4 (1.32)	140	0.055
DG	3.0	20	4 (1.32)	140	0.053
DG	3.7	12	4 (1.32)	140	0.055
DG	3.7	20	4 (1.32)	140	0.055
DG (low profile)	2.0	20	4 (1.32)	140	0.044
J	3.0	20	4 (1.32)	140	0.053
J	3.7	20	4 (1.32)	140	0.055
DJ	3.0	20	4 (1.32)	140	0.053
DJ	3.7	20	4 (1.32)	140	0.055

municates with two distal side holes. This allows for contrast injection and pressure measurement. The other lumen communicates with the balloon and allows for balloon inflation and deflation. A 0.018-in. 9 mm fixed wire, either straight (G) or curved (J), extends from the tip of the catheter. The DG and the DJ catheters are reinforced with a forming wire through the balloon lumen. This allows for shaping of the tip of the catheter. The G and J dilatation catheters have no such shaping wire. To assist with positioning at the stenosis, there are radiopaque gold markers proximal and distal to the balloon. The 2.0 balloon has a gold marker only at the proximal portion of the balloon. These catheters are available in different balloon diameters and lengths.

The 3-mm balloon catheter was the most commonly used, the 3.7-mm one being reserved for very large vessels. The 2-mm low-profile balloon catheter may be useful in very tight stenoses. If the balloon catheter persistently enters side branches, a J-wire-tipped balloon catheter, or a DG or DJ balloon catheter with a forming stylet through the balloon lumen, can be tried. The stylet in the DG and DJ allows the balloon portion to be preshaped.

The original balloon catheters have been largely replaced by over-the-wire systems, the so-called steerable catheters.

Steerable Dilatation Catheters

The concept of the steerable catheter is explained in Fig. 1, which shows a Schneider-Medintag system. Basically, the steerable system allows the placement of a movable Teflon-coated guidewire passing through the balloon catheter and out at its tip. The length of the protruding tip and the direction in which the J-shaped tip points can be altered by manipulating the other end of the wire. The ability to shape and direct guidewires makes it possible to reach almost any branch of the coronary arterial tree that has a significant stenosis. An important point to mention is that the wire must be kept free of kinks and bends to maintain free movement through the dilating catheter. Once the guidewire has been passed into the artery across the lesion to be dilated, the dilatation catheter is moved forward over the wire and through the stenosis with no risk of entering side branches or creating a false lumen. The over-the-wire system provides additional support

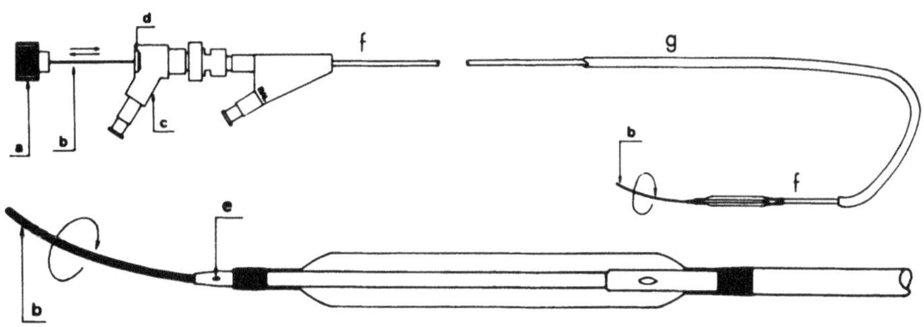

Fig. 1. A steerable catheter system for PTCA: *a* wire rotating device; *b* steerable guidewire; *c* steerable Y connector; *d* hemostatic valve; *e* side holes; *f* dilatation catheter; *g* guide catheter. (Illustration courtesy of Schneider-Medintag)

Table 2. USCI steerable dilatation catheters

Balloon dia (mm)	Balloon length (mm)	Shaft dia (F)	Usable shaft length (cm)	Tip OD (in.)	Tip ID (in.)	Average deflated balloon profile (in.)	Recommended guide wire (in.)
2.0	25	4.3	135	0.026	0.020	0.053	0.016 or 0.014
2.5	25	4.3	135	0.026	0.020	0.055	0.016 or 0.014
3.0	25	4.3	135	0.026	0.020	0.063	0.016 or 0.014
3.7	25	4.3	135	0.026	0.020	0.063	0.016 or 0.014
4.2	25	4.3	135	0.026	0.020	0.067	0.016 or 0.014

A series of similar steerable dilatation catheters is available from Schneider-Medintag in Europe. More recently, Schneider-Medintag has introduced balloon cathethers with further reduced profile (Super-low profile, Passkey) and increased flexibility (lfx type). "Floppy" guidewires with a diameter reduced to 0.010 in. are also available from Schneider-Medintag

Table 3. USCI Lo-Profile (LPS) dilating catheters

Balloon dia (mm)	Balloon length (mm)	Shaft dia (F)	Usable shaft length (cm)	Tip OD (in.)	Tip ID (in.)	Average deflated balloon profile (in.)	Recommended guide wire (in.)
2.0	25	4.3	135	0.022	0.020	0.038	0.014
2.5	25	4.3	135	0.022	0.020	0.048	0.014
3.0	25	4.3	135	0.022	0.020	0.050	0.014
3.5	25	4.3	135	0.022	0.020	0.054	0.014
4.0	25	4.3	135	0.022	0.020	0.056	0.014

for passage across tight, resistant lesions. Injections of contrast material and pressure measurements are possible through both side holes and end holes while the guide wire is being maneuvered.

There is a range of guidewires available, each with different characteristics (Table 2). The ideal wire would combine the elements of directional control (steerability), maximum safety in crossing stenoses (flexibility), and good visual characteristics (radiopacity). However, there is a trade-off in flexibility and formability. The stiffer the tip of the guidewire, the easier it will be to impart the desired shape, while an exceedingly flexible wire, which provides for maximum safety, may defy attempts to shape its tip.

The steerable system allows exchange of balloon catheters while the stenosis remains engaged. Appropriate long exchange guidewires are available for this purpose.

The introduction of the steerable system has increased the success rate and the safety of PTCA procedures and has allowed the procedure to be greatly expanded beyond the early indications.

USCI (or Schneider-Medintag) Steerable Dilatation System

Dilatation Catheters

Gruntzig Type S Steerable balloon catheters (Fig. 2) are 4.3 F in diameter and 135 cm long. All balloon lengths are 25 mm. There are five balloon diameters, ranging from 2.0 to 4.2 mm (inflated balloon diameter). Radiopaque platinum marks the proximal and distal ends within the balloon. The type S catheter has two side holes and an end hole. Although the manufacturer recommends a maximum inflation pressure of 5 atm, most balloons tolerate pressure as high as 10–12 atm. One should be aware that balloon rupture may occur and the designated outer diameter may be exceeded by up to 40% at these levels.

The *Lo-Profile Steerable* (LPS) catheter has a low-profile balloon segment approximately 20% smaller than the steerable system (Table 3). The distal end is tapered to decrease its outer diameter. This system maintains the ability to inject contrast as well as monitor pressures. The wire used with this catheter should be no larger than 0.014 in. This catheter is intended to make it possible to cross very tight lesions that cannot be crossed with the type S steerable catheters.

Table 4 and Fig. 3 demonstrate the difference between the USCI steerable system and the USCI Lo-Profile steerable system.

USCI balloon catheters cannot be gas sterilized. Should contamination occur during the aseptic transfer, resterilization should be achieved by soaking in an approved liquid sterilant for an adequate length of time.

Steerable Guidewires

USCI offers 0.016-in. and 0.014-in. Teflon-coated steerable guidewires with either straight or J tips. The J tip contains a 30° deflection. All wires are 175 cm in length, with the distal 25 cm differing in degree of flexibility to give steerable, flexible steerable, and very flexible steerable wires (Fig. 4). All wires can be twisted to aid in tip orientation.

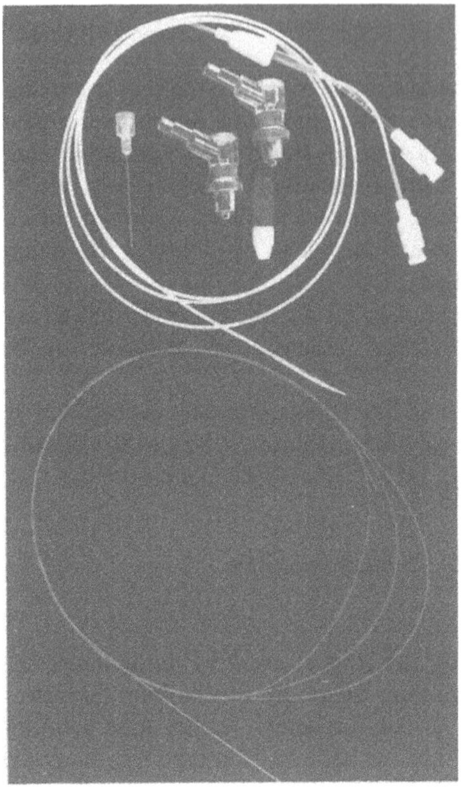

a

Fig. 2. a USCI/Schneider-Medintag Gruentzig steerable dilatation catheter, steerable guidewire, guidewire insertion tool, steerable and guiding Y connectors, and twisting device; **b** schematic of assembled USCI Gruentzig steerable dilatation catheter. (Illustration **b** provided by USCI Division, C. R. Bard, Inc.)

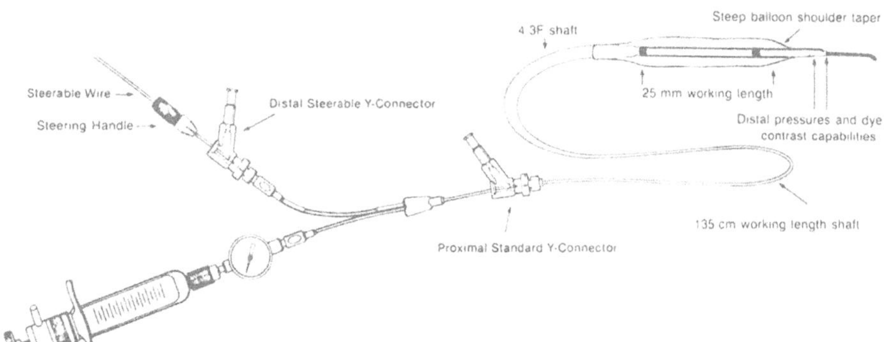

b

Table 4. Reduced dimensions of balloon catheters: comparison of USCI steerable vs low-profile steerable catheters (dimensions in inches)

Type s (Steerable)		Type LPS (Low-profile steerable)	
2.0		2.0	
1. Tip OD	0.026	1. Tip OD	0.022
2. Tip ID	0.020	2. Tip ID	0.020
3. Maximum deflated profile	0.053	3. Maximum deflated profile	0.038
2.5		2.5	
1. Tip OD	0.026	1. Tip OD	0.022
2. Tip ID	0.020	2. Tip ID	0.020
3. Maximum deflated profile	0.055	3. Maximum deflated profile	0.048
3.0		3.0	
1. Tip OD	0.026	1. Tip OD	0.022
2. Tip ID	0.020	2. Tip ID	0.020
3. Maximum deflated profile	0.063	3. Maximum deflated profile	0.050
3.7		3.5	
1. Tip OD	0.026	1. Tip OD	0.022
2. Tip ID	0.020	2. Tip ID	0.020
3. Maximum deflated profile	0.063	3. Maximum deflated profile	0.054
4.2		4.0	
1. Tip OD	0.026	1. Tip OD	0.022
2. Tip ID	0.020	2. Tip ID	0.020
3. Maximum deflated profile	0.067	3. Maximum deflated profile	0.056

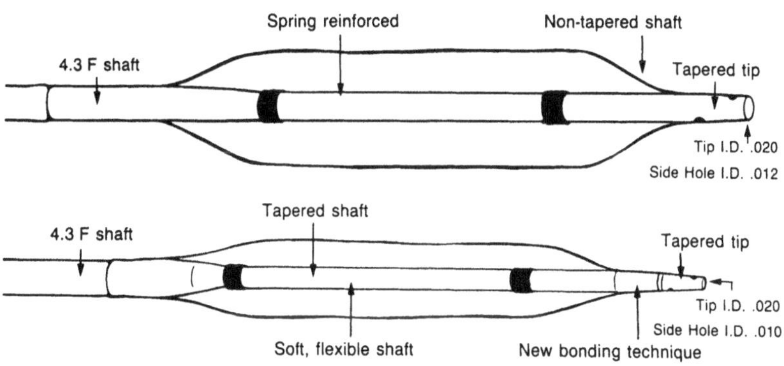

Fig. 3. USCI standard steerable and low-profile steerable dilatation catheters. (Illustration provided by USCI Division, C. R. Bard, Inc.)

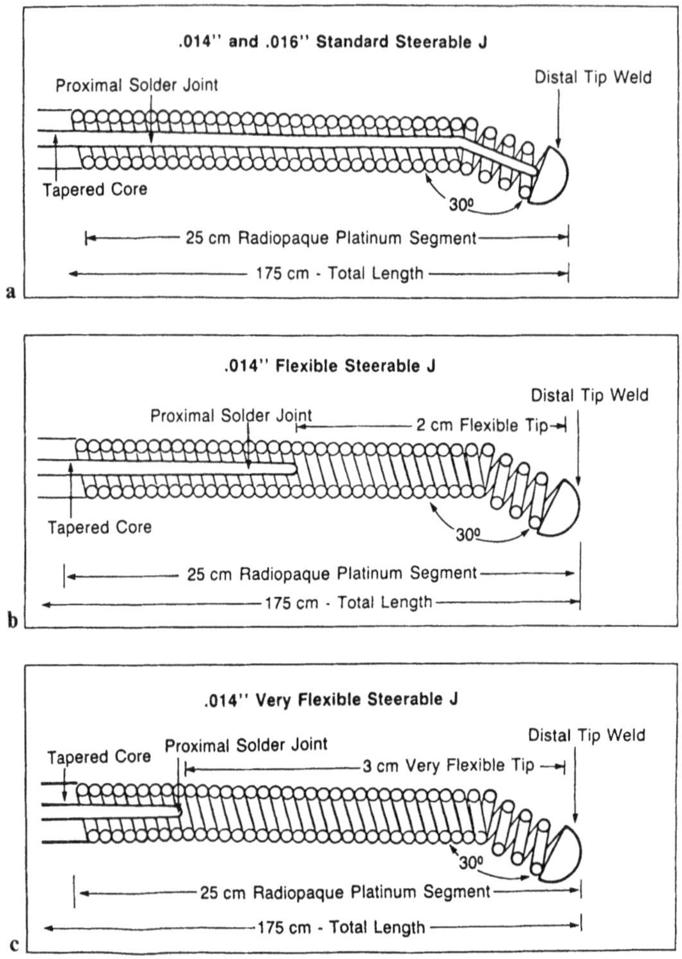

Fig. 4. a USCI standard steerable J guidewire; **b** USCI flexible steerable J guidewire; **c** USCI very flexible steerable J guidewire. (Illustration provided by USCI Division, C. R. Bard, Inc.)

Steerable Guidewire (Fig. 4a)
0.016 in. × 175 cm J tip
0.014 in. × 175 cm J tip

Available in J tip only. Highly formable spring tip. Excellent when maximum steerability is needed to reach a lesion or when good axial support is needed to cross tight lesions.

Flexible Steerable Guidewire (Fig. 4b)
0.014 in. × 175 cm straight tip
0.014 in. × 175 cm J tip

A flexible 2.0 cm tip offers a degree of flexibility that is not present in the steerable guidewire. Excellent choice for general use in most PTCA procedures.

Very Flexible Steerable Guidewire (Fig. 4c)
0.014 in. × 175 cm straight tip
0.014 in 175 cm J tip
A 3-cm flexible tip is the longest available from USCI. Good choice when softness and flexibility are a paramount concern (tortuous vessels, complex lesions, previously dilated segments).

Exchange Wire
0.014 in. × 300 cm straight tip
This exchange wire can be passed through both the USCI steerable and the USCI low-profile steerable dilatation catheters. It allows for exchange of balloon catheters while the stenosis remains engaged.

Schneider-Medintag or USCI Dilatation Catheter Preparation
Proper catheter preparation is essential for the safe performance of PTCA. The following steps will aid in balloon catheter preparation.

1. Prepare the desired mixture of saline and contrast. Contrast material should be diluted, as the viscosity of full-strength contrast may inhibit balloon inflation and deflation. A 60% contrast/40% saline mixture provides for adequate balloon visualization and proper balloon inflation and deflation. A mixture of 50 cm^3 contrast plus 20 cm^3 saline usually provides a large enough volume to prepare several catheters (if more than one is needed).
2. Prepare the inflation device by filling with 5 cm^3 contrast. Remove all air.
3. Place 3–4 cm^3 of the prepared solution in a 10-cm^3 Luer lock syringe. The Luer lock will prevent the syringe from slipping off during the preparation. Attach the syringe to the balloon port of the dilating catheter. Apply negative pressure by fully retracting the syringe plunger. Hold the negative pressure for 1–2 min, gently tapping the catheter hub to expel trapped bubbles from the catheter into the syringe.
4. Release the negative pressure. Gently inflate the balloon. Check to see that no air remains in the balloon. If there is too much air, repeat the above process. If satisfied with the balloon, remove the syringe. Place a couple of drops of contrast/saline on the inflation port hub to form a meniscus.
5. Attach the inflation device to the balloon port, expelling some of the contrast/saline mixture while making the connection. This will prevent air from entering the balloon lumen upon connection.
6. Inflate to 4 bar and then deflate. Check deflation time. Deflation times may vary depending on balloon size. When deflation time is greater than 15 s the catheter's integrity should be questioned. Larger balloons will increase deflation time.

Advanced Cardiovascular Dilatation Systems

Dilatation Catheters
The *Simpson-Robert Dilatation Catheter* is available in five balloon diameters ranging from 2.0 to 4.0 mm (Table 5 and Fig. 5). All catheters are 135 cm in

Table 5. Simpson-Robert dilatation catheters

Balloon size (mm)	Usable length (cm)	Shaft p.a. dia (F)	Deflated profile (in.)	Balloon length (mm)	Catheter/ balloon material
2.0	135	4.3	0.045	20	Polyethylene
2.5	135	4.3	0.050	20	Polyethylene
3.0	135	4.3	0.055	20	Polyethylene
3.5	135	4.3	0.065	20	Polyethylene
4.0	135	4.7	0.070	20	Polyethylene

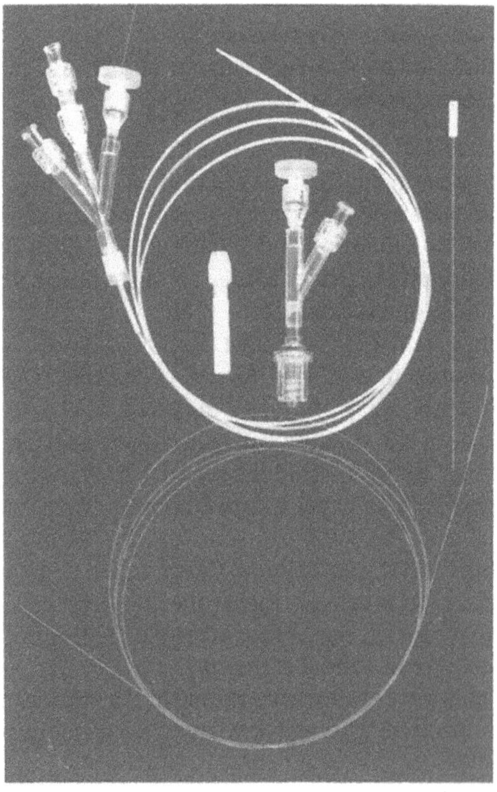

a

Fig. 5. a ACS Simpson-Robert dilatation catheter, movable guidewire, wire-rotating device, rotating hemostatic valve, guidewire insertion tool; **b** schematic of Simpson-Robert dilatation catheter. (Illustration **b** courtesy of Advanced Cardiovascular Systems)

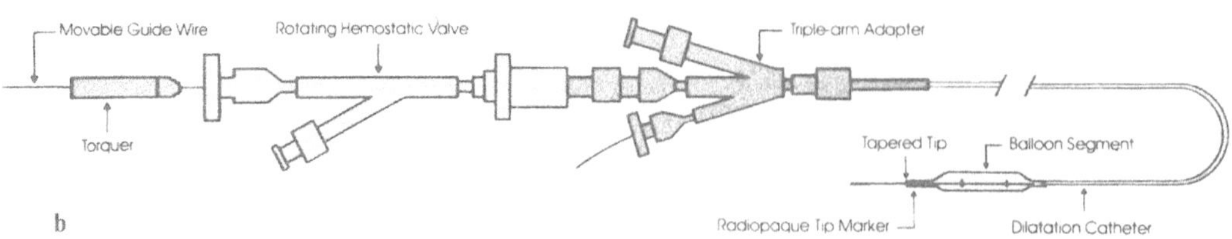

b

length and all have a balloon length of 20 mm. The shaft diameter of the 2.0-mm, 2.5-mm, 3.0-mm, and 3.5-mm catheters is 4.3 F. The 4.0-mm balloon has a shaft diameter of 4.7 F. Three radiopaque gold markers are used to mark the distal tip of the catheter and the proximal and distal portions of the balloon.

The balloon catheter has a double lumen coaxially arranged. The outer portion of the catheter forms the balloon inflation channel and the inner portion forms the central lumen. The balloon lumen opens into two ports. One port is the inflation port. The other balloon lumen port contains a 0.006-in. hollow-vent tube, which aids in the expulsion of air from the balloon. The central lumen runs the length of the catheter and allows the guidewire to pass out at the tip of the catheter (Fig. 6). It should be noted that good pressure measurements and good contrast injections can be made through the central lumen only if the wire is removed or if an ACS PDT wire is used. Luminal size makes this impossible if any other wire is used. The catheter is made of polyethylene and can be gas sterilized with ethylene oxide.

The *Simpson Ultra-Low-Profile Balloon Dilatation Catheter* has a very low crossing profile (ranging from 0.040 in. to 0.049 in. collapsed profile) and is highly flexible. It has radiopaque balloon and tip markers. It is available in 2.0 mm, 2.5 mm, and 3.0 mm balloon diameters (Fig. 7). It accepts a variety of

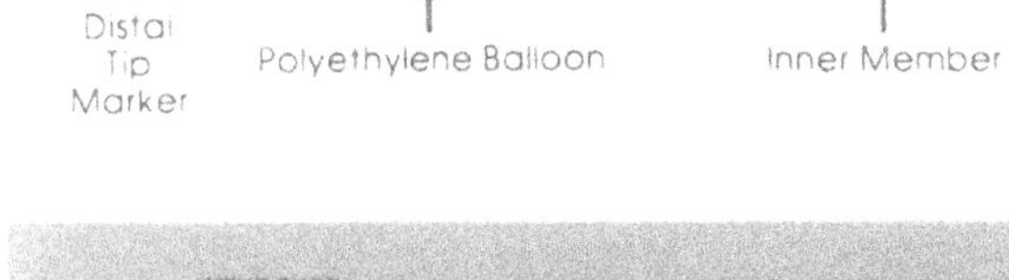

Fig. 6. Schematic of distal tip of ACS Simpson-Robert dilatation catheter. (Illustration courtesy of Advanced Cardiovascular Systems)

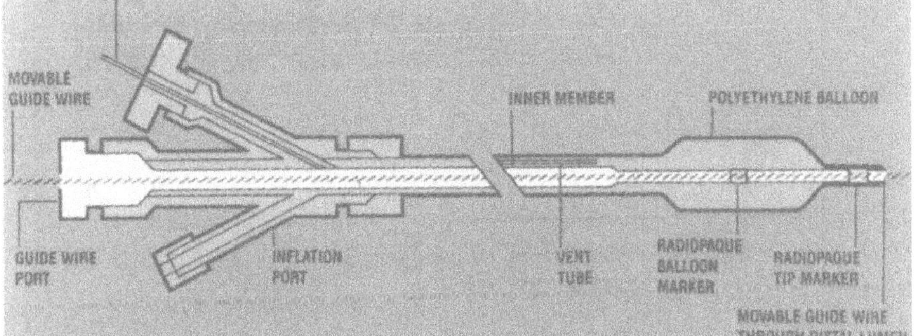

Fig. 7. Schematic of ACS Simpson extra-low-profile dilatation catheter. (Illustration courtesy of Advanced Cardiovascular Systems)

ACS 0.014-in. movable guidewires. This catheter is particularly flexible, allowing performance of complex procedures such as those with tortuous anatomy and tight eccentric lesions.

The *Hartzler Low-Profile Steerable Dilatation Catheter* is available with 2.0-mm, 2.5-mm, and 3.0-mm balloons that have an exceptionally low balloon profile segment (Table 6). These catheters have only a single lumen, in which a 0.017-in. guidewire passes through the entire length of the catheter. Extending from the distal tip of the catheter is a 1-cm length of soft platinum wire. The wire connects to a "proximal rotator knob." Manipulation of the rotator knob causes the catheter and soft wire tip to turn simultaneously and makes the catheter tip steerable (Fig. 8).

There is single gold marker equidistant from the proximal and distal ends of the balloon to aid in balloon placement. This single-lumen catheter does not allow contrast injection or pressure measurements.

Table 6. Hartzler low-profile steerable dilatation catheters

Balloon size (mm)	Usable length (cm)	Shaft dia	Deflated profile (in.)	Balloon length (mm)
2.0	135	2.5 F	0.030	20
2.5	135	2.9 F	0.037	20
3.0	135	3.2 F	0.043	20

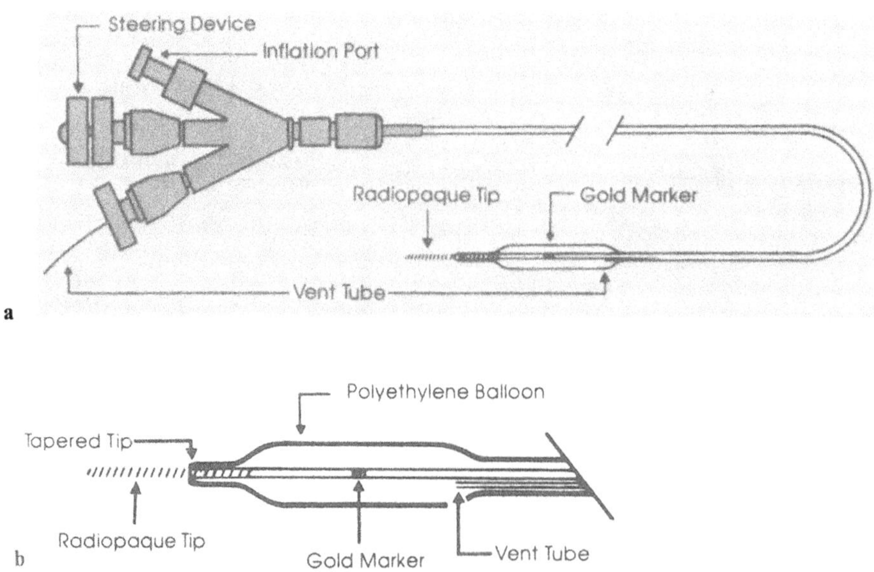

Fig. 8. a Schematic of ACS Hartzler LPS dilatation catheter; **b** schematic of distal tip of ACS Hartzler LPS dilatation catheter distal tip. (Illustration courtesy of Advanced Cardiovascular Systems)

This catheter may make the procedure easier when very tight lesions are approached. We have never used this catheter as a first choice, but only when it has proved impossible to cross the lesion with a low-profile movable guidewire system. Currently the only balloon catheter that matches these requirements is the Passkey catheter from Schneider-Medintag.

Guidewires
ACS offers a variety of intracoronary guide wires that are compatible with their dilatation catheters. All guidewires are Teflon coated, which allows for ease of movement through the dilatation catheter. The following is a brief description of the guide wires available from ACS.

PDT-S (straight): PDT stands for pressure, dye, and torque. The body of this wire tapers from 0.012 in. to a 0.006-in. mandrel. The last 3 cm is a 0.014-in. safety ribbon tip that allow both formability and flexibility. It is the taper to 0.006 in. that leaves room in the catheter lumen for pressure measurements and contrast injections through the dilatation catheter with the wire in place. The total length of this wire is 175 cm (Fig. 9 a).

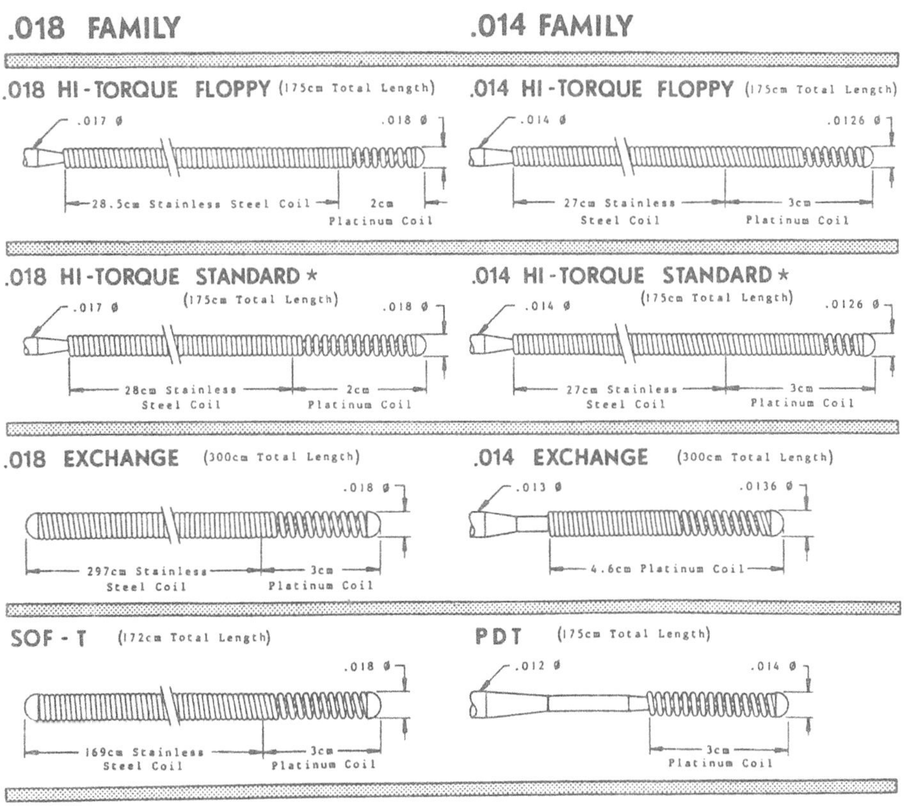

Fig. 9. Schematic of the ACS family of wires

High-Torque Standard Guidewire 0.018 in. diameter × 175 cm length: Provides a torque characteristic to facilitate negotiation of tortuous vessels. Incorporates a formable radiopaque tip and good directional control.

High-Torque Floppy Guidewire 0.018 in. × 175 cm: Offers a degree of steerability with a 2-cm "floppy" tip.

High-Torque Floppy 0.014 in. × 175 cm: Has a smaller shaft diameter and a 3-cm floppy but formable platinum tip; its torque response is high and radiopacity good (Fig. 9 b).

Standard Guidewire: One of the original ACS wires; 0.018 in. × 175 cm. Can be curved to enter desired vessels and to negotiate acute directional changes.

Floppy Guidewire 0.018 in. × 175 cm: Has a 5-cm very "floppy-flexible" tip that may prove less traumatic in eccentric tortuous lesions. Added flexibility minimizes the possibility of dissection but also limits its directional control. This wire has poor radiopaque characteristics.

Floppy Wire with Gold Tip: Same as the above, but with a radiopaque gold tip. Offers better visualization.

Sof-T 0.018 in. × 175 cm: Offers a 3-cm soft tip. Possesses a degree of torque control which allows for tip orientation. Its flexibility makes it ideal for crossing eccentric lesions (Fig. 9 c).

Exchange Wire is 0.018 in. × 300 cm: Same characteristics as the simple floppy, except for its length. Extra length allows for dilatation catheter exchanges while the wire remains beyond the lesion. This wire has poor radiopaque characteristics.

High-Torque Exchange Wire: This is a 0.014-in. × 300-cm exchange wire that possesses a 5-cm formable platinum tip. Offers torque characteristics for tip orientation and may be useful in cases where tip orientation and catheter exchanges are necessary.

Balloon Catheter Preparation

ACS has available a system that allows for the evacuation of air from the balloon by use of a tiny hollow vent tube. This small wire-like tube can be advanced into the balloon portion of the catheter. As the contrast/saline mixture is forced into the balloon, air is expelled through the vent tube. A step-by-step description of the correct method for ACS Simpson-Robert balloon preparation follows:

1. Prepare contrast saline mixture (60% contrast, 40% saline).
2. Close the O ring around the vent tube.
3. Attach a 10-cm^3 syringe and fill the balloon with 1–2 cm^3 air.
4. Loosen the O ring and advance the vent tube into the distal portion of the balloon. Keep the tip of the vent tube as close to the balloon wall as possible without actually touching it.
5. Prepare the indeflator by filling with the contrast/saline mixture. Place a three-way stopcock at the end of the indeflator tubing.

6. Attach the indeflator to the balloon port of the dilatation catheter.
7. Hold the triple hubbed end of the dilating catheter so that the inflation port is down. With the O ring still loose around the vent tube, slowly inject contrast until all air is removed from the clear yoke fitting of the catheter. If more contrast is needed in the indeflator it can be added through the side port of the three-way stopcock on the end of the indeflator tubing.
8. When satisfied that the catheter hubs are free of air, close the knurled knob to tighten the O ring around the vent tube.
9. Slowly fill the balloon port by maintaining constant pressure on the indeflator. Maintain the pressure until all air is gone from the balloon. The balloon should be held vertically and held higher than the inflation device.
10. When satisfied with the balloon, loosen the O ring and pull the vent tube approximately 5 cm from the balloon tip. Reinsert the end of the vent tube in the vent port and tighten the knurled knob.
11. Remove any air in the indeflator at this time. Again, this can be done through the stopcock on the end of the indeflator. Be sure to close the stopcock to the catheter so that air cannot enter the balloon lumen. A 5-cm^3 volume should remain in the indeflator.
12. Give the catheter a test inflation and deflation. Note deflation time to be sure that deflation is occurring in an acceptable period of time. (Balloon integrity should be questioned if deflation time is longer than 12 s.)
13. Deflate the balloon and replace the protective sheath over it until ready to start the procedure.
14. Place the guide wire of choice into the guidewire port. Be careful not to kink the wire. The catheter is now ready to use.

Guide Catheters

The guide catheter is designed to provide a conduit through which the balloon catheter is passed and to achieve coronary ostial engagement. Guide catheters have been designed with a form similar to that of the diagnostic coronary angiographic catheters.

Guide catheters are different from routine angiographic catheters in that the lumen is large enough to accept up to a 4.3-F dilating catheter. The tips are nontapered. Since it has a larger inner luminal diameter and the outer shaft diameter is kept at either 8 or 9 F, the guide catheter has thinner walls than a routine angiographic catheter. Thus, the feel and torque characteristics of a guide catheter will be different than those of a diagnostic catheter. Catheter kinking becomes a problem due to the thinner wall, especially if torque on the catheter is too high. Gentle turning and use of a rotating adapter are recommended in attempts to engage the guide catheter in the coronary orifice.

Guiding catheters with side holes near the tip, which provide blood flow from the aorta via these side holes, can also be used when the guide catheter wedges the orifice. Sometimes a coronary ostium cannot be properly engaged by any commercially available catheter. In this very rare circumstance, heating of the catheter using a hot air blower (or hot saline or steam) may make it possible to reshape the catheter in an attempt to obtain a configuration which will engage the orifice.

USCI Guide Catheters

The catheter is a bonded composite of three layers. The outer layer is made of polyurethane for memory, the middle layer is a woven mesh for torque control, and the inner surface is Teflon, which is used because its low coefficient of friction allows easy passage of the balloon catheter. For the femoral approach, guide catheters are available in modified Judkins and Amplatz left and right forms. Amplatz-type catheters can be helpful in directing the guidewire downward into circumflex coronary arteries, taking off a short main stem. They also provide better backup support to cross tight lesions. Better backup support in right coronary areries and bypass grafts can be obtained by cannulating the orifice with an El Gamal or a multipurpose guide catheter. The guide catheters are available in two sizes, 8 F and 9 F. The 9-F guide catheters are excellent in terms of backup power and torque control, but they tend to obstruct blood flow at the orifice engaged. The 8-F guide catheters appear to have good torque control. They may be preferred to avoid the problem with blood flow obstruction in patients with small arteries.

The guide catheters used for the brachial approach are made of a woven Dacron cover over a Teflon lining. Various tip curves (small, medium, and large) are designed for different aortic root configurations and sizes (modified Sones technique). They are manufactured with or without side holes. They are available with 8.3-F diameter. They have a relatively flexible tip, which permits superselective engagement into the artery to give good support when the balloon catheter cannot traverse a tight lesion or negotiate a sharp bend. The guide catheter is introduced over both a guidewire and a 3-F lead catheter, which facilitates the entry of the nontapered tip into the arteriotomy site.

N. B.: A similar series of catheters is available from Schneider-Medintag

Femoral Approach Guide Catheters

Left Coronary – Judkins Type (Table 7 and Fig. 10): Three styles of left femoral coronary guiding catheters of the Judkins type are available. The FL design was derived from Judkins style of coronary arteriography catheters. This catheter facilitates left coronary artery ostial engagement when the ostium has a "normal" take-off. The FLG is similar to the FL but its tip is oriented 30° anteriorly. This may be useful if subselective anterior descending engagement is necessary. The FLP has a tip that is oriented 30° posteriorly, which may aid in subselective circumflex engagement. All these catheters are available in 3.5-, 4-, and 5-cm curve sizes.

Right Coronary – Judkins Type (Table 8 and Fig. 10): The FR coronary guiding catheters are designed in the Judkins style of right coronary catheters. They are manufactured with or without side holes.

Table 7. Femoral left coronary guide catheters: Judkins type

Curve style	Shaft diameter (F)	Shaft diameter (mm)	Shaft diameter (in.)	Usable shaft length (cm)	Minimum tip opening ID (in.)	Guide wire for introduction (in.)
FL 3.5	8	2.67	0.104	100	0.067	0.063
FL 4	8	2.67	0.104	100	0.067	0.063
FL 4.5	8	2.67	0.104	100	0.067	0.063
FL 5	8	2.67	0.104	100	0.067	0.063
FL 6	8	2.67	0.104	100	0.067	0.063
FL 3.5	9	3.00	0.117	100	0.071	0.063
FL 4	9	3.00	0.117	100	0.071	0.063
FL 4.5	9	3.00	0.117	100	0.071	0.063
FL 5	9	3.00	0.117	100	0.071	0.063
FL 6	9	3.00	0.117	100	0.071	0.063
FL G 30° out of plane (anterior)						
FL 3.5G	8	2.67	0.104	100	0.067	0.063
FL 4G	8	2.67	0.104	100	0.067	0.063
FL 4.5G	8	2.67	0.104	100	0.067	0.063
FL 5G	8	2.67	0.104	100	0.067	0.063
FL 4G	9	3.00	0.117	100	0.071	0.063
FL 5G	9	3.00	0.117	100	0.071	0.063
FLP 30° out of plane (posterior)						
FL 4P	8	2.67	0.104	100	0.067	0.063
FL 5P	8	2.67	0.104	100	0.067	0.063
FL 4P	9	3.00	0.117	100	0.071	0.063
FL 5P	9	3.00	0.117	100	0.071	0.063

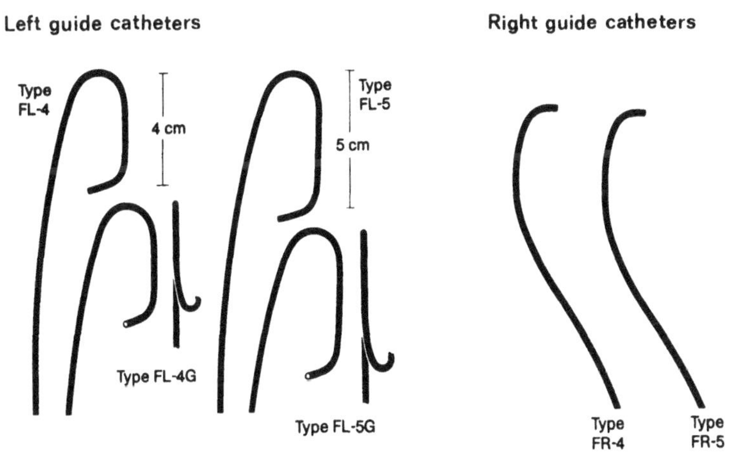

Fig. 10. Schneider-Medintag or USCI Judkins-type femoral approach left and right coronary guide catheters. (Illustration provided by USCI Division, C. R. Bard, Inc.)

Table 8. Femoral right coronary guide catheters: Judkins type

Curve style	Shaft diameter (F)	Usable shaft length (cm)	Minimum tip opening ID (in.)	Guidewire for introduction (in.)
FR 4	8	100	0.067	0.063
FR 5	8	100	0.067	0.063
FR 6	8	100	0.067	0.063
FR 4	9	100	0.071	0.063
FR 5	9	100	0.071	0.063
FR 6	9	100	0.071	0.063

Table 9. Femoral right coronary guide catheters: Reverse Amplatz type, FRS

Curve style	Shaft diameter (F)	Usable shaft length (cm)	Minimum tip opening ID (in.)	Guidewire for introduction (in.)
FRS	8	100	0.067	0.063
FRS	9	100	0.071	0.063

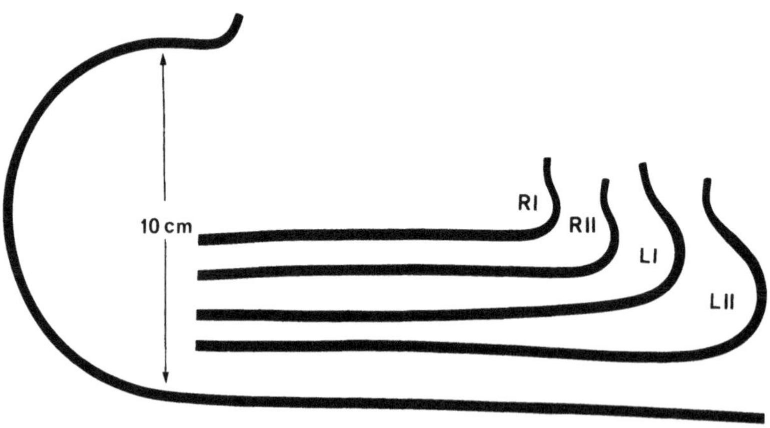

Fig. 11. Amplatz-type femoral approach left and right coronary guiding catheters. (Illustration provided by USCI Division, C. R. Bard, Inc.)

Right Reverse – Amplatz Type FRS (Table 9 and Fig. 11): This catheter provides a 10-cm reverse loop of the Amplatz curve. It may prove beneficial when it is difficult to engage the right coronary due to superior take-off.

Left and Right Amplatz Type (Table 10 and Fig. 11): These catheters are available in both left and right Amplatz-type curves and provide an alternative when ostial engagement or guide catheter support is difficult due to unique anatomy.

Table 10. Femoral approach coronary guide catheters: Amplatz type, left and right

Curve style	Shaft diameter (F)	Usable shaft length (cm)	Minimum tip opening ID (in.)	Guidewire for introduction (in.)
RI	8	100	0.067	0.063
RII	8	100	0.067	0.063
LI	8	100	0.067	0.063
LII	8	100	0.067	0.063
RI	9	100	0.071	0.063
RII	9	100	0.071	0.063
LI	9	100	0.071	0.063
LII	9	100	0.071	0.063

Table 11. Femoral approach coronary guide catheters: Multipurpose and El Gamal coronary bypass

Curve style	Shaft diameter (F)	Usable shaft length (cm)	Minimum tip opening ID (in.)	Guidewire for introduction (in.)
FMP	8	100	0.067	0.063
FMP	9	100	0.071	0.063
CB	9	100	0.071	0.063
CB	8	100	0.067	0.063

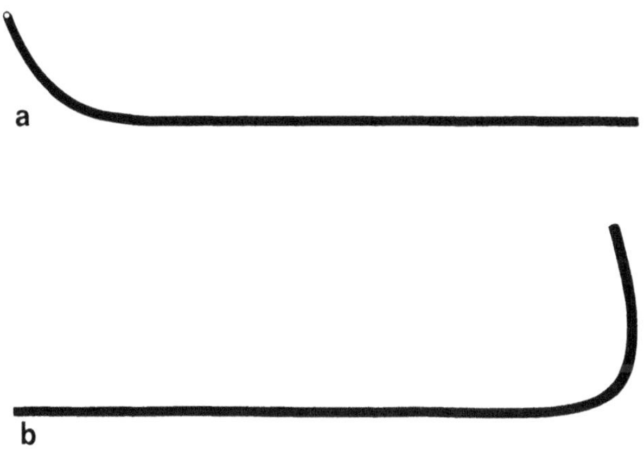

Fig. 12 a, b. USCI femoral approach coronary guide catheter: Multipurpose (**a**) and El Gamal (**b**) types. (Illustration provided by USCI Division, C. R. Bard, Inc.)

Femoral Approach – Multipurpose (Table 11 and Fig. 12): With this catheter it is possible to engage both the left and the right coronary arteries. It may be a useful tool when dilatation of bypass grafts is considered or when reshaping of a tip is necessary due to unique anatomy.

El Gamal Catheter (Table 11 and Fig. 12): This catheter provides an 80° curve 4 cm proximal to the tip of the catheter. Its design may prove beneficial in cannulation of bypass grafts or high take-off coronary ostium.

Table 12. Stertzer brachial approach coronary guide catheters

Curve style	Shaft diameter (F)	Usable shaft length (cm)	Minimum tip opening ID (in.)	Guidewire for introduction (in.)
Small No side holes	8.3	90	0.071	0.035
Small 2 side holes	8.3	90	0.071	0.035
Medium No side holes	8.3	90	0.071	0.035
Medium 2 side holes	8.3	90	0.071	0.035
Large No side holes	8.3	90	0.071	0.035
Large 2 side holes	8.3	90	0.071	0.035

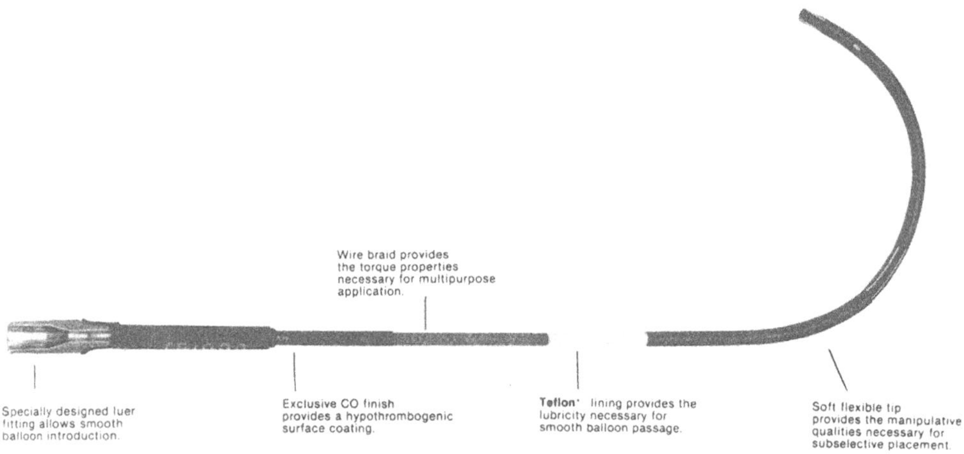

Fig. 13. USCI brachial approach Stertzer coronary guide catheter. (Illustration provided by USCI Division, C. R. Bard, Inc.)

Brachial Approach – Stertzer Guide Catheters

This catheter (Table 12 and Fig. 13) is used for the brachial approach in the performance of PTCA. It is available in three curve types, with or without side holes. These catheters are a woven Dacron construction with an inner luminal lining of Teflon and are supplied with a Teflon introducing catheter which aids in placement into the brachial artery.

ACS Guide Catheters

ACS guide catheters (Tables 13–16) are available with shaft diameters of 8 F and 8.8 F. In the case of the 8-F model the inner diameter of the tip is 0.072 in. The

Table 13. ACS guide catheters: Femoral approach to left coronary artery 8.8 F

Type	Description	Shaft length (cm)	Shaft diameter (F)	Tip ID (in.)
SRJL 3.5	Judkins curve STD	100	8.8	0.076
SRJL 3.5	Judkins curve LCX	100	8.8	0.076
SRJL 3.5	Judkins curve LAD	100	8.8	0.076
SRJL 4.0	Judkins curve STD	100	8.8	0.076
SRJL 4.0	Judkins curve LCX	100	8.8	0.076
SRJL 4.0	Judkins curve LAD	100	8.8	0.076
SRJL 4.5	Judkins curve STD	100	8.8	0.076
SRJL 4.5	Judkins curve LCX	100	8.8	0.076
SRJL 4.5	Judkins curve LAD	100	8.8	0.076
SRJL 5.0	Judkins curve STD	100	8.8	0.076
SRJL 5.0	Judkins curve LCX	100	8.8	0.076
SRJL 5.0	Judkins curve LAD	100	8.8	0.076
SRJL 6.0	Judkins curve STD	100	8.8	0.076
SRJL 6.0	Judkins curve LCX	100	8.8	0.076
SRJL 6.0	Judkins curve LAD	100	8.8	0.076
SRAL 1	Amplatz Curve 1	100	8.8	0.076
SRAL 2	Amplatz Curve 2	100	8.8	0.076
SRAL 3	Amplatz Curve 3	100	8.8	0.076
SRAL 4	Amplatz Curve 4	100	8.8	0.076

LAD, anterior curve for left anterior descending coronary artery; LCX, posterior curve for left circumflex coronary artery; STD, standard (in plane)

Table 14. ACS guide catheters: Femoral approach to right coronary artery, 8.8 F

Type	Description	Shaft length (cm)	Shaft diameter (F)	Tip ID (in.)
SRJR 3.5	Judkins curve 3.5	100	8.8	0.076
SRJR 3.5 s	Judkins curve 3.5 s	100	8.8	0.076
SHJR 3.5[a]	Judkins curve 3.5	100	8.8	0.076
SHJR 3.5 s[a]	Judkins curve 3.5 s	100	8.8	0.076
SRJR 4	Judkins curve 4	100	8.8	0.076
SRJR 4 s	Judkins curve 4 s	100	8.8	0.076
SHJR 4[a]	Judkins curve 4	100	8.8	0.076
SHJR 4s[a]	Judkins curve 4s	100	8.8	0.076
SRJR 5	Judkins curve 5	100	8.8	0.076
SRJR 5 s	Judkins curve 5 s	100	8.8	0.076
SRJR 6	Judkins curve 6	100	8.8	0.076
SRAR 1	Amplatz curve 1	100	8.8	0.076
SRAR 2	Amplatz curve 2	100	8.8	0.076

s, Short (3 mm) tip
[a] RCA Side-hole guide catheter

Table 15. ACS guide catheters: Femoral approach to left coronary artery, 8 F

Description	Shaft length (cm)	Shaft diameter (F)	Tip ID (in.)
Amplatz I	100	8	0.072
Amplatz II	100	8	0.072
Amplatz III	100	8	0.072
Amplatz IV	100	8	0.072
Judkins 3.5 STD	100	8	0.072
Judkins 4 STD	100	8	0.072
Judkins 4.5 STD	100	8	0.072
Judkins 5 STD	100	8	0.072
Judkins 6 STD	100	8	0.072

Table 16. ACS guide catheters: Femoral approach to right coronary artery, 8 F

Description	Shaft length (cm)	Shaft diameter (FR)	Tip ID (in.)
Amplatz I	100	8	0.072
Amplatz II	100	8	0.072
Amplatz III	100	8	0.072
Judkins 3	100	8	0.072
Judkins 3.5	100	8	0.072
Judkins 3.5 side holes	100	8	0.072
Judkins 4.0	100	8	0.072
Judkins 4.0, side holes	100	8	0.072
Judkins 5	100	8	0.072
Judkins 6	100	8	0.072

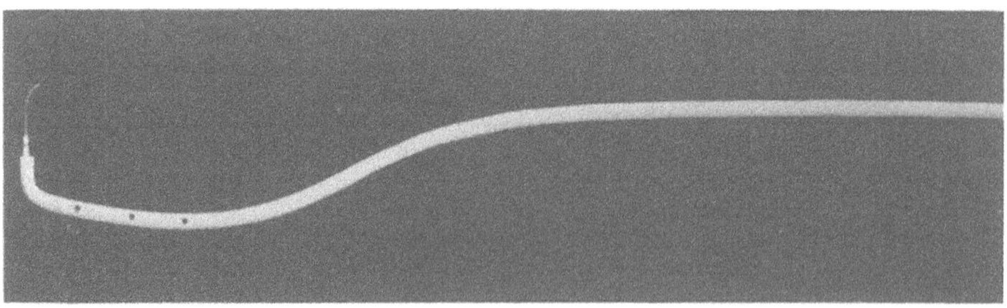

Fig. 14. ACS Judkins-type right coronary guide catheter with side holes

inner diameter of the tip is 0.076 in. in the 8.8-F catheter. All catheters are 100 cm in length. They are made of polyethylene with a Teflon inner core to allow smooth passage of dilatation catheters. Catheter tips are manufactured with either Judkins or Amplatz configurations. Judkins left coronary guide catheters are reformed with either a posterior or an anterior tip deflection to permit semiselective access to the left circumflex or left anterior descending coronary artery, respectively. A right coronary artery guide catheter with side holes is available to avoid any damping effect of the catheter in the right coronary artery (Fig. 14).

System Accessories and Angioplasty Tray

To facilitate setting up of the PTCA procedure, a prepackaged angioplasty tray should be prepared. Everything necessary for the performance of a "routine" angioplasty should be included. If more than one system is being used in a particular laboratory, essential accessories of each system should be included on the tray. The operator may often wish to switch from one system to another during a procedure. If this happens, all the necessary accessories are then available and do not need to be fetched to the sterile field individually. This will save time and aggravation. At the beginning of the procedure, take the accessories of the system that will not be used, wrap them in a sterile towel, and place them to the side of the sterile stand. If they are not used, they may be repackaged and placed on the next angioplasty tray.

The following is a list of items included on the angioplasty tray at St. Louis University Medical Center. Guide catheter introducers, guiding catheters, dilatation catheters, and guidewires are not included in this list as these items vary from case to case.

Angioplasty Tray

1 Bowl for heparinized saline, 7 in. dia.
1 Bowl for contrast/saline mixture, 5 in. dia. for balloon preparation
1 Manifold set or PTCA kit
2 Glass syringes (Socorex), 2 cm^3
1 Guide catheter Y connector/USCI
1 Steerable dilating catheter Y connector/USCI
1 ACS guiding catheter Y connector
1 Inflation device and gauge
1 Insertion tool/ACS
1 Insertion tool/USCI
1 Wire-rotating device (torquer)
1 Pacing lead extention cable
1 Medicine cup (glass or metal), 10 cm^3
1 Glass syringe (Socorex), 10 cm^3
1 Guidewire (J or straight), 0.063 in.
1 Small piece of fine emery paper. Include desired syringes, needles, blades and other accessories of choice

Manifold System

Use of a dual manifold system is necessary in the performance of PTCA. The guide catheter is connected to one manifold and the dilatation catheter to another. The system provides a means of monitoring pressure and of injecting flushing solution and contrast medium through the coaxial system. This is essential for documentation of proper dilatation catheter placement. Prior to the start of the procedure, the manifold system should be prepared in the following way:

- Tighten all connections. Connect the pressure connecting line to the transducer, connect the flush connecting line to the flush bag, and connect the contrast line to the contrast bottle.

- Purge all lines of air.
- Connect syringes that will be used.
- Flush the transducer line, remove all air. Check that all lines are tight, and that air has been removed from the entire system.

There are several manifold systems commercially available, including both disposable and reusable systems. System characteristics that one should consider when selecting a system include:

- Ease of stopcock manipulation.
- Incorporation of a quality rotating adaptor on the catheter port.
- Clear lumens for air bubble visualization.
- Possibility of an undamped pressure wave form.

Our experience has been with a disposable kit commercially available from the North American Instrument Co. (Fig. 15). The kit includes the two manifolds with all necessary tubing attached. This is convenient and facilitates quick set-up.

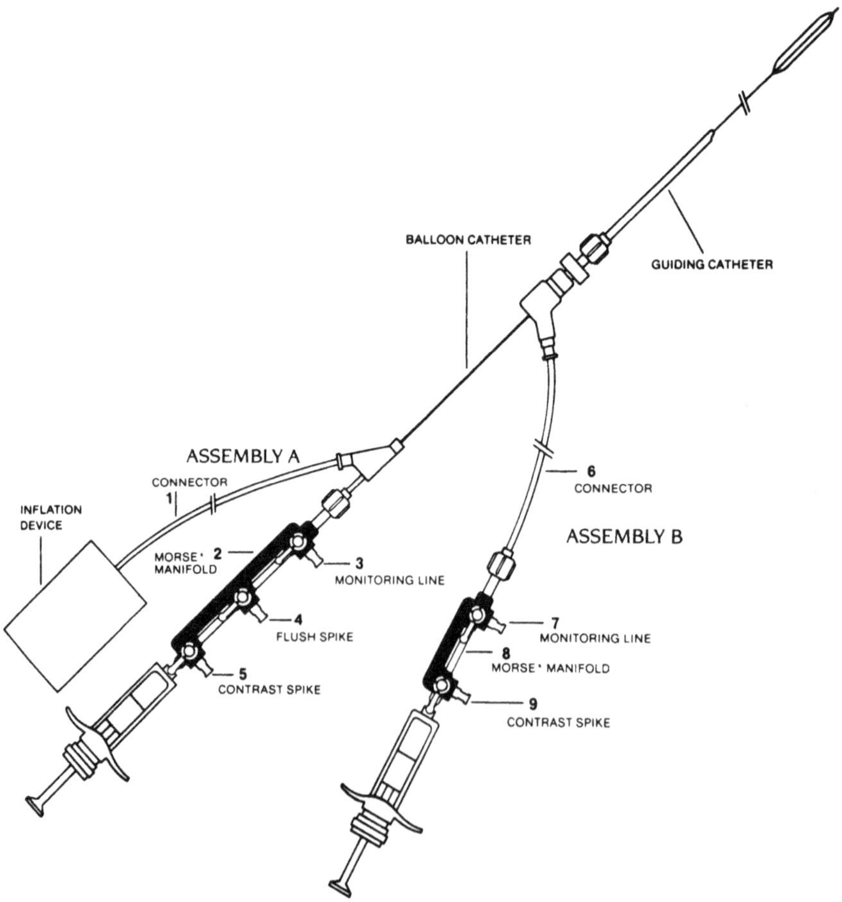

Fig. 15. Manifold system: *Assembly A* for dilatation catheter and *Assembly B* for guide catheter. (Illustration provided courtesy of North American Instrument Company)

Glass Syringes (Socorex)

There are several reasons for using glass syringes (Fig. 16) during PTCA. The limited size of the dilatation catheter flush lumen increases the resistance through the injection port. One way to overcome this resistance is to use a syringe that provides as little resistance as possible. A 2-cm^3 glass syringe seems to work the best. A 10-cm^3 glass syringe should be provided on the tray for the initial tracking angiograms and for injections through the guide catheter. Some caution should be used during the injection, as very high pressures can be generated with these small syringes. Several technical considerations to be borne in mind with glass syringes are:

- The barrels are easily broken, so keep plenty of replacements on hand.
- Be careful with the male Luer lock syringe tips. If they are dropped and dented the glass may not fit perfectly, and the syringe will leak.
- If the plunger feels tight and hard to move, try a different glass barrel.
- There should be no need to lubricate the barrel. They should be cleaned and dried prior to resterilization.
- The glass withstands 200 °C. Keep this in mind when considering sterilization technique. Leave the syringe components unassembled until after sterilization. If the plunger is in the glass the barrel may break owing to expansion and contraction during the sterilization cycles.
- Be sure the locking nut on the syringe holder is tight prior to the start of the procedure and that the syringe is put together properly and operates without leaks.

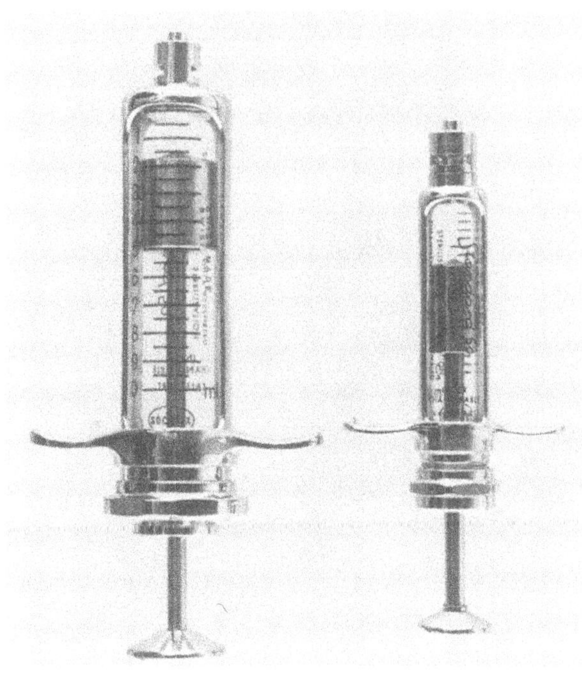

Fig. 16. Glass syringes. *Left* 10 cm^3; *right* 2 cm^3

Y Connectors
The Y connector (Fig. 17) allows for placement of a dilating catheter through the lumen of the guiding catheter, yet maintains the ability to inject contrast and monitor pressure through the guiding catheter lumen. In steerable systems, a Y connector on the dilating catheter allows placement of a steerable wire through the dilating catheter lumen yet maintains the ability to inject contrast and monitor pressure through the dilating catheter.

Schneider-Medintag and USCI Y Connectors for Steerable and Guide Catheters (Fig. 17). The guide catheter Y connector can be differentiated from the steerable Y connector in that the guiding Y connector is a clear plastic and the steerable Y connector has a yellow tint. The rotating adapter portion of each type can be reused. The plastic part, or "replacement body" must be changed after each use. This part contains a plastic membrane which prevents backbleed when a catheter or wire is placed through the Y connector. Replacement kits are offered for this purpose. The replacement kit contains a plastic replacement body and an O ring.

Technical considerations with respect to USCI Y connectors:

Prior to the *start* of the procedure, make sure the connection is tight between the plastic body and the metal rotating adapter. Do not trust the connection made

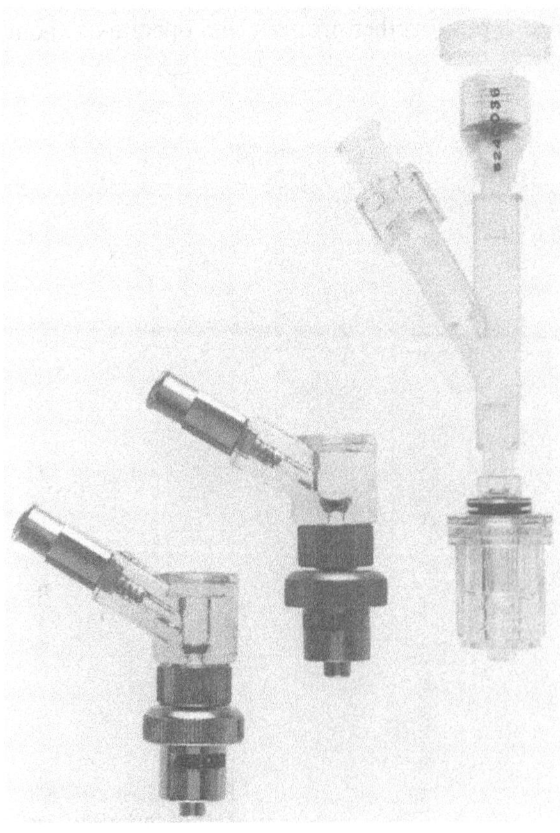

Fig. 17. Schneider-Medintag and USCI Y connectors (*left*); ACS rotating hemostatic valve (*right*)

by the manufacturer. A quick check prior to the start of a procedure will save much time and aggravation should a Y not have been put together properly.

If *pressure damping* occurs, check for a proper connection between the plastic Y and the rotating adapter. A loose connection will cause inaccurate pressures.

If *pressure damping* occurs and the *connection* seems *tight,* loosen the connection and reconnect. This may alleviate the damping. If not, replace the entire Y connector.

If too much *pressure* is applied during the injection of contrast medium a Y connector membrane may rupture. This will cause reflux of the contrast around the catheter during subsequent injections, as well as pressure damping, making the Y connector useless. The replacement body must be changed at this point. The use of the small 2-cm^3 glass syringe may increase the occurrence of Y connector membrane rupture, as greater pressures can be exerted with these syringes. The advantages of good contrast injection with 2-cm^3 syringes must be weighed against the chance of Y membrane rupture when this system is used.

When *cleaning* the reusable rotating portion, clean well with an approved detergent. Subject the item to ultrasonic cleaning for 30 min. Rinse well.

When *reconstructing* the body with the rotator, make sure the O ring is properly seated.

ACS Guide Catheter Y Connector (Fig. 17). The ACS Y connector system incorporates a Tuohy-Borst type of hemostatic valve through which the dilating catheter is placed. A knurled knob can be turned, which tightens an O ring around the catheter, thereby eliminating backbleed from the guide catheter around the dilating catheter. ACS offers two types of Y connectors:

- Hemostatic valve with a rotating adapter
- Standard hemostatic valve without a rotating adapter

The rotating adapter allows for independent movement of the guide catheter.

Technical considerations with respect to use of ACS Y connectors:

- The knurled knob must be turned clockwise prior to contrast injection through the guide catheter. Failure to tighten this knob will allow contrast to reflux through the back port of the Y rather than going through the guide catheter and into the coronary.
- Pressure damping will occur if the knob is too tight or too loose.
- If the knob is too tight, inflation of the balloon may be impossible.
- If the knob is tightened after inflation is made and is tightened too much, deflation of the balloon may be impossible.
- Proper tightening of the connections between catheters and Y connectors during the PTCA procedure is important, to maintain an air-free system without leaks and to allow accurate pressure monitoring.

Inflation Device and Gauges

The inflation device and gauge provide a means of exerting a known pressure through the balloon lumen of the dilatation catheter. Following is a brief dis-

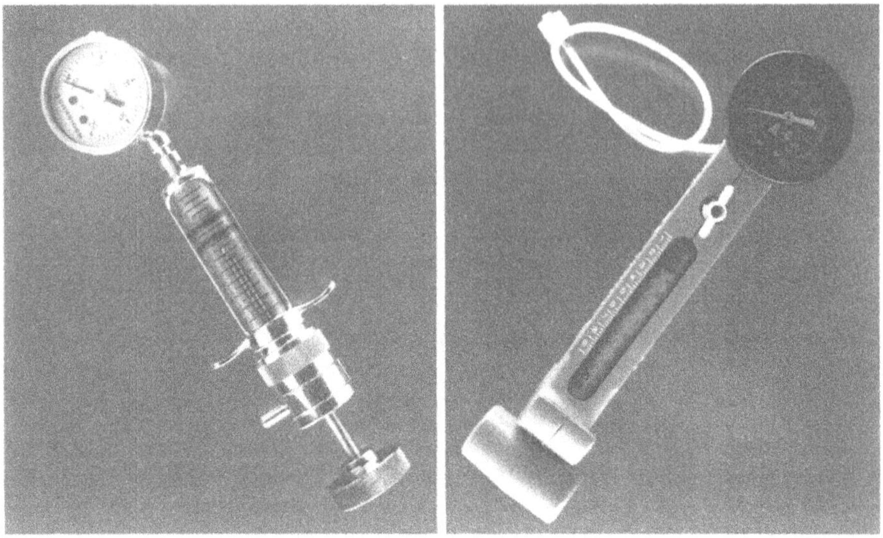

a b

Fig. 18. a USCI angioplasty balloon inflation device; **b** ACS indeflator

cussion of the technical aspects of the ACS indeflator and the USCI balloon inflation device (Fig. 18).

ACS Inflation Device. The ACS indeflator is a hand-held device that incorporates a syringe for inflation, a gauge for pressure monitoring, and a stopcock to hold either positive or negative pressure. It is supplied sterile, and it can be used on the sterile field during the procedure. The gauge has a maximum range of 11 bar/160 psi.
Technical considerations regarding the ACS indeflator:

- It is compact and can be placed on the sterile field.
- Its simple design makes this system easy to operate.
- The gauge is easy to see and read.
- It is nonreusable. The cost per procedure is approximately $75.00.
- Maintenance of a consistent positive pressure is sometimes difficult owing to a slow leak when the stopcock is closed. This varies from one device to another. Continuous physical application of pressure may be needed for maintenance of a steady pressure if a leak develops.

USCI Inflation Device. The USCI inflation device is made of stainless steel and is a reusable system. A glass Socorex syringe is placed in a stainless steel holder. A threaded piston rod, plunger, and locking device are attached to the back of the syringe holder. When the locking device or the actuator is not in place the plunger can be pushed forward or retracted in the usual manner. Inflation is achieved by screwing the plunger knob clockwise until the desired pressure is achieved. Pressure can be gradually increased by turning the knob clockwise or gradually decreased by turning it counterclockwise. To release pressure the lock-

ing device is slipped out of position and the plunger is retracted manually. When the plunger is fully retracted the locking device is flipped back into position and it will hold the plunger in a retracted position to maintain a negative pressure. A manometer is not included with this device and must be ordered separately. These manometers have a range of –1 to 20 atm.
Technical considerations with respect to the USCI inflation device:

- This is a reusable system.
- It can be sterilized with ethylene oxide gas or autoclaved.
- It can be handheld or put on the sterile field.
- Allows exertion of high pressures without physical exertion by the operator and maintenance of stable pressures.
- "O" rings and gaskets, if not handled properly, may cause the device to malfunction.
- The actuator knob is sometimes difficult to engage on the piston rod. If they are not engaged properly, damage to the device and threads on the piston rod may result. If there is difficulty in engaging the actuator or locking device, turn the piston rod slightly. The actuator will then fall into place.
- Plunger lubrication may be necessary. Cordis Syringe Lubricant works well. A small amount on the piston O ring is all that is necessary.

Several other systems are available for the purpose of balloon inflation that are not mentioned in this chapter. When selecting a system, one should consider the following:

- Physical size of the device
- Airtightness of the system
- Accuracy of the manometer
- Overall ease of operation

The two systems that have been discussed are comparable in the above characteristics.

Insertion Tools

Insertion tools (Figs. 2 and 5), facilitate placement of the guidewire into the dilatation catheter through the steerable Y connector (USCI) or the rotating hemostatic valve (ACS). Any attempt to place wires without the use of this tool may result in wire kinking. When using a USCI steerable system it is impossible to place the guidewire through the steerable Y connector without an insertion tool. Place the insertion tool through the membrane of the yellow Y connector. Once the tool is in place, the distal (stiff) end of the guide wire can be placed through the Y connector. The insertion tool can then be removed.

Wire-Rotating Device

This device (Figs. 2 and 5) can be placed on the distal end of the guidewire and used for turning or steering the guide wire. Some workers may prefer to put a 90° bend in the end of the wire and use the end of the wire as a handle instead of using a totating device.

Pacing Lead Extension Set

If a temporary pacing catheter is placed prior to the start of PTCA, a lead extension with alligator clips is convenient. The extension cable can be sterilized and placed on the catheter table connected to the pacing catheter. The external pacing control unit can then be placed off the sterile field and under the drape. It can now be handled by the circulating personnel. The sets available are: Cordis Universal Lead Extension with alligator clips; Medronic Lead Extension.

Medicine Cup (Glass or Metal)

This is used to dilute 1 mg nitroglycerin in 9 cm^3 saline to make a solution of 100 $\mu g/cm^3$. This is then kept on the sterile field for easy accessibility and can be used at any point as needed during the procedure.

Guide Wire (J or Straight)

This Teflon-coated guidewire is available from USCI and can be placed through the guide catheter to straighten the catheter during the insertion. A 0.038-in. wire can also be used.

Small Piece of Fine Emery Paper

Should a catheter need to be reshaped or the tip cut for proper fit into the coronary ostium, the availability of a fine emery paper for smoothing the cut edge is desirable. If this technique is used, caution is urged to insure a smooth edge on the tip of the catheter, as well as flushing the catheter to remove any debris from the catheter tip. If guide catheter reshaping is necessary, insertion of the stiff end of the 0.063-in. guidewire into the catheter lumen is recommended to prevent kinking at the point of the catheter being reshaped.

Guide Catheter Insertion Instruments – Sheath Introducers

There are a number of reasons for using a sheath introducer for the introduction of the guiding catheters used in PTCA:

1. Guide catheters are stiffer, less pliable, than routine angiographic catheters. It is felt that a longer introducer provides a safety factor when the stiffer guide catheter is introduced through the femoral artery and iliac vessels.
2. It allows for a quick exchange of the catheter systems.
3. The introducer can be left in place following the procedure until the patient stabilizes from an anticoagulated state.
4. It facilitates quick access to the femoral artery if problems develop later in the day and recatheterization becomes necessary.

Our experience has been with the sheath introducer commercially available from USCI and Schneider-Medintag. It is referred to as a USCI Insertion Instrument and is available in 8-F and 9-F diameter. This system is made up of three components (Fig. 19): the inner dilator, the secondary dilator, and the sheath itself. Both the 8-F and the 9-F sheath contain a hemostatic valve and a side flush port with a three-way stopcock.

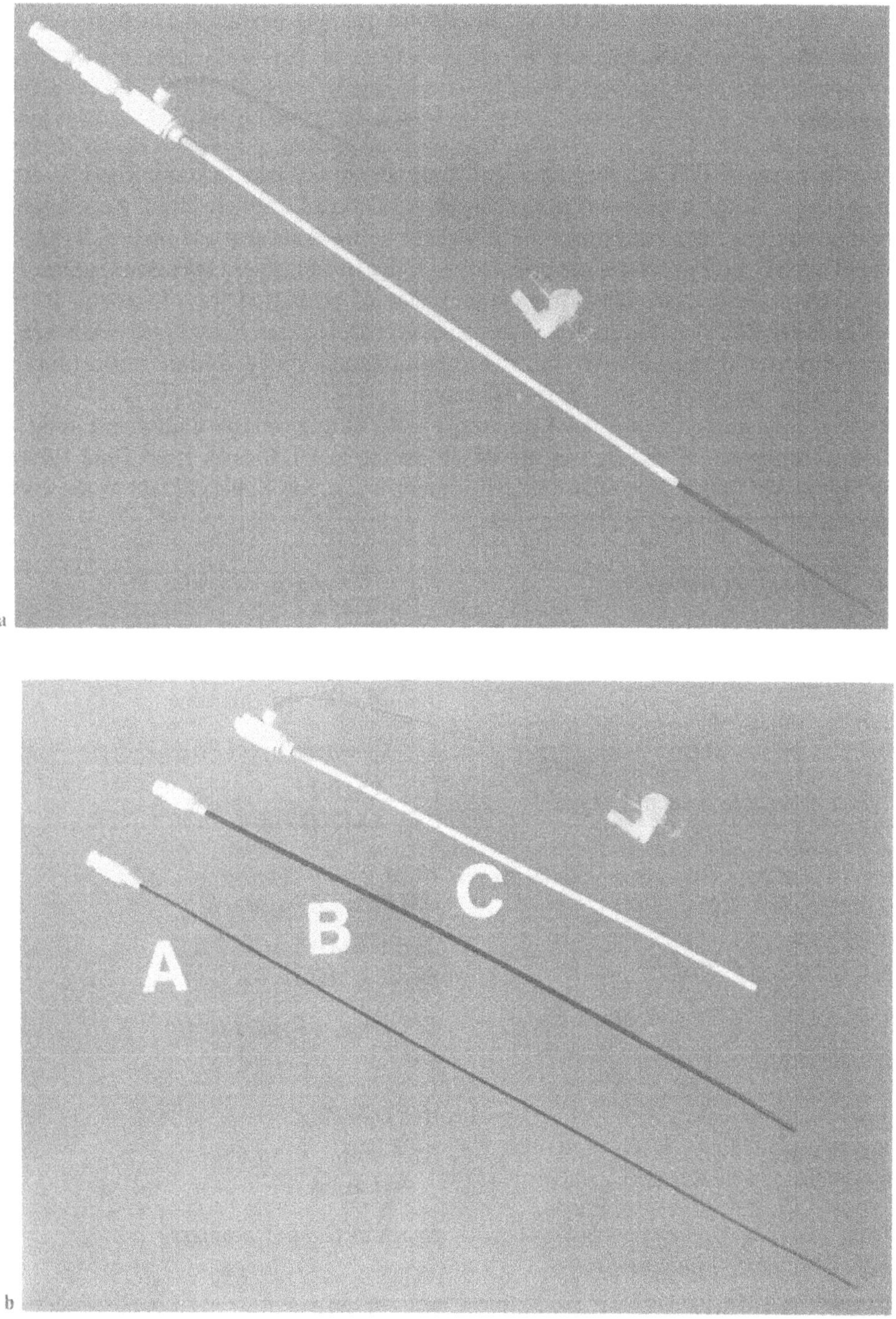

a

b

Fig. 19. a USCI guide catheter insertion instrument; **b** inner dilator (*A*), secondary dilator (*B*), and sheath introducer with hemostatic valve and side port (*C*)

Note that these sheaths are much longer than conventional introducers (22.7 cm vs 11 cm). This length puts the sheath opening beyond the aortoiliac bifurcation.

Inventory

A wide range of PTCA accessories and supplies should be stocked in the PTCA laboratory. Often a different approach or selection of another guiding catheter or dilatation catheter may make the difference between success and failure. Stocking of several systems offers the operator a choice in equipment selection that may vary from case to case, depending on the lesion to be dilated.

Because PTCA equipment is expensive, inventory control and overheads are very important issues. Most of the PTCA equipment is dated, and the importance of rotating the stock cannot be overstressed.

The following is a survey of the usage rates of angioplasty equipment at St. Louis University. These figures are based on the last 100 cases from June 1984 to September 1984. This record of equipment usage will hopefully aid in the selection of system types and quantities.

ACS Dilatation Catheters

2.0/20 mm	12%
2.5/20 mm	8%
3.0/20 mm	27%
3.5/20 mm	4%
4.0/20 mm	0.6%

USCI Steerable Systems (Type S)

2.0/25 mm	3%
2.5/25 mm	7%
3.0/25 mm	20%
3.7/25 mm	4%
4.2/25 mm	0%

USCI Low-Profile System (LPS)

2.0/25 mm	0.6%
2.5/25 mm	0.6%
3.0/25 mm	7%
3.5/25 mm	2%
4.0/25 mm	0%

USCI Guiding Catheters – 8 F
Left Coronary – Judkins Style

FL 3.5	0.8%
FL 4	48%
FL 4.5	0%
FL 5	4%
FL 6	0%

Right Coronary – Judkins Style

FR 4	21%
FR 5	0.8%

0% on other of this type

Left Coronary – AMPLATZ Style – 8 F

Left AMP I	5%
Left AMP II	4%

Right Coronary – AMPLATZ Style – 8 F

Right AMP I	2%
Right AMP II	0.8%

El Gamal – Bypass Graft

8 F	1.6%

ACS Guiding

Rt 4 with side holes	1.6%

Brachial Guide Catheters

SM No side holes	1.6%
MED No side holes	4%
LG No side holes	0.8%

Guidewires – USCI

Standard 0.016 in. J	3.9%
Standard 0.014 in. J	3.2%
Flexible 0.014 in. J	0%
Very flexible 0.014 in. J	52%

Guidewires – ACS

Floppy with gold tip	16%
SOF-T	16%
Exchange wire	6%

Although many items have not been used over the last 100 cases, very small quantities of the lower volume items are still maintained in the inventory (one or two of each).

PTCA equipment is constantly being refined. As new equipment becomes available, some of the items that have been discussed may become obsolete. It would prove prudent to keep up with new trends in PTCA and to make inventory adjustments as necessary. For example, the availability of the Schneider-Medintag and USCI low-profile steerable dilatation catheters and the ACS ultra-low profile dilatation catheters now decreases usage of the original "steerable" catheters.

It is important to note that some of the angioplasty equipment available from the various companies can be interchanged. For example, ACS dilatation catheters have been used with USCI guide catheters and vice versa. Certain guidewires can also be interchanged. There are several technical points one should be aware of when combining components of one company with those from another.

- The balloon of the ACS dilatation catheter tends to inflate during the injection of contrast through the 8-F USCI guide catheter. This can be alleviated by using a 9-F guide from either company, or by using the 8-F guide catheter recently released by ACS [8].
- Be sure that the guidewire size is compatible with the central lumen of the dilatation catheter.

Final Comments and Perspective

Since PTCA is still developing as a therapeutic method, new technical advances can be expected. Some of the information provided in this chapter could be out of date by the time it is published, and the reader is therefore referred to the most recent literature published by the various manufacturers.

As mentioned at the beginning, it was not our intention to provide an extensive review of all the equipment available for the performance of PTCA, but rather to describe the instrumentation currently in use at our own institution.

Over the last 2 years the development of high-pressure balloons, lower profile balloon catheters, and over-the-wire steerable systems has contributed tremendously to the increased success and safety of PTCA procedures. This continuing refinement of PTCA techniques has allowed the applications of the procedure to be expanded far beyond those earlier envisaged.

As PTCA becomes more widely practiced, it will be essential to develop catheter systems to meet the challenge of increasingly more complex PTCA procedures. Further improvements in materials and methods will no doubt lead to even wider application of PTCA as a therapeutic modality in the presence of complex coronary anatomy and in high-risk medical situations.

Finally, newer technology may develop, such as the use of laser energy, so that the angioplasty catheter will make it possible to attack the atherosclerotic plaque directly in several ways at once [9].

Appendix

List of vendors supplying angiographic equipment and supplies [a]

Company	Supplies/accessories
Schneider-Medintag CH-8052 Zurich, Switzerland Telephone (From U.S) 011-41-1-301-2350 Telex 822 482 HSCZ CH	Entire dilatation catheter system (Europe, and US as of 1986) 2-cm^3 Syringes Manometer/gauges
USCI (licensée of Schneider-Metintag) P.O. Box 566 Billerica, MA 07821, USA 1-800-225-0898	Entire dilatation catheter system
Advanced Cardiovascular Systems 1500 Salado Drive Mountain View, CA 94043, USA 1-800-227-9902 In Calif. 1-800-227-7203	Entire dilatation catheter system
Universal Medical Instrument Corp. Box 100 Balston Spa, NY 12020, USA 1-800-833-6237	10-cm^3 Glass syringes 2-cm^3 Glass syringes Replacement barrels
North American Instrument Box 350 Hudson Falls, NY 12839, USA 1-800-833-9973	PTCA manifold kits Luer locking stopcocks
Interventional Medical P.O. Box 2186 Danvers, MA 01923-5186, USA 617-777-0042	Hand-held inflation device Guide catheters

[a] Balloon catheters have more recently become available from additional manufacturers: Meditech, American Edwards, Scimed, Cook

References

1. Williams DO, Gruentzig AR, Kent KM, Myler RK, Stertzer SH, Bentivoglio L, Bourassa M, Block P, Cowley M, Detre K, Dorros G, Gosselin A, Simpson J, Passamani E, Mullin S (1982) Guidelines for the performance of percutaneous transluminal coronary angioplasty. Circulation 66:693
2. Gruentzig AR, Senning A, Siegenthaler WE (1979) Nonoperative dilatation of coronary artery stenosis. Percutaneous transluminal coronary angioplasty. N Engl J Med 301:61–68
3. Myler RK, Gruentzig AR, Stertzer SH (1981) Technique and clinical indications for percutaneous transluminal coronary angioplasty. In: Mason DT, Collins JJ Jr (eds) Myocardial revascularization. Yorke Medical, New York, pp 431–444
4. Dorros G, Stertzer SH, Bruno MS, Kaltenbach M, Myler RK, Spring DA (1982) The brachial artery method to transluminal coronary angioplasty. Cathet Cardiovasc Diagn 8:233
5. Gruentzig AR (1982) Technique of percutaneous transluminal coronary angioplasty. In: Hurst JW (ed) The heart. New York, pp 1904–1908
6. Simpson JB, Baim DS, Robert EW, Harrison DC (1982) A new catheter system for coronary angioplasty. Am J Cardiol 49:1216–1222
7. Gruentzig AR, Hollman J (1982) Improved primary success rate in transluminal coronary angioplasty using a steerable guidance system. Circulation 66 [Suppl II]:II-330 (abstract)
8. van Gelder LM, van der Krieken AM, El Gamal MIH, Bonnier JJRM, Michels HR (1984) Cathet Cardiovasc Diagn 10:253–258
9. Ischinger T (1985) Anwendung von Laserstrahlen im kardiovasculären System. Herz Gefässe 7:343–345

Chapter 8. Technique of PTCA – Femoral Approach

THOMAS ISCHINGER

Typical Procedure

Before PTCA

Patients are admitted on the day before that scheduled for angioplasty. A medical history is taken and a physical examination performed upon admission. In addition to chest X-ray and ECG, the routine laboratory tests performed upon admission include a complete blood count, chemistry profile, and coagulation battery. Any drugs being taken prior to hospital admission are usually continued. Additional medication given on the day of admission includes aspirin 500 mg or 650 mg per day (Table 1).

Table 1. Checklist for reference during preparation of patients for PTCA

Patient: ______________________ Date: ______________

1. ECG (on admission or on day before procedure)
2. Complete blood count, PT, PTT, platelets, potassium, chemistry profile, fibrinogen and chest X-ray
3. Blood type and screen with one tube for matching
4. Schedule for treadmill exercise

   Yes ____________ No ____________ Date ____________
5. Diet: After midnight before PTCA only water and oral medication. No other oral intake. The patient is not classed NPO for water
6. Medication (to be started the day before the procedure):
   a) Aspirin 500 mg or 650 mg per day
   b) Persantine 75 mg every 8 h
   c) Nifedipine 10 mg every 8 h
   d) Other ______________________

   ____

   e) Premedication ______________________
7. Shave and scrub both groins and legs
8. Give patient the PTCA information form
9. Consent forms for PTCA and coronary bypass surgery must be signed
10. Reserve bed in CCU

____

Signature

An exercise test is usually performed on the day of admission. If the patient has had a recent exercise test, or if there has been evidence of unstable angina no exercise test is performed. On admission patients are given a booklet explaining the procedure in detail. A member of the angioplasty team visits the patient on the day of admission and obtains informed consent for coronary angioplasty and potential coronary surgery.

Beginning 8 h before the angioplasty procedure, the patient is not permitted to eat. No restriction is placed on moderate water intake, to avoid dehydration, and medication is continued as prescribed.

The PTCA Procedure

When the patient arrives in the cardiac catheterization laboratory on the day of the angioplasty procedure, an IV line is placed in the forearm by nursing personnel. An infusion of 500 cm^3 dextran 40 is started before the procedure and continues over a period of 5 h. Before the procedure, the patient may receive medication for sedation (e.g., meperidine 25 mg and diphenhydramine 25 mg). Patients with a history of contrast medium allergy are pretreated with oral hydrocortisone starting the day before the procedure and receive 100 mg hydrocortisone IV on the day of the procedure. Nitroglycerin 0.4 mg and nifedipine 10 mg are administered sublingually immediately before the angioplasty procedure is started, to prevent coronary artery spasm. Local anesthesia is administered with 1% lidocaine and the femoral vein is punctured percutaneously using the Seldinger needle. A 0.035-in. or 0.038-in. safety J guidewire is then inserted through the needle and a 6-F sheath is placed into the femoral vein. A 6-F bipolar pacing lead is advanced and positioned in the right ventricular apex. Proper functioning of the pacemaker is confirmed and this is then left in the standby mode.

The femoral artery is punctured percutaneously in the same fashion and an 8-F sheath is placed. When both the venous and arterial sheaths are in place the patient is given heparin 10000 units IV. If the duration of the procedure is longer than 1 h an additional IV bolus of heparin 5000 units is given to ensure full anticoagulation. PTT is measured at 15 min and at 1 h after administration of heparin. It should be noted that after removal of the dilatation system we frequently find fibrin deposits on the distal portion of the angioplasty guidewire, despite adequate anticoagulation. Routine administration of urokinase (100000 units/h) during coronary angioplasty might be warranted in view of these observations [1].

We usually select guide and balloon catheters on the basis of the diagnostic arteriogram and prepare them before the procedure. The guide catheter is inserted over a 0.063-in. J-tipped wire and then used for the coronary arteriogram of the PTCA vessel immediately before PTCA ("guide shots"). The angiographer can thus judge whether the guide catheter is fitted well into the ostium of the PTCA vessel and whether pressure damping occurs. When a left coronary lesion is to be dilated it is also possible to assess whether the left coronary guide catheter is directed selectively toward the anterior descending or circumflex artery. Those of the preangioplasty diagnostic angiograms that best demonstrate the lesion to be dilated are chosen as guide shots and stored for reference. Particularly if biplane angiography is not available it is important to note the precise degree of projection at which the guide shots were taken, so that these projections can be reproduced during the angioplasty procedure and for the post-PTCA control angiograms. We usually obtain the pre-PTCA angiograms while the patient is breathing normally. This enhances their usefulness for orientation in the coronary tree and identification of stenoses when they are compared with the repeat angiograms taken during the procedure. Continuous replay and still frame disk capacity are extremely helpful for orientation and exact positioning of the dilatation catheters.

Prior to insertion of the balloon catheter into the guide catheter the angioplasty guidewire is checked for steerability and easy maneuverability inside the balloon catheter. If the distal J tip of the wire cannot be smoothly rotated through 360° in a 1 : 1 fashion steerability is inadequate and the wire is exchanged. For insertion into the guide catheter, the wire tip is withdrawn into the central lumen of the balloon catheter.

With the USCI and Schneider-Medintag systems the (deflated) balloon catheter is flushed as it is inserted into the guide catheter, which at this point should be in the descending aorta. After checking all lines and connectors for air bubbles, the guide catheter and balloon catheter are flushed under fluoroscopic control.

It is important to verify that the pressure tracing from the guiding catheter is an accurate reflection of aortic pressure. With the USCI and Schneider-Medintag systems separate pressure tracings are recorded from the balloon and the guide catheter (Fig. 1). The two pressure tracings should be equal prior to introduction of the balloon catheter into the coronary artery. Before the guide catheter is advanced to the coronary ostium the distal tip of the balloon catheter is positioned approximately 5 cm from the tip of the guide catheter. The guidewire is then advanced beyond the tip of the balloon catheter to a position just within the tip of the guide catheter. The guide catheter is then enganged in the coronary ostium. Correct positioning of the catheter is confirmed by injection of small amounts of contrast medium through the guide catheter. It should also be confirmed that there is no pressure damping through the guide catheter. If damping does occur careful repositioning of the catheter or use of a guide catheter with distal side holes may solve the problem (see below).

Wedging of the coronary ostium with the guide catheter for a few seconds can be accepted if the dilatation system is successfully placed in position during this time span. Once the dilatation system is in position the guide catheter can be pulled back over it into a free position. These maneuvers are more likely to be successful with dilatation in the left coronary artery.

The steerable guidewire should be advanced gently and independently of the balloon catheter under continuous fluoroscopic visualization in both RAO and LAO projections, and should never be advanced when resistance is encountered. Injection of small amounts of contrast through the guide and/or balloon catheter allows the position of the guidewire within the coronary artery to be ascertained. The tip of the steerable guidewire can be directed by slowly rotating its proximal portion, either by using a rotator or by bending the proximal end of the wire. Fre-

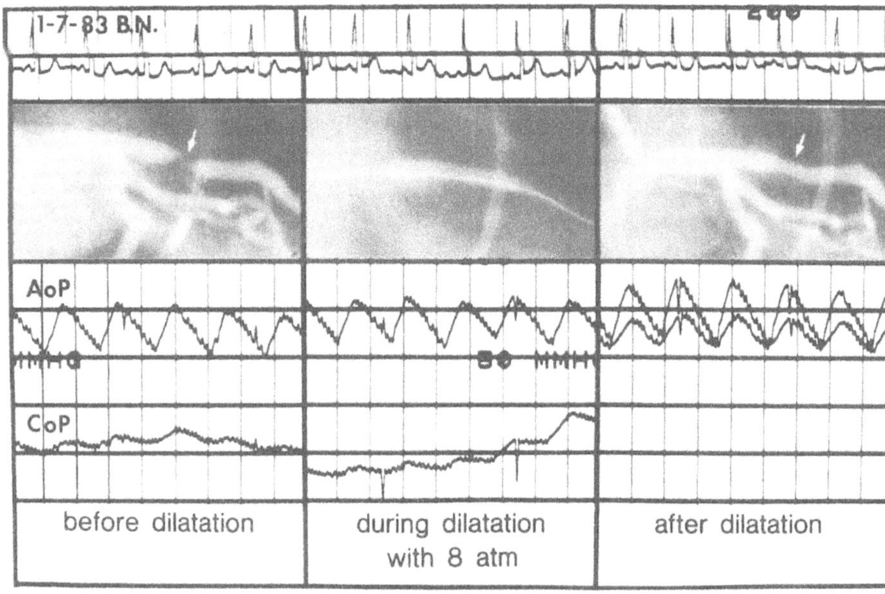

Fig. 1. Coronary angiogram and pressure gradient before, during, and after balloon dilatation of a stenosis in the proximal left anterior descending artery. After successful dilatation the poststenotic intracoronary pressure (*COP*) is almost equal to the aortic pressure (*AOP*), and the pressure gradient across the stenosis is abolished. The angiograms before and after dilatation were taken without the balloon catheter in place

quent confirmation in at least two projections that the guidewire is positioned within the true lumen of the PTCA vessel is important.

Prior to passage of the lesion with the guidewire, 0.3 mg nitroglycerin or 0.1 mg nifedipine is injected into the vessel to be treated by PTCA. The guidewire is then threaded through the coronary lesion and its tip placed in the very distal segments of the vessel to be dilated (Fig. 2). The balloon catheter is then advanced over the guidewire to the area of stenosis, while the wire position has to be maintained. This maneuver usually involves three components: (a) Maintenance of adequate backup position of the guide catheter, which is accomplished by cautious advancement of the guide catheter; (b) advancement of the balloon catheter over the prepositioned guidewire; and (c) maintenance of the guidewire position by slight withdrawal of the wire while the balloon catheter is advanced.

Before placement of the balloon within the stenosis the precise location of the lesion must be known. Review of the initial angiograms is helpful at this juncture, as are injections of contrast medium through the balloon catheter for selective visualization of the PTCA vessel. If thc balloon catheter is just proximal to the stenosis a wedge position with arrested flow (contrast medium) may result. Slight withdrawal of the balloon will then allow the contrast to wash out. This "washout sign" usually indicates proper positioning of the dilatation system within the true lumen of the artery. Prolonged total obstruction of coronary flow should be

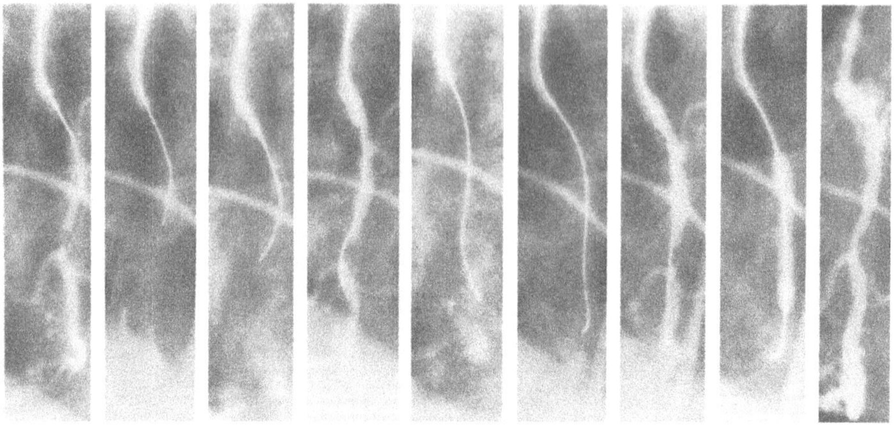

Fig. 2. From left to right: Use of an over-the-wire balloon dilatation system for an irregular stenosis in the middle portion of the right coronary artery. The wire is independently threaded through the stenotic segment and placed in the distal artery. Then the balloon catheter is advanced over the wire and dilatation is performed

avoided in a coronary vessel filled with contrast, as this may increase the risk of ventricular fibrillation.

Once the balloon is positioned within the stenosis the pressure gradient across the lesion is measured (USCI / Schneider-Medintag systems) (Fig. 1). Balloon inflation is then carried out with a hand-held inflator, using incremental pressures starting at 1–2 atm. The balloon should be visualized on fluoroscopy during inflation. As the balloon inflates an indentation in the configuration of the balloon caused by the coronary stenosis is often discerned. Disappearance of this indentation is a sign of successful dilatation.

During each balloon inflation, the patient is monitored closely for angina pectoris, changes in blood pressure, heart rate, and the development of electrocardiographic ST segment changes or arrhythmias. Following each balloon inflation time is allowed for the patient's chest pain to resolve and for any electrocardiographic changes to normalize before another dilatation is performed. After each dilatation the residual pressure gradient across the lesion is measured. Injections of contrast through the guide and/or balloon catheter permit evaluation of the angiographic result and of the blood flow through the dilated artery. However, the presence of the balloon in the area of the stenosis will often preclude adequate angiographic evaluation of the result of dilatation. The balloon catheter is therefore withdrawn to a position proximal to the coronary artery lesion and contrast is injected through the guide and the balloon catheter simultaneously. If the result is unsatisfactory the balloon can safely be repassed across the lesion over the wire, which has been left in place. The same procedure can be repeated with subsequent dilatations. If a larger balloon appears necessary for complete dilatation of the stenosis the balloon is placed distal to the lesion and a long exchange wire advanced into the distal artery. Then the initial balloon can be removed over the wire and replaced with a more adequately sized balloon. If the result of the dilatation seems satisfactory the balloon catheter is withdrawn into the guide catheter while the guidewire is still held in place. An angiogram through the guide and balloon catheters is then repeated, and if the angiographic situation is unchanged and the patient stable the dilatation system is removed under fluoroscopic control. The entire dilatation system should be withdrawn at once, to avoid scraping off fibrin deposits from the segment of the guidewire protruding from the balloon catheter. A control angiogram through the guide catheter in the same projections as were used for the pre-PTCA angiograms is performed. The patient is then kept in the catheterization laboratory for another 15 min while the film is being developed. If review of the coronary angiogram confirms a satisfactory result the patient is moved to the unit.

After PTCA

The venous and arterial sheaths are secured in place following the procedure. The sheaths are usually removed 2 h after the angioplasty. Direct manual pressure fol-

Table 2. Checklist for reference during supervision of patients after PTCA

Patient: ____________ Date: ____________ Time: ____________

1. Check vital signs, punctured groin, and pedal pulses every 15 min until removal of sheaths. Keep punctured leg straight
2. Sheaths are removed (if anticoagulation is not continued) 2–3 h after PTCA. Check PTT before removal

   Removal of sheaths at ____________ h

   by ____________
3. After removal of sheaths bed rest for at least 6 h. Check vital signs, puncture site, and pedal pulses every 30 min. Be with patient when first allowed up (usually morning after PTCA)
4. ECG daily until discharge
5. Check CPK and MB isoenzymes immediately and at 6 and 12 h after PTCA
6. Restrict PO intake to clear liquids for 2 h after PTCA. Liquid diet for first meals, then usual diet
7. When IV fluids are finished maintain heparin lock for 12 h
8. Medications: Nifedipine 10 mg every 8 h
   Aspirin 325 mg per day
   Persantine 75 mg every 8 h
   Other: ____________
9. If patients complains of angina, order ECG and NPO, and notify

Dr. ____________, phone ____________

10. Schedule control exercise test (usually 2nd day after successful PTCA)

____

Signature

lowed by the application of a pressure dressing are applied to the puncture site to prevent hemorrhage. The 2- to 3-h delay before removal of the sheaths allows time for the effect of the heparin to wear off and allows the patient to be returned to the ward with less chance of hematoma formation at the puncture site. In addition, arterial and venous sheaths provide ready access to the femoral artery and vein for repeat coronary angiography or right ventricular pacing in the event of acute myocardial ischemia during the initial hours after PTCA.

If patients need continued anticoagulation after PTCA the sheaths remain in place until anticoagulation is stopped and PTT normalizes.

The patient is allowed to eat 2 h after the angioplasty procedure. Vital signs, puncture site, and pedal pulses are checked frequently during the first few hours after PTCA. The patient is required to lie flat in bed until 6 h after removal of the venous and arterial sheaths. The post-PTCA procedure is summarized in Table 2.

The medication after PTCA includes nifedipine 10 mg every 8 h and low-dose aspirin for 4–6 months if the patient tolerates this medication. A repeat exercise test is routinely performed on the 2nd or 3rd day after a successful coronary angioplasty procedure. If the result of the exercise test is satisfactory the patient is discharged from the hospital. The patient is advised to notify a physician immediately in the case of recurrent chest pain, which requires prompt repeat coronary angiography. Particularly sedentary patients are advised to undergo a monthly exercise test to help in early detection of recurrent stenosis. We do not routinely schedule asymptomatic patients for repeat coronary angiography after PTCA.

Selection of the Appropriate Dilatation System

Guide Catheter

We have found that 8-F guide catheters are almost always satisfactory. In selecting the type and size of guide catheter we consider the vessel to be dilated and the catheters that proved suitable for coronary arteriography at the previous diagnostic study. It should be noted, however, that subtle "stretching" of the primary and secondary curves, resulting from the presence of the balloon catheter within the thin-walled guide catheter, can often make cannulation of the coronary ostium rather more difficult.

"Shaping" (bending of the secondary curve) of the guide catheter in the aortic sinus is sometimes helpful in these situations.

The guide catheters for femoral PTCA are of three general configurations, as shown in Fig. 3: Judkins type, Amplatz types, and multipurpose types.

For dilatation of the left anterior descending artery a Judkins-type left coronary catheter is commonly used. A no. 4 catheter is initially selected if the aortic arch appears normal in width and size. Counterclockwise rotation and advancement of the guide catheter mostly allow for selective cannulation of the left anterior descending artery (see below). Occasionally, it is worthwhile to try an off-

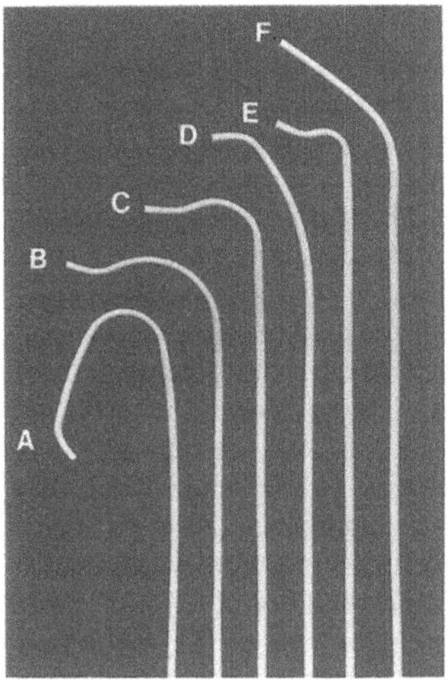

Fig. 3. Frequently used guide catheters. For the left coronary artery: *A*, Judkins type no. 4; *B*, Amplatz type no. 2; *C*, Amplatz type no. 1. For the right coronary artery: *D*, Judkins type no. 4; *E*, Amplatz type no. 1; *F*, multipurpose type

plane Judkins-type left coronary catheter (G type, see Fig. 10, chapter: "Angioplasty Equipment and Supplies: Technical Considerations.") for difficult selective cannulation of the anterior descending artery.

For dilatation within the left circumflex system a left Judkins-type guide catheter is also the instrument of choice. The purpose of the guide catheter is not only to guide the balloon catheter into the PTCA vessel, but also to provide sufficient backup for exertion of pressure on the balloon catheter to advance it through the coronary artery and across tight stenoses. The Amplatz-type guide catheter usually facilitates selective cannulation of the left circumflex system *and* provides increased stability when dilatation of high-grade stenoses is attempted. It is important to achieve stable positioning of the guide catheter prior to the dilatation attempt. An inadequate fit of the guide catheter may complicate the procedure unnecessarily: if it is impossible to cross the stenosis because of inadequate backup of the guide catheter, withdrawal of the whole system, including the guidewire, is necessary before the guide catheter can be exchanged. During this exchange procedure, total occlusion of the lesion that had already been crossed with the wire may develop, in which case recanalization cannot be attempted at once, since selection of a new, more adequate guide catheter takes time and ready access to the PTCA vessel has been lost.

Although use of the Amplatz-type guide catheter may sometimes be unavoidable, we usually consider this catheter the second choice. Cannulation of the left coronary artery with the Amplatz guide catheter carries an increased risk of trauma to the coronary ostium. We therefore never use it when a lesion is present in the left main stem.

A Judkins-type right coronary guide catheter (no. 4) is the usual choice for dilatations within the right coronary artery. If a stable position within the artery and an adequate backup for angioplasty are not achieved with this catheter, multipurpose guide catheters (USCI, Interventional Medical) or Amplatz-type guide catheters can be used. The multipurpose guide catheter usually allows for deeper cannulation of the right coronary artery and can provide excellent backup, particularly for right coronary arteries with a high upward takeoff.

For these anatomic situations of the right coronary artery the *left* Amplatz-type guide catheters (no. 1 and no. 2) may also be useful.

For dilatations within a saphenous vein graft the catheters used are generally the same as for the right coronary artery, but in most cases multipurpose, El Gamal, and Amplatz-type guide catheters are needed to ensure adequate backup.

With experience and cautious manipulation of the guide catheter stable cannulation of the PTCA vessel can usually be achieved (see below); shaping of the guide catheter (over the proximal, stiff end of the 0.063 guidewire) with the aid of a heat gun or boiling water is time consuming, often unsuccessful, and rarely necessary. The 9-F guide catheters can sometimes have an advantage in that they may provide better torque control and backup for angioplasty. Also, 9-F guide catheters allow better pressure recordings and contrast injections when loaded with the balloon dilatation system. Potential disadvantages of the 9-F guide catheters are that they require larger puncture holes (use of 9-F introducer sheaths) and are more likely to cause pressure damping due to a wedge position in the coronary ostium.

This wedging problem occurs mostly with cannulation of the right coronary artery and can often be solved by making two or three side holes (perpendicular to the curvature) in the distal section of the guide catheter (perforation trepane no. 00036/00037, A.D. Krauth, Hamburg, W. Germany) approximately 2 or 3 cm from the distal tip of the guide catheter. Catheters with side holes can be wedged into a coronary orifice without pressure damping, as antegrade flow through the side holes and out the distal opening in the catheter can be maintained. Guide catheters with side holes are commercially available.

Balloon Catheter

The most important consideration in selecting the balloon catheter is matching the inflated diameter of the balloon as closely as possible to the size of the non-diseased arterial segments adjacent to the target stenosis. Use of a balloon that is larger than the dilated vessel may result in mechanical overdistension of the artery and undue vessel injury. Use of balloon that is not as large as the dilated artery may result in inadequate stenosis dilatation. The diagnostic angiogram should be carefully studied and the pre- and poststenotic diameter of the vessel lumen measured using the known diameter of the diagnostic catheter as a gauge.

Features of some of the currently available balloon catheters have already been discussed in the chapter: "Angioplasty Equipment and Supplies: Technical Considerations." Today we use low-profile over-the-wire dilatation systems exclusively (Fig. 4). Currently, the most commonly used balloon catheters are the Schneider-Medintag, USCI, and ACS dilatation systems.

Selection of the balloon catheter will be largely determined by operator experience. However, there are differences between the currently available systems,

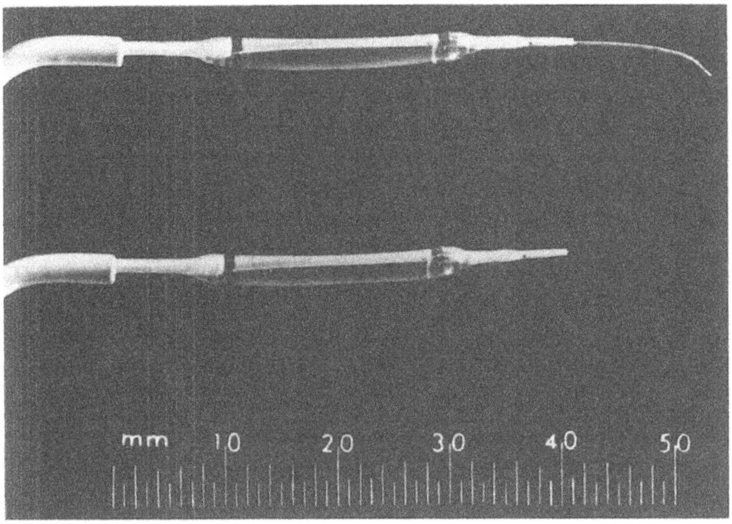

Fig. 4. Steerable balloon catheter (3 mm inflated balloon diameter) with and without movable, J-tipped angioplasty guidewire. The guidewire is protruding from the central lumen of the balloon catheter

which may have practical implications. The Schneider-Medintag and USCI balloon catheters are somewhat stiffer than the ACS balloon catheters. For lesions that are situated at vessel curves or for tortuous vessels the more flexible catheter shaft of the ACS dilatation system may offer some advantage in allowing for smooth advancement with less mechanical trauma to the vessel wall. To date, measurements of the poststenotic coronary pressure via the balloon catheter with the guidewire in place have only been satisfactory with the Schneider-Medintag/USCI balloon dilatation system. We believe in measuring the pressure gradient as one means of assessing the PTCA result and therefore feel more comfortable using dilatation systems that allow for adequate measurement of intracoronary pressure.

Guidewire

Features of the guidewires currently available have been described in the chapter on equipment and supplies. In selection of the guidewire two properties need to be considered: flexibility of the distal guidewire tip and steerability (torque control) of the guidewire. Generally, the guidewires that are most flexible distally (floppy wires) are the least steerable. However, most of the angioplasty guidewires of the latest generation exhibit a satisfactory combination of the characteristics "steerability" and "flexibility." The 0.012-in. (or 0.014-in.) steerable wires from Schneider-Medintag (or USCI) and the 0.016 in. (or lately 0.014-in.) high-torque floppy guidewires from ACS are the ones we currently use most frequently. It is desirable to cross the coronary stenosis with the softest and most flexible guidewire possible, as this will reduce the likelihood of producing mechanical injury of the vessel intima or the atherosclerotic plaque.

This is particularly important if the stenosis is very tight or if the morphology of the lesion is irregular or eccentric. It is not always possible to predict from the diagnostic coronary arteriogram whether the guide and dilatation catheters can be directed toward the vessel to be dilated. Often maneuvers using both the guide catheter and the steerable angioplasty guidewire are necessary to enter the target vessel with the balloon dilatation system. Manual shaping (bending) of the distal guidewire tip is frequently required to negotiate acute angles or side branches.

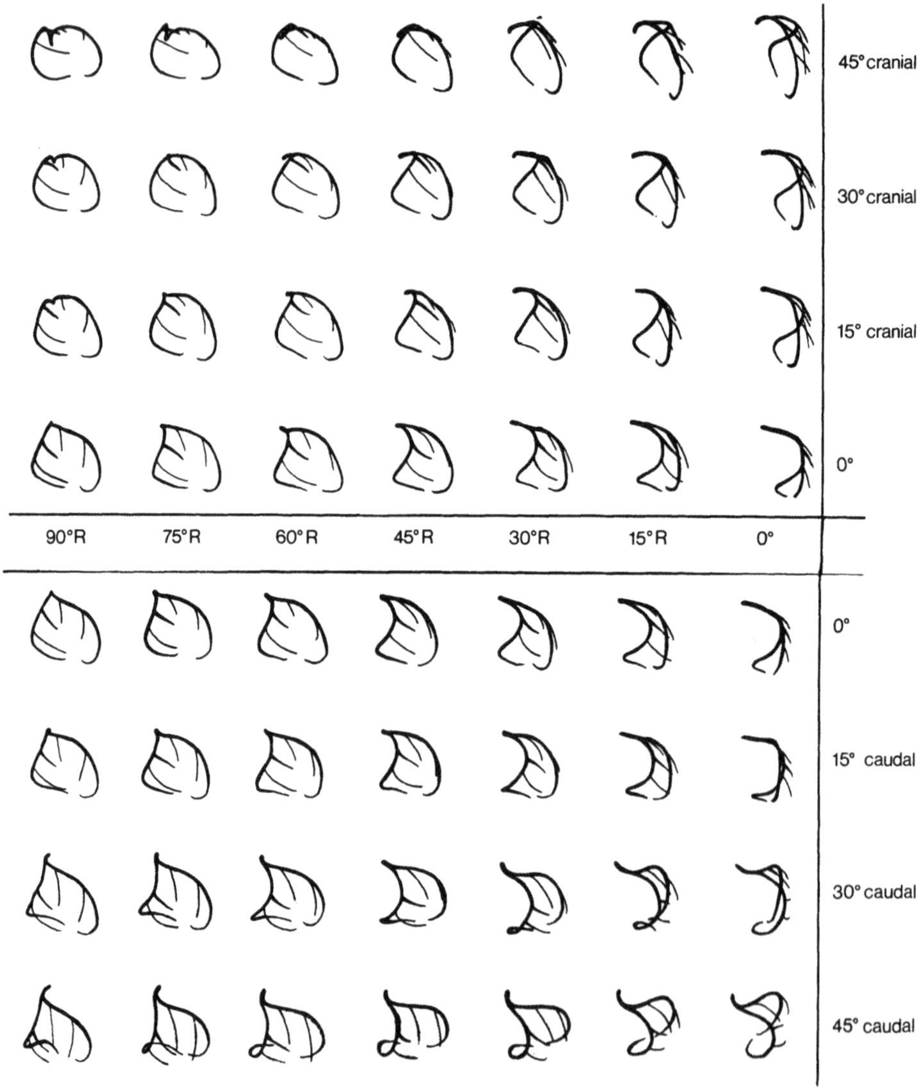

Fig. 5 a. Left coronary artery in right oblique views with cranial and caudal angles; **b** left coronary artery in left oblique views with cranial and caudal angles; **c** right coronary artery in right oblique views with cranial and caudal angles; **d** right coronary artery in left oblique views with cranial and caudal angles. [32]

While a significant bend in the guidewire tip may be useful at one point of the procedure, it may be a disadvantage later, e.g., for passage of a tight, complicated stenosis. In that case, the shaped guidewire would be used to gain access to the PTCA vessel with the balloon catheter and then exchanged for a straight floppy guidewire to accomplish passage of the stenosis more safely.

A long (3 m) exchange guidewire is needed to exchange the balloon catheter and leave the angioplasty guidewire in place for ready access to the PTCA vessel. Recently, a technique using a long, steerable (exchange) guidewire routinely from the onset of the procedure has been described [1].

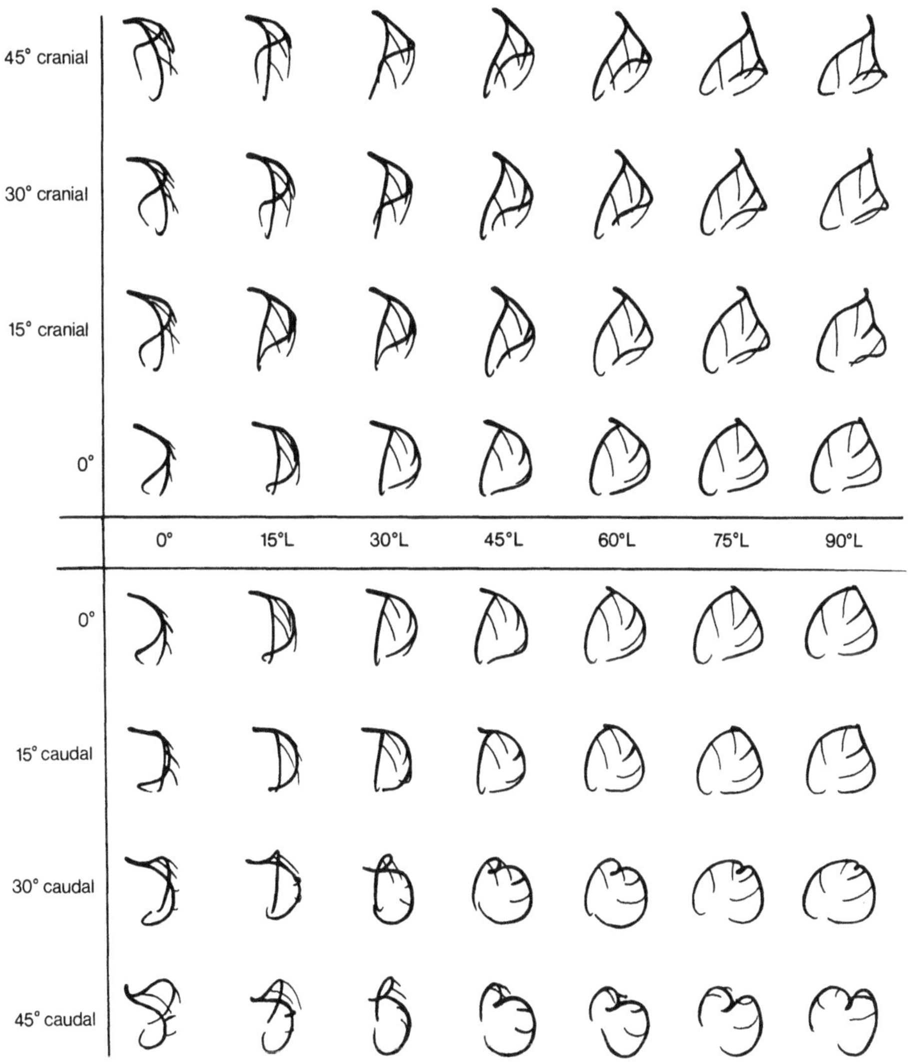

Fig. 5b

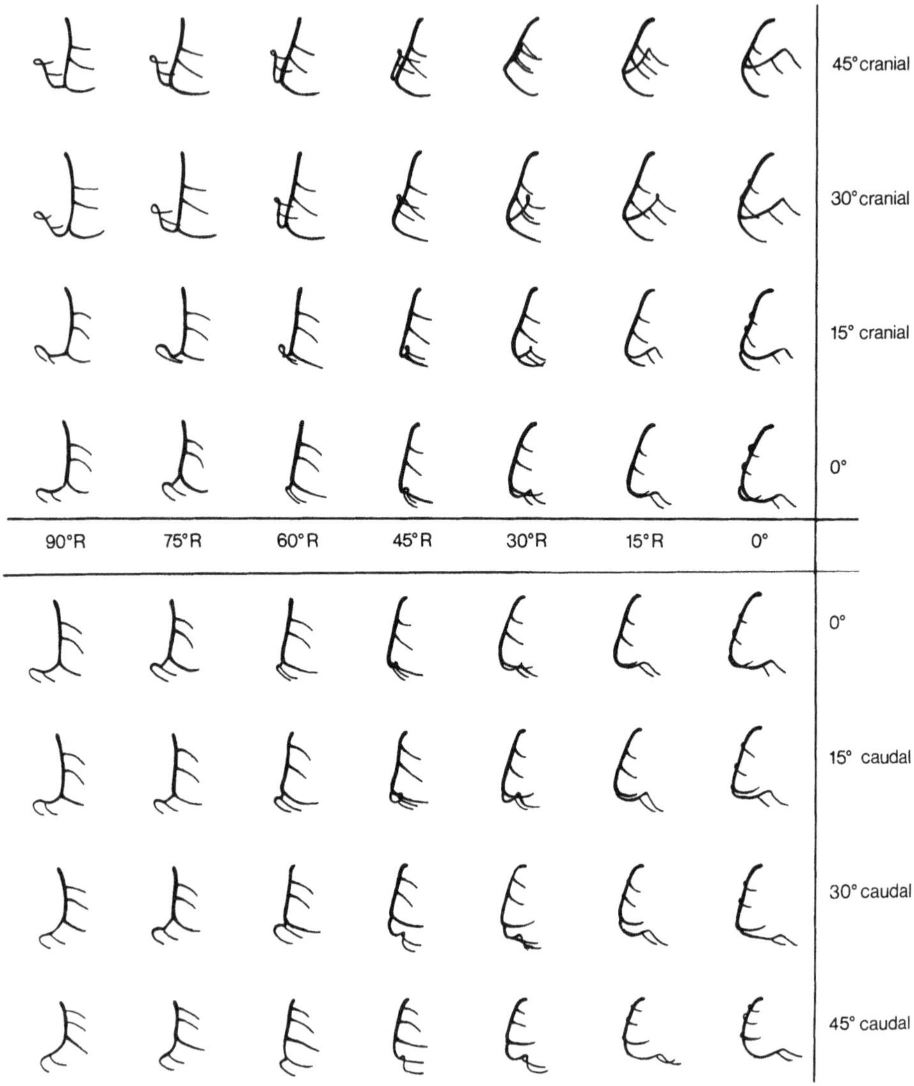

Fig. 5c. (Legend see p. 138)

The advantage of this technique is that the guidewire can be advanced independently through the stenosis without the balloon catheter being already inserted into the guide catheter, thus permitting better contrast injections through the guide catheter and – if necessary – faster and safer exchange of balloon catheters. It should be noted at this point that withdrawal and reinsertion of guidewires through the balloon catheter may carry a risk of intracoronary thromboembolism. We have not yet encountered complications with angioplasty guidewire exchange; however, we have frequently seen fibrin deposits on the guidewire after PTCA. We therefore avoid withdrawal of the angioplasty guidewire through the balloon catheter whenever possible.

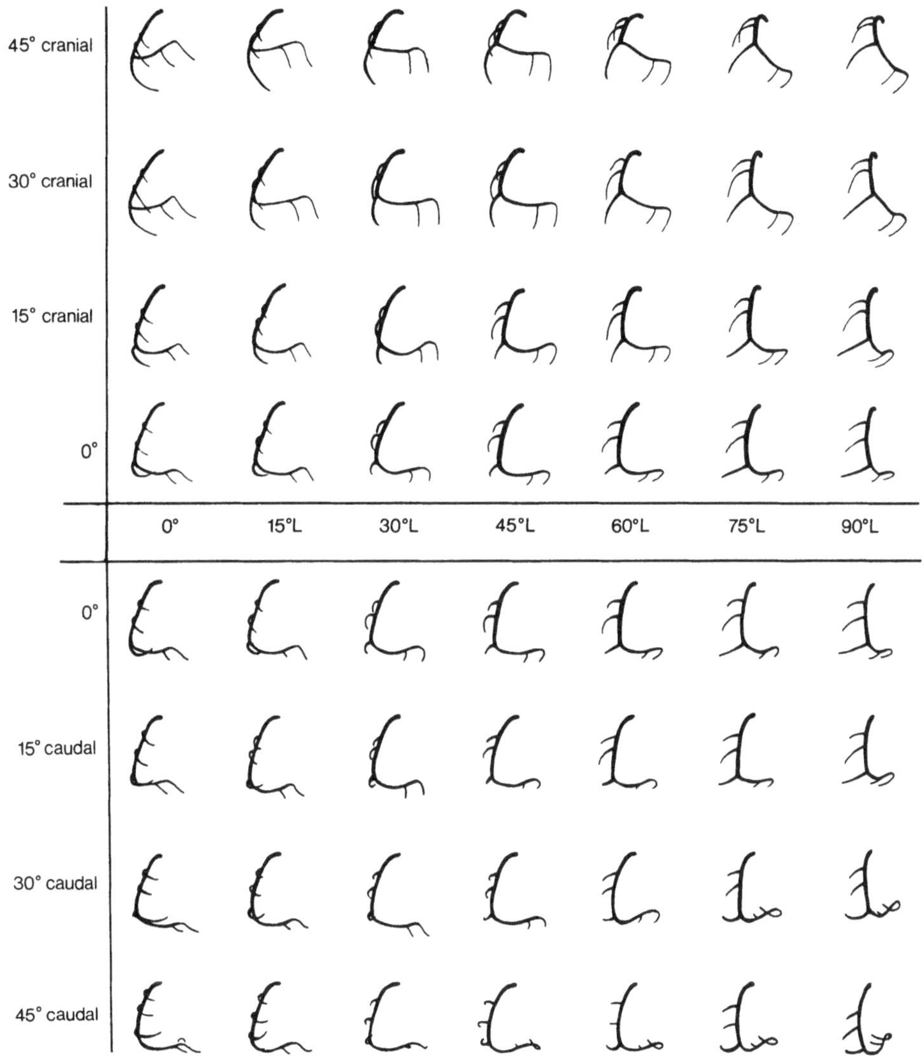

Fig. 5d. (Legend see page 138)

Special Technical Problems

Angiographic Views

Safe and effective performance of coronary angioplasty requires accurate angiographic visualization of the coronary arteries. A high-resolution X-ray system and high-quality video tape or video disk systems for immediate replay are prerequisites for coronary angioplasty. However, proper selection of multiple angiographic views is equally important, for accurate identification of the course of the coronary artery, its bifurcations, and the configuration of the stenosis. Overlapping vessels, foreshortening, and end-on visualization of the coronary segments are frequent problems, which can lead to misinterpretation of the arteriogram and complicate the angioplasty procedure. From multiple views of the diagnostic angiogram the operator will choose two or three that show the course of the PTCA vessel accurately and without overlap (Fig. 5). "Circumferential" visualization of coronary stenoses is important to detect the "true" morphology.

For angioplasty of tight eccentric or ulcerated stenoses the operator must choose the projection that allows the best appreciation of the residual lumen and pass the guidewire safely.

Visualization of the *left main coronary artery* is best accomplished using a frontal or 5°–10° RAO (right anterior oblique) view (i.e., with the image intensifier over the right side of the chest). As a second view a 30°–50° LAO (left anterior oblique) view (i.e., with the image intensifier over the left side of the chest) can be used with a 20°–30° cranial or a 10°–20° caudal angulation.

A left anterior oblique caudal view is usually best to visualize the left main and the origin of the left anterior descending and left circumflex arteries (Fig. 9). Additional projections (e.g., frontal cranial view, "chin shot") may be necessary for a definite assessment of the left main coronary artery prior to coronary angioplasty.

For dilatation in the *left anterior descending artery* a 20°–30° RAO with 20°–30° cranial angulation is usually best, in combination with a 45° LAO view with 20°–30° cranial angulation. The LAO cranial view with 20°–30° cranial angulation. The LAO cranial view avoids foreshortening of the proximal and middle parts of the LAD and allows excellent evaluation of the course of the LAD and its bifurcations into diagonal and septal branches. If selective cannulation of the LAD with the dilatation system is difficult the LAO cranial and the LAO caudal projections are most helpful in finding the proper direction (Figs. 6 and 9). The RAO cranial view is helpful in avoiding overlap of the LAD with diagonal branches.

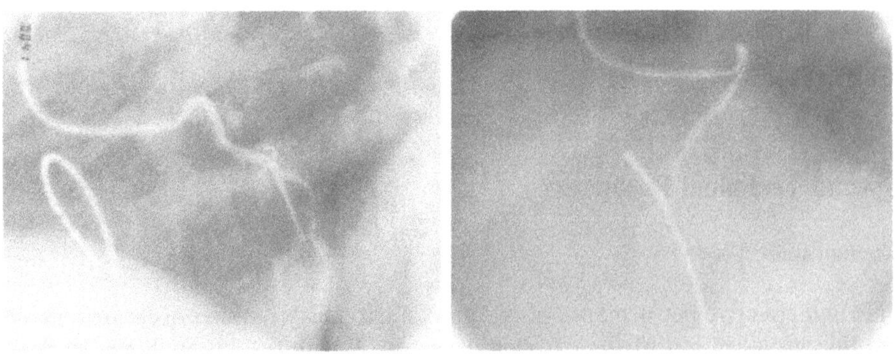

a b

Fig. 6 a. A left Judkins type guide catheter is selectively cannulating the left circumflex artery (cranial LAO projection during inspiration). **b** Counterclockwise rotations and gentle advancement of the guide catheter allowed entry of the left anterior descending artery. (Cranial LAO projection, as in **a**)

The *left circumflex coronary artery* is often best visualized in RAO views. However, the proximal segment of the left circumflex artery may be visualized end-on in the standard RAO view. Caudal or cranial angulation may permit better visualization. As a second projection an LAO cranial view is used. This view "unfolds" the middle section of the left circumflex artery, which is often foreshortened in RAO views. An LAO caudal view separates the origin of the left circumflex and the left anterior descending arteries. This view is most helpful when selective cannulation of either artery with the guiding catheter or guidewire is attempted (Figs. 10 and 13).

For dilatation of the *right coronary artery* we mostly use standard RAO 30° and LAO 45°–60° projections. In the LAO view the ostium and the proximal portion of the right coronary artery are usually well visualized. RAO views or cranially angulated LAO views are needed to avoid overlap with right ventricular branches and end-on visualization of the posterior descending artery or the left ventricular branches.

Entering the Left Anterior Descending Artery

Usually a left Judkins-type guide catheter is chosen for the left anterior descending artery. After the guide catheter has been engaged in the left main coronary ostium the angioplasty guidewire is advanced independently. The LAO cranial view shows best whether the wire is entering the LAD or the left circumflex artery. If gentle steering movements (rotation in both directions) with the guidewire do not bring the guidewire tip into the LAD the tip of the guiding catheter needs to be pointed more toward the LAD (Fig. 6). Prior to reorientation of the guide catheter the guidewire is withdrawn into the guide catheter.

When the tip of the Judkins catheter is in the left coronary orifice, counterclockwise rotation of the catheter will direct the tip in an anterior direction to-

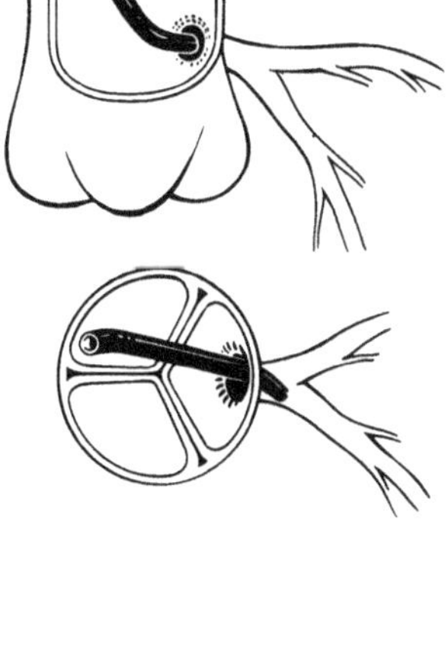

Fig. 7. Tip of left guide catheter (Judkins type) in left coronary ostium. Counterclockwise rotation of guide catheter directs tip more towards left anterior descending artery (anterior direction). RAO view (*above*) and theoretical view from above the aortic valves (*below*)

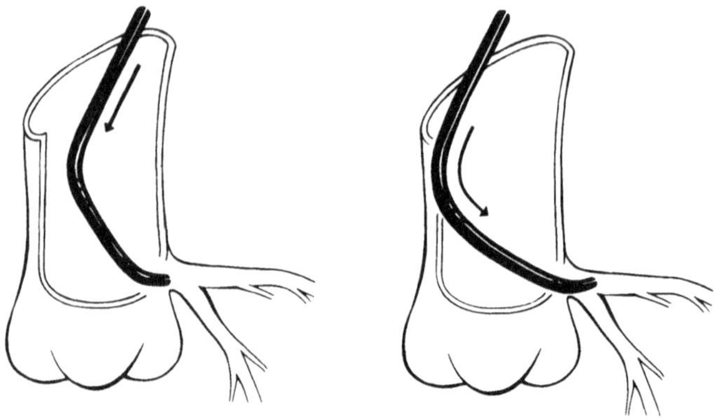

Fig. 8. Right anterior oblique view of left guide catheter (Judkins type) engaged in the left coronary ostium. Advancement of the guide catheter leads to deeper engagement into the left main stem and directs the catheter tip upward toward the left anterior descending artery. (Adapted from [26])

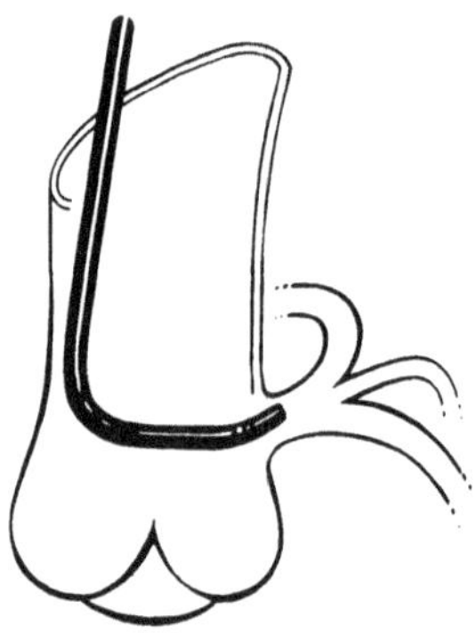

Fig. 9. Left anterior oblique caudal view with a left Judkins type guide catheter in the left main stem. This view gives the best separation between the origin of the left anterior descending and that of the left circumflex artery and intermediate branches. (Adapted from [26])

ward the LAD "due to the fulcrum effect on the tip in the left coronary orifice" [2]. This is illustrated in Fig. 7 by means of an RAO view (above) and a theoretical view from above the aortic valves (below). Counterclockwise rotation with simultaneous advancement of the guide catheter usually directs the tip of the guiding catheter towards the orifice of the anterior descending coronary artery (Fig. 8). This maneuver is best monitored in the cranial LAO view, as shown in Fig. 6. The LAO caudal view is helpful when selective cannulation of the left anterior descending or left circumflex artery is difficult, as it allows good visualization of the origin of either artery (Fig. 9). The advancement of the guide catheter tip deeper into the left main stem represents a potential risk of left main stem injury, particularly in the presence of left main stem disease. Therefore, even very slight left main stem disease should be ruled out prior to these maneuvers, and only gentle pressure should be applied, to minimize complications. There are two anatomic situations which do not allow the guide catheter to be directed toward the LAD: A very long left main stem and an acute angle of takeoff of the LAD from the left main coronary artery. In these situations entry of the LAD requires use of the steerable guidewire in addition to the maneuvers described with the guide

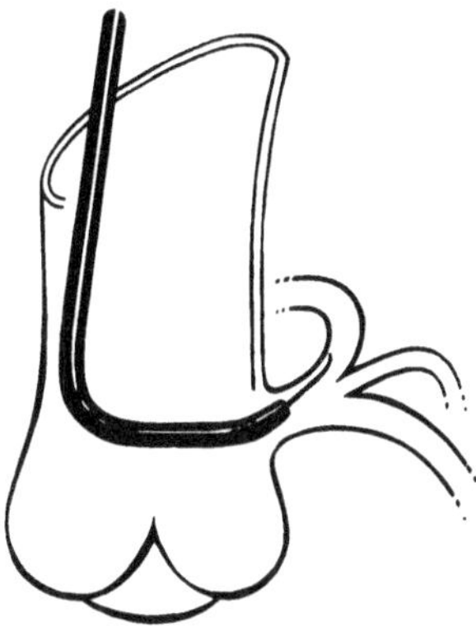

Fig. 10. Left anterior oblique view of the left Judkins type guide catheter in the left coronary ostium (same view as in Fig. 8). The J-tipped guidewire is directed toward the left anterior descending artery, following the terminal curve of the Judkins catheter. (Adapted from [26])

catheter. The J-tipped angioplasty guidewire usually follows the final curve of the Judkins catheter and is therefore directed toward the LAD. This is best visualized in the LAO caudal views (Fig. 10). In the case of an acute takeoff from the left main stem a very pronounced and long curve on the distal wire is needed to enter the LAD. As mentioned earlier, such pronounced curves at the wire tip may hinder further advancement of the guidewires down the artery or crossing of the lesion. In this event it may seem desirable to exchange the guidewire once the balloon catheter has entered the PTCA vessel and reached the area of stenosis. Prolonged manipulation of the guidewire may reduce its steerability and movability inside the balloon catheter lumen. It is therefore important to keep the balloon dilatation system as straight as possible, in order to avoid unnecessary bends in the guidewire. The angioplasty guidewire is maneuvered by the operator or the assistant. Constant rotation of the guidewire in one direction is undesirable; rather it should be turned back and forth, because this minimizes the potential risk of unraveling the spring coil of the distal guidewire. If rotation of the proximal end of the guidewire is not transmitted to the tip of the guidewire in a one-to-one fashion – this is mostly due to bends in the shaft – the guidewire must be exchanged. Optimally functioning dilatation tools are absolutely essential for success and safety.

Crossing the Lesion

The wire is independently advanced across the lesion and placed as far distal as possible in the LAD (usually near the apex). Crossing of the lesion requires accurate visualization of its configuration, particularly in the case of tight asymmetric stenoses, to allow direction of the J tip of the guidewire in a controlled manner toward the residual lumen of the stenosed segment. Hopes that the wire will "float" through the lesion by itself can be disappointed. While the assistant pulls gently back on the guidewire to maintain its position in the distal coronary, the balloon catheter is introduced over it and across the lesion. Gentle pressure on the balloon catheter will usually cause it to cross the lesion. If pressure on the balloon catheter causes the guide catheter to come out of the coronary ostium, a bet-

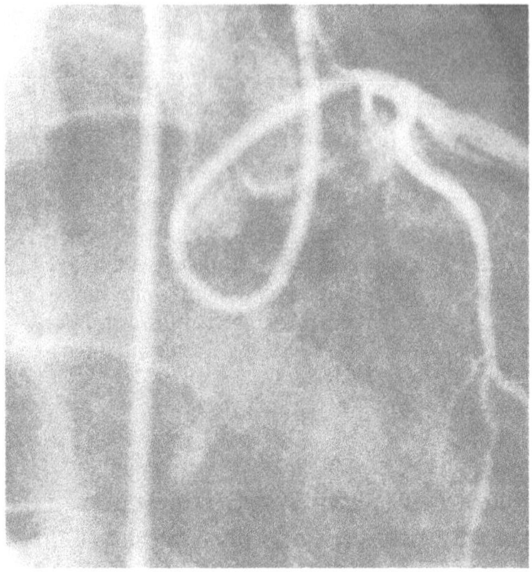

a

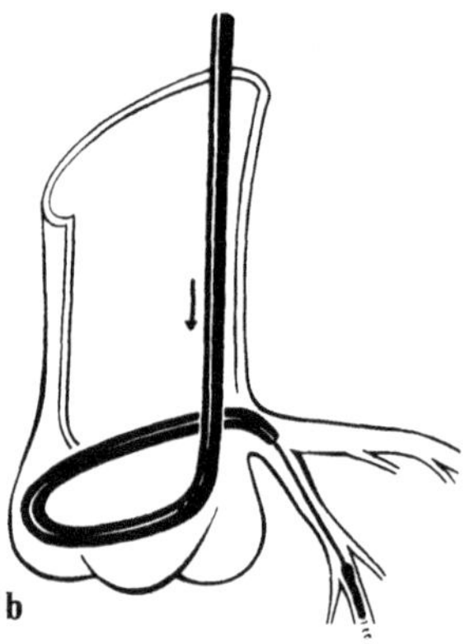

b

Fig. 11 a, b. Unusual but helpful backup position of the left Judkins type guiding catheter in the left coronary ostium (RAO view). This maneuver with the guide catheter should only be attempted when the dilatation system is already engaged into the PTCA vessel. It is helpful for crossing tight stenoses

ter backup position of the guide catheter is needed. This is achieved by pulling the balloon catheter back slightly while advancing the guide catheter over it further into the left main stem.

The combined maneuver with the guide and dilatation catheters may result in formation of a guide catheter loop that rests at the opposite wall of the aortic root and provides excellent backup (Fig. 11). Once the lesion is crossed the guide catheter is pulled back from the left main coronary ostium while the balloon catheter is advanced slightly to maintain its position within the coronary stenosis.

If the coronary stenosis still cannot be crossed the balloon catheter may be exchanged for a lower profile balloon catheter.

Entering the Left Circumflex Artery

The left circumflex artery takes off from the left main stem in a more posterior and inferior direction, as shown in Fig. 12. A left Judkins-type catheter usually

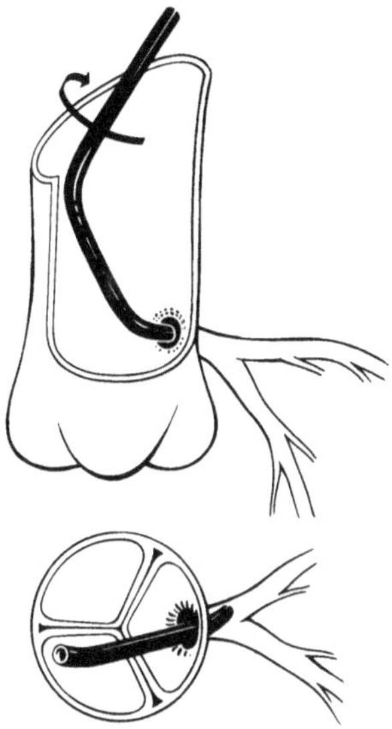

Fig. 12. Tip of left guiding catheter (Judkins type) in left coronary ostium. Clockwise rotation moves tip in a more backward direction toward the left circumflex artery. RAO view (*above*) and theoretical view from above the aortic valves (*below*)

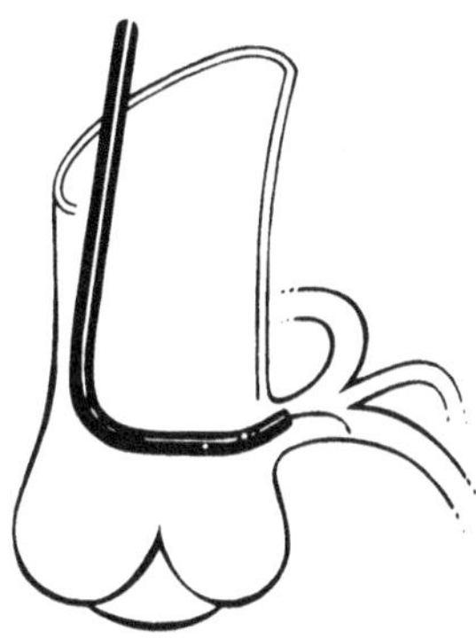

Fig. 13. Left anterior oblique caudal view of the left Judkins-type guide catheter in the left coronary ostium. An S curve (double curve) of the guidewire is needed to bring the tip of the wire downward (opposite direction to the terminal curve of the Judkins catheter) into the left circumflex artery. (Adapted from [26])

permits entry into the left circumflex artery, but clockwise rather than counterclockwise rotation of the guide catheter is required to orient the tip of the guide catheter toward the left circumflex artery. However, the guidewire is often needed for entry of the artery.

With good steerability of the guidewire a marked bend in its distal tip is often enough to bring the guidewire into the left circumflex artery. If the left circumflex artery takes off at a sharper downward angle a double-S-type curve of the distal end of the guidewire may be needed for selective circumflex cannulation (Fig. 13) [1].

If the left circumflex artery cannot be entered with the guidewire using a left Judkins-type guide catheter a left Amplatz-type guide catheter should be selected. The tip of the Amplatz catheter is oriented in a downward direction toward the left circumflex artery and the J-tipped angioplasty guidewire can usually be steered into the left circumflex artery (Fig. 14a, b). The Amplatz catheter has the additional advantage of providing stable backup for advancing the dilatation sysa

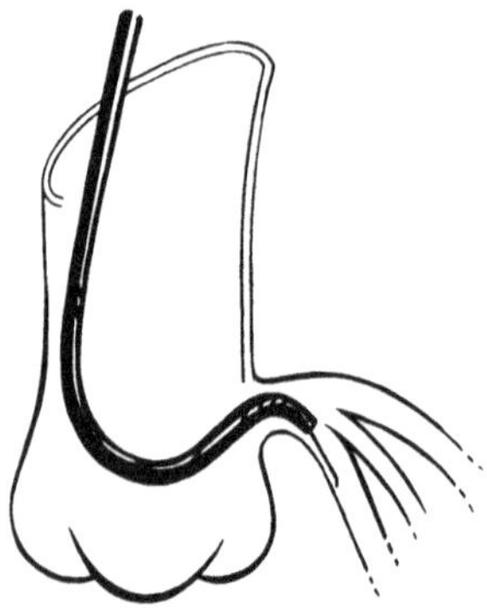

b

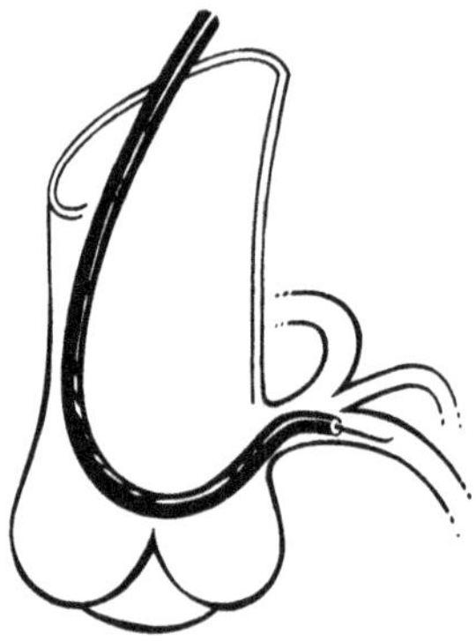

Fig. 14. a Right anterior oblique view showing the Amplatz-type guide catheter engaged in the left coronary ostium. The tip of the catheter is pointing toward the left circumflex artery (downward), facilitating selective advancement of a straight or slightly curved guidewire. **b** Same situation in a left anterior oblique view. (Adapted from [26])

tem and crossing the lesion. The disadvantage of the Amplatz catheter is the potential risk of increased trauma to the left main stem. The Amplatz catheter usually engages firmly into the left main coronary ostium because the curve of the catheter is supported against the opposite aortic wall. Also, abrupt withdrawal of the Amplatz catheter may result in transient deeper engagement of the catheter tip, which constitutes a potential hazard. We therefore use Amplatz-type guide catheters only as a second choice and if the left main stem is free of disease. *Crossing of the lesion* is accomplished in essentially the same fashion as described for the left anterior descending artery.

Entering the Right Coronary Artery

For the right coronary artery the Judkins-type guiding catheter is usually the instrument of choice (Fig. 15). The rather frequent wedging problem with guide catheter cannulation of the right coronary artery can be minimized by using 8-F guide catheters or guide catheters with side holes, as described above. If advancement of the dilatation system can be accomplished quickly, a transient wedge position might be acceptable until the balloon dilatation system is in place, which then allows withdrawal of the guide catheter from its wedge position. This maneuver must be done with great caution as the right Judkins-type guide catheter has the tendency to "snap back," once it is pulled out from the coronary ostium, and disengage the entire dilatation system.

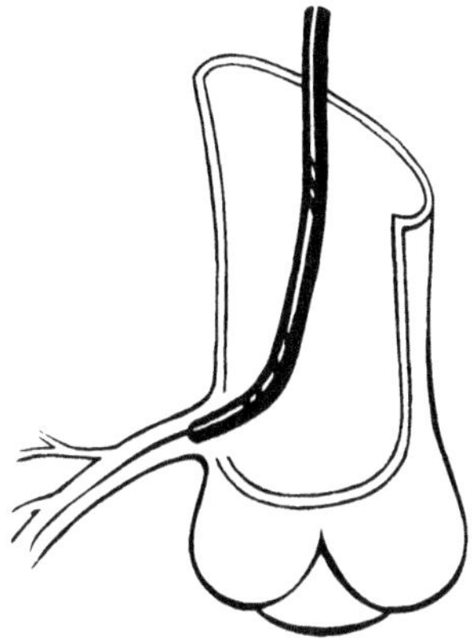

Fig. 15. Left anterior oblique view showing the right Judkins-type catheter entering a right coronary artery with a downward course

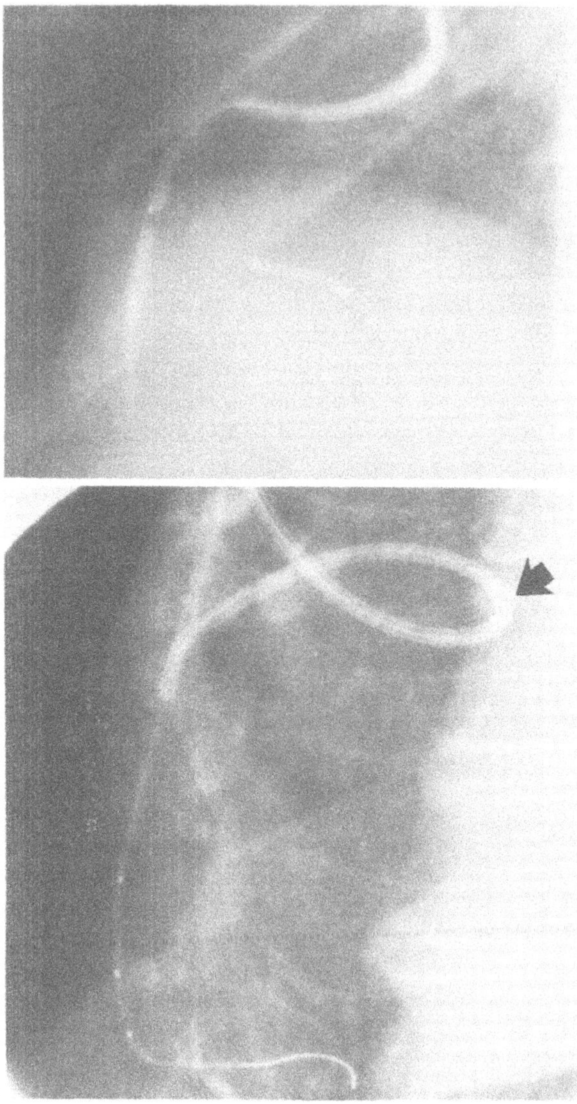

a

b

Fig. 16. a Deep engagement of the right Judkins-type guiding catheter into the right coronary artery with the catheter being propped against the opposite aortic wall. **b** Further advancement of the guiding catheter (over the guidewire) may result in formation of a loop and cannulation of the proximal to middle portion of the right coronary artery. (Hartzler, this volume)

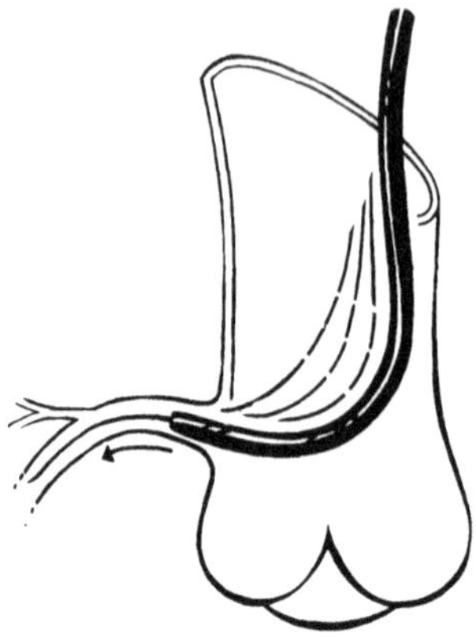

Fig. 17. Left anterior oblique view of a multipurpose guide catheter engaged in the right coronary ostium. This catheter often permits stable engagement of ascending right coronary arteries and provides better backup for advancement of the dilatation system

For negotiation of tight stenoses or vessel tortuosities the right Judkins-type guide catheter does not provide sufficient backup in its usual position (Fig. 15). A maneuver similar to the one described for dilatation in the left coronary artery is used to achieve a better backup position of the Judkins guide catheter: The operator pulls the balloon catheter back slightly while advancing the guide catheter over it to cause it to engage more deeply in the proximal segment of the right coronary artery. This maneuver may bring the catheter into a position where it is supported against the opposite wall of the aorta and lead to a stable backup position (Fig. 16A). Further advancement (over the dilatation system) of the guide catheter into the middle portion of the right coronary artery can be accomplished by forming a loop with the guide catheter, which directs the tip of the catheter downward following the course of the right coronary artery (Fig. 16B).

If the right coronary artery starts in an upward direction and then turns downward at a sharp angle (shepherd's crook), cannulation with the guide catheter and advancement of the dilatation system may be very difficult. A multipurpose (Fig. 17) or a left Amplatz-type guide catheter may be useful in these situations. Both catheters usually provide adequate backup for advancing the balloon catheter through tight lesions. The multipurpose type guide catheter is also helpful in right coronary arteries with a descending proximal segment, as it permits deep cannulation and exertion of pressure along the axis of the guide catheter.

Any attempt to *cross* tight coronary lesions is facilitated by placing the angioplasty guidewire as far distal as possible (Fig. 16A and B). We always try to place the tip of the guidewire beyond the crux cordis or in the posterior descending branch.

Entering Saphenous Vein Grafts

The catheters used for the right coronary artery may also be suitable for dilatation of vein grafts. The multipurpose guide catheter (or the El Gamal guide catheter) are often best from the aspect of deep cannulation of the graft and provision of adequate backup for angioplasty. It may be necessary to bend the distal end of the multipurpose catheter to an angle of 90° or more to enter saphenous vein grafts that start in a upward direction.

Aspects of Balloon Inflation

Number of Inflations

The total number of inflations performed for dilatation of the lesion is determined by assessing the anatomic and hemodynamic results following each inflation. When the pressure gradient across the lesion can be monitored inflations are usually continued until the pressure gradient is less than 20 mmHg. If the pressure gradient is not measured, termination of the procedure will be based largely on the angiographic result. In a recent analysis published by the National Heart, Lung, and Blood Institute PTCA Registry the total number of inflations was identified as a factor associated with successful angioplasty [3]. Uncomplicated dilatation of single and localized lesions usually requires two or three balloon inflations. However, we sometimes terminate a procedure after a single long balloon inflation (more than 60 s) if the angiographic and hemodynamic results are satisfactory.

Duration of Inflations

We generally attempt to maintain balloon inflation for 40–60 s (sometimes longer), as there is evidence that prolonged pressure can improve the results of coronary angioplasty [4]. The inflation time is usually limited by the degree of chest pain experienced by the patient or electrocardiographic signs of myocardial ischemia (ST segment depression, ST segment elevation, arrhythmias). In most patients chest pain begins within 10 s of balloon inflation, but is usually tolerated for longer than 30 s. There is evidence that intracoronary administration of nitrates or calcium antagonists improves the tolerance of balloon-catheter-induced myocardial ischemia [5]. ST segment elevations during balloon occlusion of the coronary artery do not necessarily indicate immediate deflation, whereas ventricular extrasystole does. If signs of myocardial ischemia are induced by balloon inflation repeat dilatation should be performed after a recovery period of about 3 min. Angina pectoris often resolves within 30 s of balloon deflation, whereas electrocardiographic signs and parameters of left ventricular function may take longer to normalize [6, 7, 33].

Inflation Pressure

We generally perform an initial inflation at 1–2 atm to assess the configuration and position of the inflated balloon and to monitor the coronary wedge pressure (distal occlusion pressure) (see Chap. 4). Then the inflation pressure is increased by stepwise increments up to 6 or 7 atm, and is usually held at this level during the initial inflation. We tend to use the lowest pressure that yields satisfactory angiographic and hemodynamic results.

If the result of dilatation is not satisfactory higher pressures may be used at the second balloon inflation. In particular, if the indentation produced on the inflated balloon by the coronary stenosis does not disappear during balloon inflation higher pressures are more likely to achieve successful stenosis dilatation [8]. It should be noted that the shape of the balloon may change during inflation and the outer diameter may increase at pressures greater than 5–7 atm [9]. This may be turned to advantage if the selected balloon catheter appears to be somewhat undersized. In that case, inflation pressures of 9–10 atm may slightly increase the diameter of the inflated balloon and improve the result. On the other hand, use of excessively high pressures is a potential hazard, in that overdistension of the artery or balloon rupture may occur.

Measurement of Intracoronary Pressure

We routinely record intracoronary pressure during PTCA via the balloon catheter. Determination of the translesion pressure gradient with the balloon catheter is inaccurate and leads to overestimation of the hemodynamic significance of a coronary lesion [10, 11], because the balloon catheter itself contributes to the coronary obstruction and artifactually increases the gradient.

However, assessment of the intracoronary pressure allows to make a judgement about the hemodynamic result of balloon dilatation. If the angiographic result is equivocal or if angiographic visualization of the dilated segment is poor, recording of the intracoronary pressure may be of great practical value and further guide the procedure. Significant reduction (usually more than 20 mmHg) of the translesional pressure gradient following balloon dilatation mostly signals an acceptable dilatation result; a reduction of the pressure gradient to less than 20 mmHg almost invariably corresponds to angiographically insignificant lesions.

Measurement of the distal coronary artery pressure during balloon occlusion allows for estimation of the status of collateral circulation to the PTCA vessel (see Chap. 4).

Furthermore, intracoronary pressure recording represents a safety factor in that it helps to continuously verify intraluminal placement of the dilatation catheter. These advantages, in our experience, outweigh the little effort that is usually needed to achieve a reliable and stable pressure tracing through the narrow lumen of the balloon catheter. This usually requires thorough checking of the guiding and dilatation system for air bubbles, leaks or loose connections.

Standby Pacing

It is still common practice to insert a bipolar pacemaker lead into the right ventricle, permitting immediate pacing of the heart in the case of bradyarrhythmia. The pacing catheter is usually inserted through the femoral vein at the arterial puncture site by means of a sheath. Pacing leads with a central lumen (e.g., Myler catheter, Zucker catheter, Swan-Ganz catheter with pacing capacity) have the advantage of also allowing assessment of hemodynamics and central administration of drugs during the angioplasty procedure. Pacing leads, particularly those positioned in the pulmonary outflow tract, can also be used as a reference point, giving better orientation during the procedure.

The use of nonionic contrast material with low osmolality has markedly decreased the incidence of arrhythmic complications during coronary angioplasty and thus the need for temporary cardiac pacing.

Intracoronary or left ventricular pacing via the angioplasty guidewire has recently been described as a method that obviates the necessity for separate placement of a pacemaker in the right ventricle [12].

Coronary Angioplasty of Bifurcational Lesions

THOMAS ISCHINGER and PAUL ZACK

A relative contraindication to the performance of PTCA is the presence of a large side branch arising from the primary coronary artery stenosis. Such bifurcational lesions have been associated with a significant risk of iatrogenic side branch occlusion during coronary angioplasty [13, 14] (see Fig. 2b of Chap. 4). To increase the safety of coronary angioplasty in patients with bifurcational lesions a technique involving the simultaneous use of two over-the-wire dilatation systems can be applied. This section describes the technique for dilatation of an LAD/diagonal branch bifurcational stenosis.

With the Seldinger method, 8-F arterial sheaths are placed in both the right and the left femoral arteries. Two 8-F Judkins-type guide catheters are inserted and left in the descending aorta. Medical treatment is as described earlier for a typical angioplasty procedure. Both guide catheters are then loaded with steerable balloon dilatation catheters of the same size. The balloon size is selected according to the smallest nondiseased vessel segment in the areas of balloon inflation. This allows both systems to be used for either artery involved in the bifurcational lesion. After flushing of the catheters, if pressure transmission through the guide and the balloon catheters is adequate (if fewer than 4 pressure channels are available pressure recordings via the guide catheters should have priority) one guide catheter (system A, Fig. 18a) is engaged in the left coronary orifice and the guidewire positioned within the major vessel distal to the origin of the side branch. Guide catheter A is then pulled back from the left coronary ostium into a free position within the aortic sinus (Fig. 18b). The second left Judkins-type guide catheter (system B) is then placed in the left coronary ostium and the guidewire is advanced into the side branch. After withdrawal of guide catheter B from the coronary ostium, guide catheter A is reengaged to advance the balloon catheter A over its wire for dilatation of the major vessel lesion (Fig. 18c). If there is no stenosis in the side branch and successful dilatation of the major vessel does not result in side branch occlusion the procedure is terminated. If, however, there is significant preexisting stenosis within the origin of the side branch or if dilata-

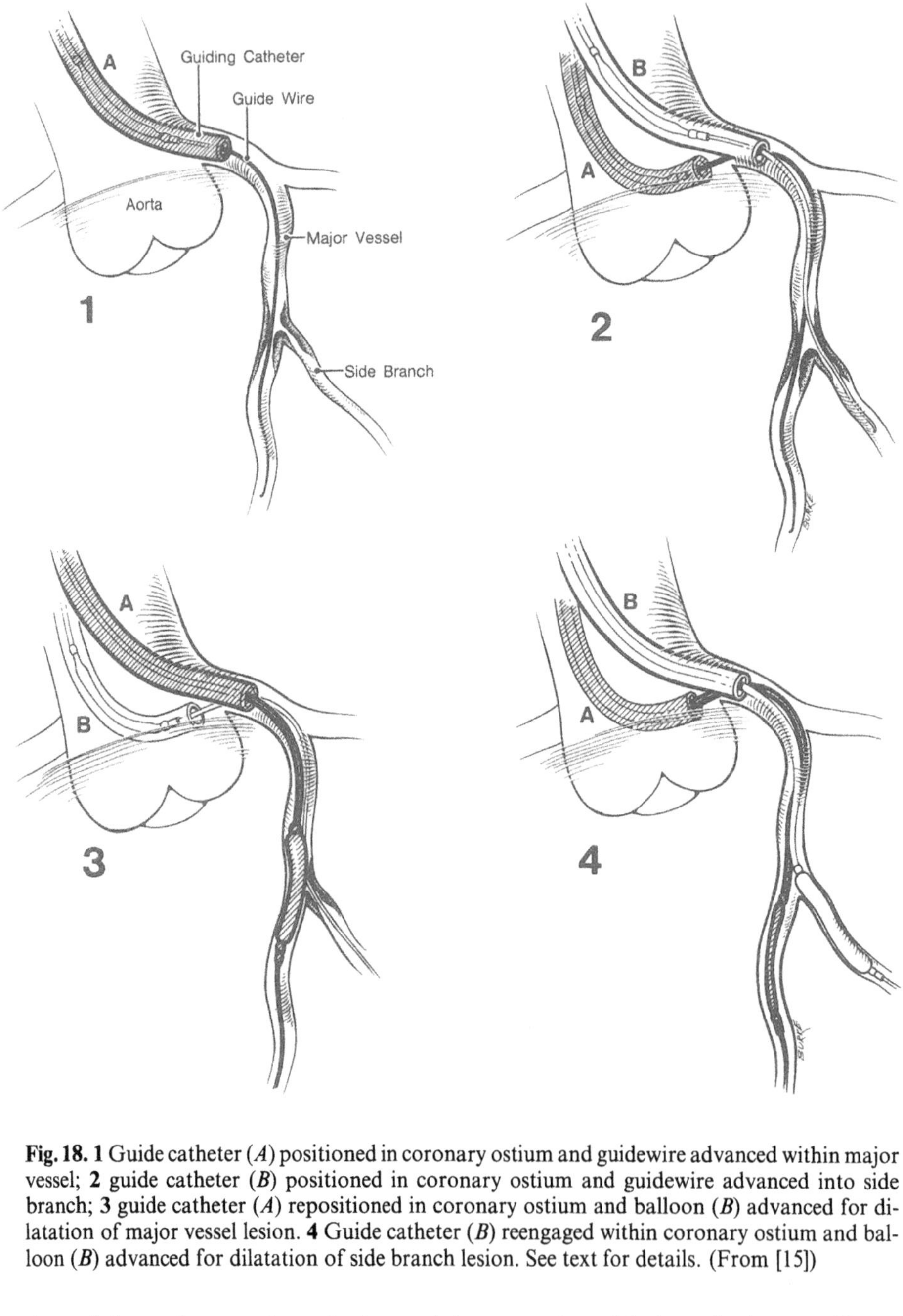

Fig. 18. 1 Guide catheter (*A*) positioned in coronary ostium and guidewire advanced within major vessel; **2** guide catheter (*B*) positioned in coronary ostium and guidewire advanced into side branch; **3** guide catheter (*A*) repositioned in coronary ostium and balloon (*B*) advanced for dilatation of major vessel lesion. **4** Guide catheter (*B*) reengaged within coronary ostium and balloon (*B*) advanced for dilatation of side branch lesion. See text for details. (From [15])

tion of the major vessel results in partial or complete side branch closure, dilatation of the side branch lesion is then performed. Guide catheter A is withdrawn from the coronary ostium while deflated balloon A is kept in position distal to the bifurcation, and guide catheter B is repositioned within the coronary ostium to allow advancement of the balloon catheter over its guidewire to the side branch stenosis (Fig. 18d).

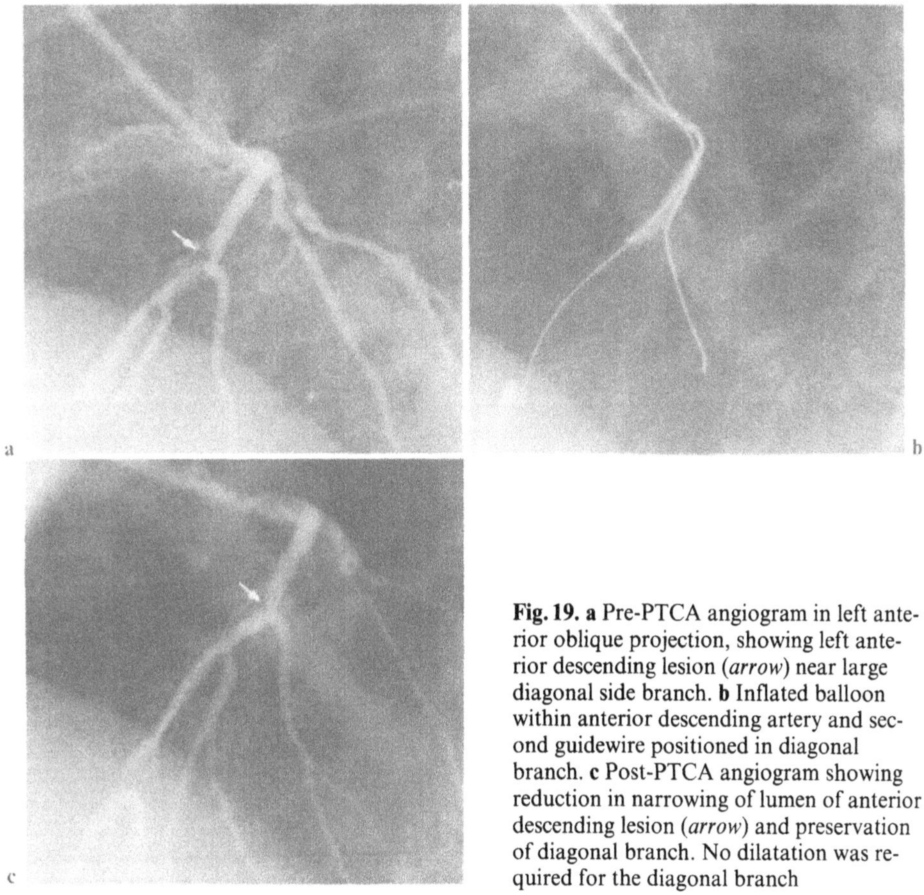

Fig. 19. a Pre-PTCA angiogram in left anterior oblique projection, showing left anterior descending lesion (*arrow*) near large diagonal side branch. b Inflated balloon within anterior descending artery and second guidewire positioned in diagonal branch. c Post-PTCA angiogram showing reduction in narrowing of lumen of anterior descending lesion (*arrow*) and preservation of diagonal branch. No dilatation was required for the diagonal branch

We have recently reported the use of this technique in patients undergoing coronary angioplasty for bifurcational lesions in the left anterior descending (Fig. 19a–c) and left circumflex coronary arteries (Fig. 20) [15]. The average time required for placement of the additional dilatation system was 15 min. No complications have occurred. In particular, no complications related to the additional arterial puncture have been encountered, and the duration of hospitalization and ability to perform exercise stress testing before discharge from hospital have remained unaffected. However, several potential risks are associated with the placement of a second balloon dilatation system. These include the risk of local complications at the arterial puncture site and the inherent risk of coronary dissection or occlusion, which may occur with manipulation of the additional dilatation system within the coronary artery.

Instead of sequential dilatations of the vessels involved in bifurcational lesions, it is possible to perform simultaneous dilatation within the two vessels. However, simultaneous dilatation may carry a risk of overdistension at the level of the kissing balloons. We therefore suggest that simultaneous dilatation be re-

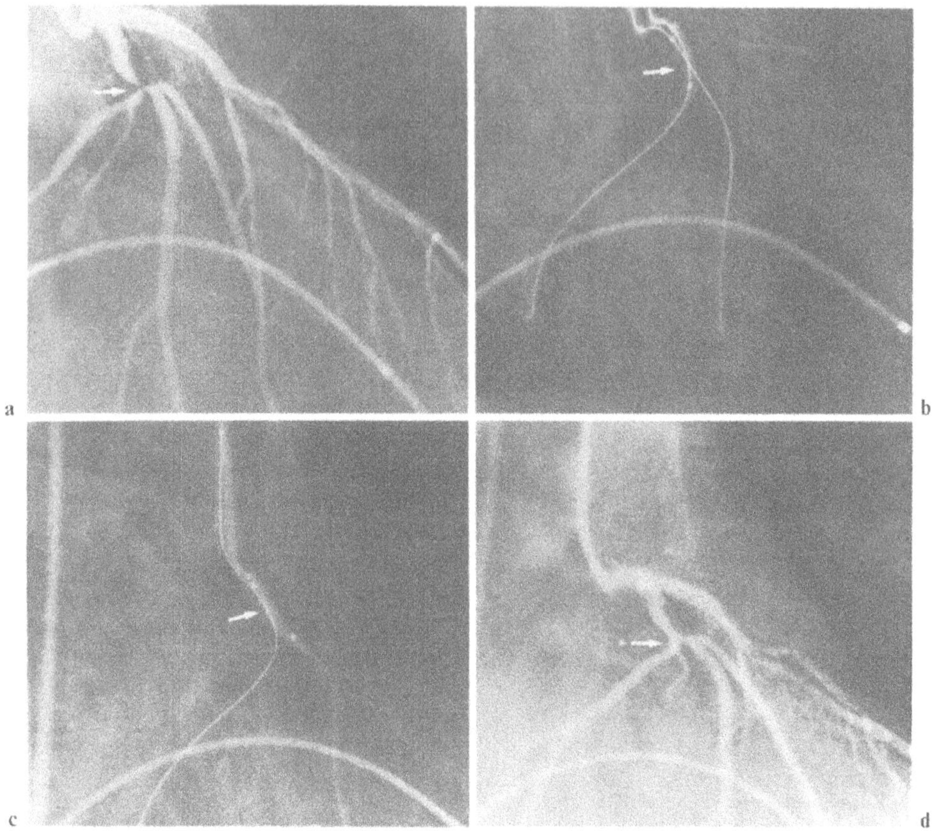

Fig. 20 a–d. Pre-PTCA angiogram in right anterior oblique projection showing left circumflex obtuse marginal lesion (*arrow*). **b** Inflated balloon within circumflex artery and second guidewire positioned in marginal branch. **c** Inflated balloon within marginal branch and first guidewire positioned in circumflex artery. **d** Successful result after PTCA

served for use exclusively in situations where the sequential method has failed to yield a satisfactory result at the branching point of the two vessels.

Iatrogenically occluded vessels may reopen spontaneously [16] or be cleared by other means than the technique described. An attempt can be made to advance the single steerable guidewire across the area of closure, and intracoronary administration of nitroglycerin or streptokinase may also lead to reperfusion of an occluded vessel [17, 18]. These measures, however, are sometimes unsuccessful and may lead to additional complications. We believe that the prepositioning of a steerable guidewire within an important side branch that is at risk for occlusion can provide a significant measure of safety during angioplasty of bifurcational coronary lesions. Because of the potential difficulty and risk associated with the placement of a second dilatation system, the technique should be used in selected patients who are judged to be at high risk for iatrogenic side branch occlusion and in whom a considerable amount of myocardial tissue is in jeopardy. PTCA was previously considered to be contraindicated in such patients, but the technique described appears to constitute an effective method of performing coronary angioplasty safely.

Management of Complications of PTCA

THOMAS ISCHINGER

Coronary Vascular Complications

Following successful coronary angioplasty, arteriography often reveals an *"intimal tear"* in the area of balloon inflation [19]. This is characterized angiographically by the extravasation of contrast medium into the vessel wall and irregular opacification of the vessel lumen (see Figs. 10 and 12c, e of Chap. 4). An intimal tear is the angiographic correlate of the actual disruption and splitting of the atheromatous plaque and vessel intima. There is evidence that plaque and intimal disruption are important mechanisms of mechanical coronary artery dilatation and that a subsequent "healing process" restores integrity of the vessel wall. An intimal tear following otherwise successful coronary angioplasty is usually considered an innocuous angiographic finding. Progression of a localized asymptomatic intimal tear to occlusive coronary artery dissection is rare [20]. However, we attempt to prevent sudden occlusion in the few hours immediately after the procedure by continuing anticoagulation with heparin (PTT twice control) for 12–24 h following the procedure if an intimal tear or any marked luminal irregularities are visualized on the post-PTCA arteriogram.

The angiographic appearance of a *coronary artery dissection* may be similar to that of an intimal tear, but dissection is distinguished clinically by evidence of myocardial ischemia and impaired coronary blood flow in the injured vessel. Acute ischemia due to dissection of the coronary artery is the most frequent complication of PTCA and accounts for approximately two-thirds of the emergency bypass operations. When the characteristic angiographic picture of coronary dissection is not demonstrated in the presence of obstruction of coronary flow in the dilated vessel the term *"total coronary occlusion"* is used. In these cases intracoronary thrombus formation and coronary artery spasm are among the possible causes of obstruction.

If occlusive coronary dissection or total occlusion occurs with angioplasty, a decision must be made as to whether and by what means recanalization of the artery should be attempted. If signs of evolving myocardial infarction become apparent preparations for surgery and insertion of the intraaortic balloon pump should be started to avoid losing time if interventions in the catheterization laboratory are unsuccessful.

If occlusion occurs with the angioplasty guidewire across the lesion then the balloon catheter can be easily and safely advanced to the lesion again and the vessel redilated. Repeated dilatation with long inflation times at moderate pressures is then performed in an attempt to reattach the dissected layer of the arterial wall. If these attempts fail emergency bypass surgery is usually required.

Whether surgical revascularization is necessary, and how urgently, is dictated by the acuteness of signs of myocardial ischemia and the amount of myocardial tissue in jeopardy. The variation among different centers in the incidence of emergency coronary bypass surgery now reflects the different philosophies of patient selection rather than mere differences in ability to perform coronary angioplasty successfully. However, despite prompt surgical revascularization, transmural ischemia following complicated PTCA is frequently associated with evidence of myocardial necrosis [21].

Although there is no definitive evidence of myocardial salvage achieved by prompt surgical revascularization, emergency bypass surgery is advocated for patients with refractory acute ischemia due to complicated PTCA. The low mortality and myocardial infarction rates of experienced centers are attributed in part to the short period (approximately 60 min) between the arterial injury and revascularization of the infarcted vessel [22]. In an effort to minimize myocardial injury before coronary flow can be restored by vein grafting, interventions that augment blood flow into the infarcted area and reduce myocardial oxygen demand should be instituted in the catheterization laboratory. With the balloon catheter still across the lesion, arterialized blood from the contralateral femoral artery can be perfused through the balloon catheter into the coronary artery distal to the obstruction, either manually or by means of a roller pump [23]. Although the flow rate through the balloon catheter is limited, we have observed resolution of chest pain and ST segment elevations with this method.

Balloon catheters with side holes communicating with the central lumen of the catheter proximal to the balloon [such balloon catheters (and intracoronary perfusion catheters) have recently become available from Schneider-Medintag and ACS] are another means of maintaining antegrade flow without the necessity for pumping blood through the balloon catheter [24]. More recently, clinical interest has been aroused in interventions sparing the myocardium, including retroperfusion and intermittent coronary sinus occlusion, which are performed via the coronary sinus. In particular, retroperfusion/infusion via the coronary sinus is hoped to be a promising mode of treatment for acute myocardial ischemia caused by coronary occlusions [25, 26].

When a large amount of myocardial tissue is at risk and patients become hemodynamically unstable, intra-aortic balloon support is indicated. Percutaneous insertion of the intra-aortic balloon catheter over a guidewire can be performed more quickly if the groin contralateral to that used for PTCA is prepared in advance. Safe and quick institution of intra-aortic balloon counterpulsation requires some experience, and it should not on any account delay prompt surgical revascularization. If surgery is not readily available intra-aortic balloon support along with other medical and mechanical interventions can provide means of stabilizing the patient during the interval.

The management of acute myocardial ischemia caused by occlusion of the vessel treated by PTCA after removal of the dilatation system from the artery is more complex and depends on the angiographic result of the PTCA attempt, the chances of reopening the occluded vessel, and the availability of surgical support. If angioplasty has been apparently uneventful and successful a new angiographic study should be carried out immediately to identify the problem. During the preparations for repeat coronary angiography any pharmacologic maneuvers that are deemed adequate to reverse the acute ischemia should be applied, including sublingual or IV administration of nitroglycerin or nifedipine but excluding systemic thrombolysis. This is not appropriate before the problem has been identified, as it may result in bleeding complications at the femoral puncture sites and perioperative hemorrhage if emergency bypass surgery is subsequently performed. If angiography shows that the PTCA vessel is reoccluded at the dilatation site small doses of nitroglycerin and/or nifedipine are injected through the diagnostic catheter into the coronary bed. If the artery remains closed and there is no angiographic evidence of coronary dissection an infusion of intracoronary streptokinase is started at 4000 IU/min through the diagnostic catheter while the equipment for repeat dilatation is being set up [18]. Figures 21–23 illustrate a case of complete restoration of vessel patency by means of drug treatment following total occlusion after PTCA.

Once the dilatation system is ready an attempt to recross the lesion with the angioplasty guidewire is made, and if this is successful repeat dilatation is performed (Fig. 24).

With the use of soft-tipped angioplasty guidewires total obstructions observed after PTCA can be safely recrossed even in the presence of coronary dissection. However, with occlusive coronary dissection the changes of achieving sustained vessel patency by repeat dilatation are lower. If the initial angioplasty has resulted in significant arterial dissection or an otherwise equivocal result that does not seem to be amenable to angioplasty we tend to have recourse to surgery more readily in the event of acute PTCA-related ischemia.

Coronary arterial spasm also is likely to play an important role in the genesis of coronary occlusion associated with PTCA [28], since arterial spasm is a known response of an artery to injury (Fig. 24). The stepwise combined medical and mechanical approach will allow many of these patients to respond and stabilize, thus obviating the need for emergency coronary bypass surgery [17, 18].

In the case of acute ischemia following multiple vessel dilatations the procedure is influenced by the confidence the operator has in the results of the dilatations performed thus far and the degree of revascularization that has been achieved by the time the ischemic complication occurs. Whether successfully dilated arteries should be grafted at bypass operation to replace the diseased artery is a moot point; reduced flow rates due to competitive flow may jeopardize the long-term patency of both the grafts and the successfully dilated coronary arteries. However, one tends to recommend complete surgical revascularization in these patients.

Coronary artery performation or rupture are rare complications of coronary angioplasty [27–30]. With incorrect use of the dilatation catheter the wire tip may function as a stiletto. In particular, this is true for the early generation balloon catheters with fixed and reinforced tip wires (D type). Correct use of an over-the-wire dilatation system will avoid arterial perforation. However, if the movable guidewire is not allowed to extend far enough out from the tip of the balloon catheter it will become less flexible and be more likely to function as a stiletto.

The risk of perforation of a coronary artery with the dilatation system is greatest in the presence of acute angles and ulcerated lesions. Independent placement

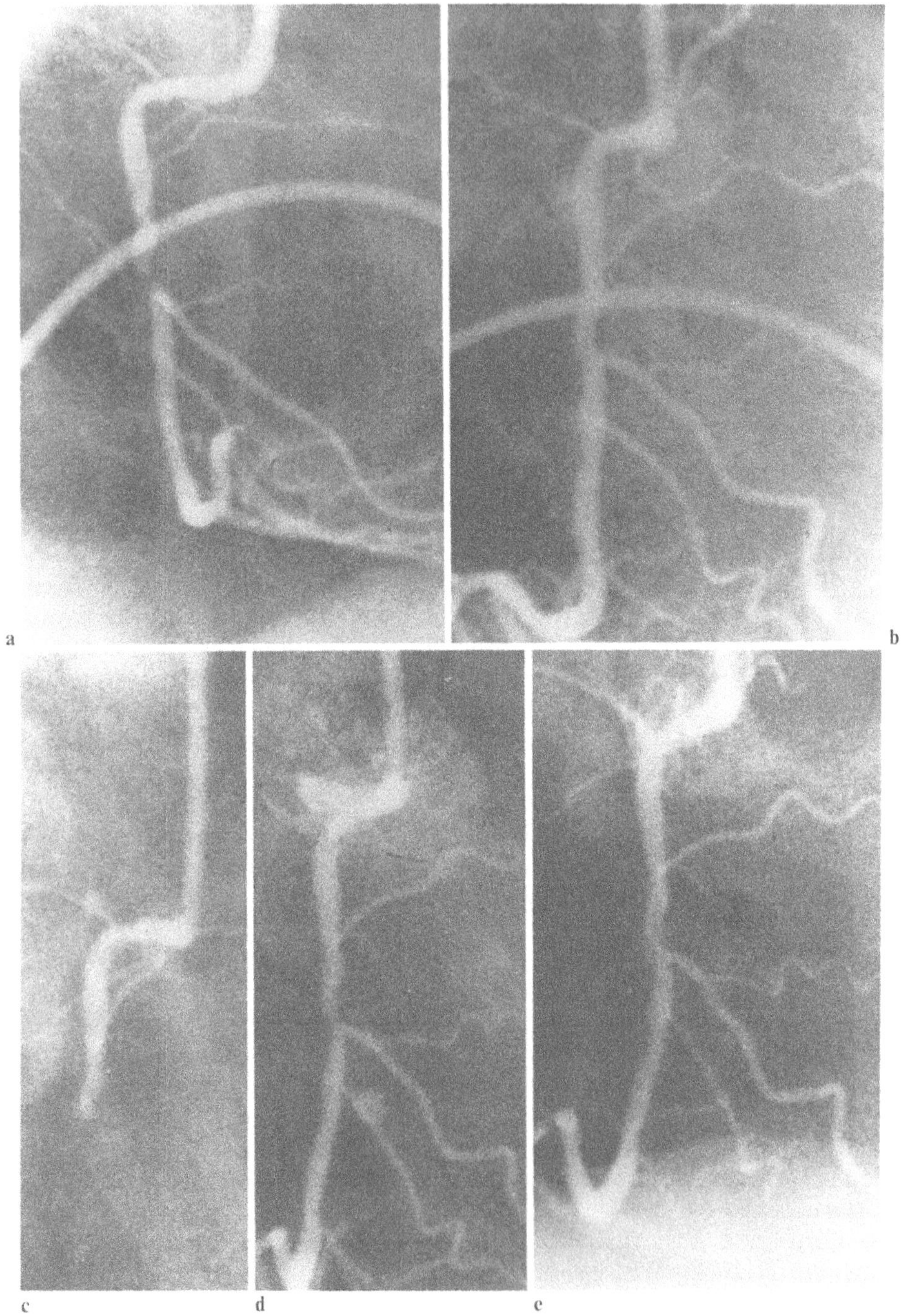

Fig. 21. a Coronary angiogram in the right anterior oblique view of the right coronary artery immediately before PTCA, showing tight stenosis below the overlying pacing catheter. b Angiographic result immediately after balloon dilatation. c 5 min later, after removal of pacing catheter, total occlusion of the artery at the dilated site. d After 10 min intracoronary streptokinase infusion recanalization occurs with residual narrowing. e After > 1 h streptokinase infusion there is further reduction of narrowing, now similar to the immediate post-PTCA result (b)

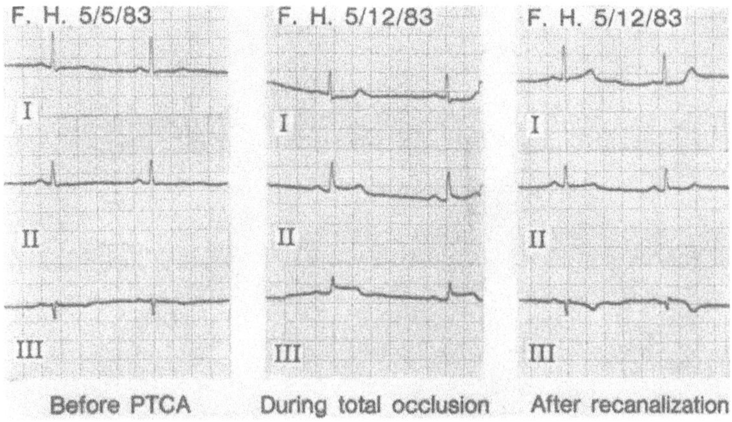

Fig. 22. ECG (limb leads I–III) of the patient whose coronary angiogram is shown in Fig. 21. *Left*, tracing made before PTCA. The ST elevation in leads II and III (*center*) during total occlusion of the right coronary artery resolved 10 min after streptokinase infusion (*right*), when partial recanalization was achieved

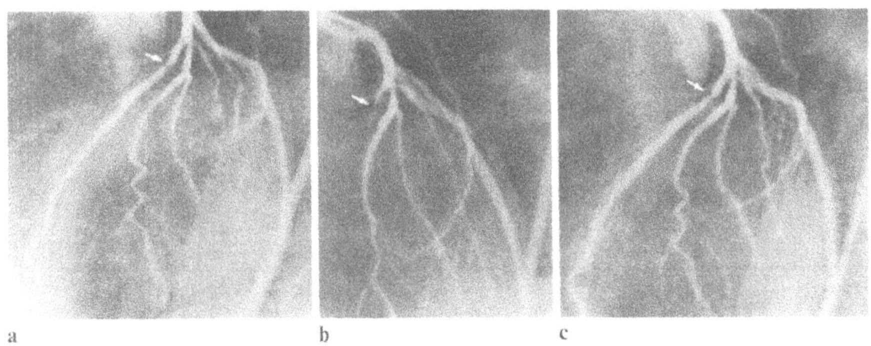

Fig. 23. a Coronary angiogram in the left anterior oblique view of the left anterior descending artery (*arrow*). **b** Total occlusion of the LAD at the level of the narrowing. This angiogram was taken immediately after the first attempt to cross the stenosis with the balloon catheter. **c** Recanalization of the artery after infusion of 200 μg intracoronary nitroglycerin

of the guidewire a good distance beyond the lesion or angle is needed for safe negotiation of tortuosities.

Monitoring of intracoronary pressure via the balloon catheter helps to determine whether the dilatation catheter is inside or outside the lumen and constitutes an additional safety factor. A small perforation caused by the tip of the angioplasty guidewire may not be of consequence, whereas advancement of the balloon catheter through the arterial wall will produce a large hole with resultant cardiac tamponade.

The most likely causes of coronary arterial rupture in these patients are inflation of the balloon within the arterial wall and the use of too-large balloons. An inadequate dilatation result often leads the operator to select a larger balloon and try again. However, failure to dilate the stenosis may be unrelated to balloon size.

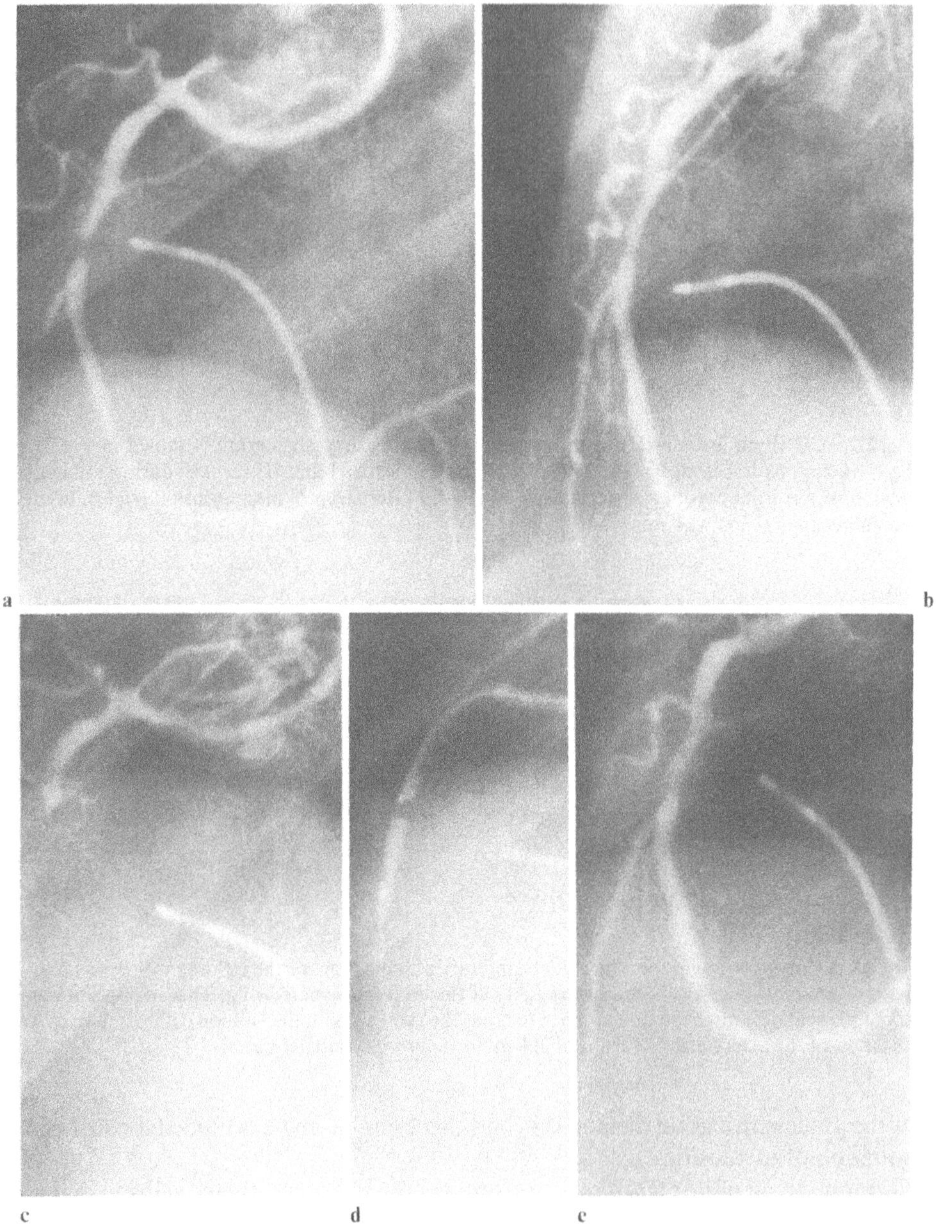

Fig. 24. a Before PTCA, subtotal occlusion of the right coronary artery. **b** After PTCA, irregular appearance of the angioplasty site. **c** At 5 min later, total occlusion. **d** Recrossing of the lesion with over-the-wire system and repeat dilatation. **e** Successful result after repeat PTCA. No reocclusion occurred

Compliant segments of the arterial wall within an eccentric lesion may dissipate most of the dilatation force without substantially altering the atheroma. If the inflated diameter of the initial balloon appeared adequate a larger balloon will be unlikely to improve the result and is a potential cause of arterial overdistension. Balloon rupture has also been implicated as a cause of arterial disruption, but seems less likely. If the complication is recognized while the dilatation system is still in place it has been suggested that the balloon catheter should not be withdrawn from the perforation, because the catheter itself may occlude it. This may prevent sudden cardiac tamponade and allow prompt location of the site of perforation by the surgeon.

Cardiac tamponade must be considered in any patient who develops hemodynamic instability during or after an angioplasty procedure. Appropriate management of cardiac tamponade is based on its early recognition and on the institution of prompt therapy, including pericardiocentesis and, if necessary, surgical drainage.

Cardiac tamponade may also be caused by perforation of the right ventricle by a pacemaker wire. The pacing catheters originally often used – Myler or Zucker pacing catheters – permit pressure measurements, fluid administration, and cardiac pacing, but are stiffer and more difficult to maneuver than the standard pacing leads. Particularly in heparinized patients these catheters must be placed with great caution. If none of the above mentioned catheter functions are utilized during angioplasty, perforation of the right ventricle may not be apparent until the catheters are removed, because they themselves occlude the right ventricular perforation.

Other complications that are more common with angioplasty than with diagnostic arteriography are bleeding from the femoral puncture site, including hematoma formation and retroperitoneal bleeding. Manual compression of the femoral artery at the puncture site until complete arrest of hemorrhage is achieved, followed by application of an adequate pressure dressing, helps prevent later bleeding complications. Mechanical compression devices should not be used. The patients should be monitored closely for bleeding during the first few hours after the procedure, and the puncture site must be inspected when the patient first gets up.

Technical Complications

Rupture of the angioplasty balloon is a complication that has occurred in almost every angioplasty operator's experience. Balloon rupture is not necessarily associated with adverse effects, other than rendering the balloon catheter useless.

Usually the balloons rupture longitudinally, and the balloon catheter can be withdrawn without further complications. Today's generation of angioplasty balloons tolerate pressures greater than 12 atm. For adequate dilatation of coronary stenoses lower inflation pressures are usually sufficient. Use of excessive inflation pressures may result in some overdistension, which can culminate in sudden rupture of the balloon. Sudden balloon rupture may generate a jet of contrast medium, which is thought to be a potential cause of arterial injury. Slow leakage of the balloon at low inflation pressures is usually due to a material defect and should be recognized when the balloon catheter is prepared.

Severance of the distal segment of the angioplasty guidewire or unraveling of the distal spring coil are rare complications, but have been reported [30]. A small (nonperforating) piece of guidewire left in a distal coronary segment will not inevitably lead to coronary surgery. Wires left in the proximal coronary circulation and those protruding from the left main coronary artery into the aorta require surgical removal unless they can be retrieved with catheter techniques [30].

Acknowledgment. I thank Egi Liebwein for preparing the illustrations.

References

1. Kaltenbach M (1984) Neue Technik zur steuerbaren Ballondilatation von Kranzgefäßverengungen. Z Kardiol 73:669–673
2. King SB, Douglas JS (1985) Coronary arteriography and angioplasty. McGraw-Hill, New York, pp 241–247
3. Faxon DP, Kelsey SF, Ryan TJ, McCabe CH, Detre K (1984) Determinants of successful percutaneous transluminal coronary angioplasty: report from the National Heart, Lung and Blood Institute registry. Am Heart J 108:1019–1023
4. Kaltenbach M, Beyer J, Walter S, Klepzig H, Schmidts L (1984) Prolonged application of pressure in transluminal coronary angioplasty. Cathet Cardiovasc Diagn 10:213–219
5. Schreiner G, Erbel R, Henkel B, Pop I, Meyer J (1984) Improved ischemic tolerance during percutaneous transluminal coronary angioplasty (PTCA) by antianginal drugs. Eur Heart J 5:39
6. Henkel B, Erbel R, Schreiner G, Clas W, Pop I, Meyer J (1984) Echocardiographic monitoring of left ventricular function during percutaneous transluminal coronary angioplasty. Eur Heart J 5:75
7. Simon R, Amade I, Lichtlein PR (1984) Coronary blood flow and hemodynamics during prolonged balloon inflation in coronary angioplasty. Eur Heart J 5:109
8. Meier B, Gruentzig AR, King SB, Douglas JS, Hollman J, Ischinger T, Galan K (1984) Higher balloon dilatation pressure in coronary angioplasty. Am Heart J 107:619–622
9. Thornton MA, Gruentzig AR, Brown JE, Arnold TC, Hesser F (1983) Characteristics of coronary balloon dilatation catheters. Circulation 68:347
10. Feldman RC, Anderson DJ (1985) Gradients at PTCA: Physiological or artifactual? J Am Coll Cardiol 5:525
11. Sigwart U, Grbic M, Goy J, Essinger A (1985) High-fidelity pressure gradients across coronary artery stenoses before and after transluminal angioplasty (PTCA). J Am Coll Cardiol 5:521
12. Meier B, Rutishauser W (1985) Coronary pacing during coronary angioplasty. Circulation 71 (in press)
13. Meier B, Gruentzig AR, King SB, Douglas JS, Hollman J, Ischinger T, Aueron F, Galan K (1984) Risk of side branch occlusion during coronary angioplasty. Am J Cardiol 53:10–14
14. Vetrovec GW, Cowley MJ, Wolfgang TC, Ducey KF (1983) Effects of PTCA on lesion-associated branches. Circulation 68:313
15. Zack PM, Ischinger T (1984) Experience with a technique for coronary angioplasty of bifurcational lesions. Cathet Cardiovasc Diagn 10:433
16. Leimgruber PP, Moldenhauer ST, Libow MA, Douglas JS, Gruentzig AR (1984) Fate of occluded sidebrances after coronary angioplasty. Circulation 70:296
17. Hollman J, Gruentzig AR, Douglas JS, King SB, Ischinger T, Meier B (1983) Acute occlusion after percutaneous transluminal coronary angioplasty – a new approach. Circulation 68:725–732

18. Ischinger T, Zack PM, Aker U (1984) Acute coronary occlusion during balloon angioplasty due to intracoronary thrombus and coronary spasm: a reversible complication. Am Heart J 107:1271–1275
19. Holmes DR, Vlietstra RE, Mock MB, Reeder GS (1983) Angiographic changes produced by percutaneous transluminal coronary angioplasty. Am J Cardiol 51:676–683
20. Zack PM, Ischinger T (1985) Late progression of an asymptomatic intimal tear to occlusive coronary artery dissection following angioplasty. Cathet Cardiovasc Diagn 11:41
21. Murphy DA, Craver JM, Jones EL, Curling PE, Guyton RA, King SB, Gruentzig AR, Hatcher CR (1984) Surgical management of acute myocardial ischemia following percutaneous transluminal coronary angioplasty. J Thorac Cardiovasc Surg 87:332
22. Akins CW, Block PC (1984) Surgical intervention for failed percutaneous transluminal coronary angioplasty. Am J Cardiol 53:108 C
23. Meier B, Gruentzig AR, Dekmezian RH, Brown JE (1985) Percutaneous perfusion of occluded coronary arteries with blood from the femoral artery: a dog study. Cathet Cardiovasc Diagn (in press)
24. Busch U, Erbel R, Pfeiffer U, Meyer J, Blümel G, Blömer H (1984) Improved tolerance of intracoronary balloon inflation with a modified Gruentzig balloon angioplasty catheter. Symposium on improvement of myocardial perfusion, 27–29 September 1984, Mainz (abstract volume)
25. Mohl W, Wolner E, Glogar D (eds) (1985) The coronary sinus. 1st International symposium on myocardial protection via the coronary sinus. 27–29 February 1984, Wien. Steinkopff, Darmstadt
26. Meerbaum S, Drury K, Corday E (1984) Coronary venous retroperfusion and retroinfusion. Symposium on improvement of myocardial perfusion. 27–29 September 1984, Mainz (abstract volume, p 3)
27. Meier B (1985) Benign coronary perforation during PTCA. Br Heart J (in press)
28. Saffitz JE, Rose TE, Oaks JB, Roberts WC (1983) Coronary arterial rupture during coronary angioplasty. Am J Cardiol 51:902
29. Kimbiris D, Iskandrian AS, Goel I, Bemis CE, Gehl L, Owens J, Segal BL (1982) Transluminal coronary angioplasty complicated by coronary artery rupture. Cathet Cardiovasc Diagn 8:481
30. Höfling B, Erdmann E (1984) Extraktion eines gebrochenen und die A. circumflexa perforierenden intrakoronaren PTCA-Führungsdrahtes mit Hilfe eines Dotter-Fangkatheters. Z Kardiol 73:663
31. King SB, Douglas JS (eds) (1985) Coronary arteriography and angioplasty. McGraw-Hill, New York
32. Bergmans RF (1976) Oblique caudal and cranial x-ray beam angulation with the poly Diagnost C. Medica Mundi 21:114
33. Antoni D, Ischinger T, Nowak F, Delins W (1985) EKG Veränderungen bei intrakoronarer und peripherer Ableitung während PTCA. Z Kardiol 74(5):11

Chapter 9. Technique of PTCA by the Brachial Approach: Practical Considerations and Comparison with the Femoral Artery Method

GERALD DORROS

Introduction

The development of a double-lumen dilatation catheter modified the original coaxial catheter technique and permitted successful dilatation of peripheral arterial stenoses [1]. The miniaturization of this double-lumen catheter permitted the dilatation of stenoses in the epicardial coronary arterial system. However, a delivery system was necessary to guide these coronary dilatation catheters into the coronary artery [2]. Initially, preshaped guide catheters were percutaneously introduced through the femoral artery to engage the coronary ostium and thereby allow passage of the dilatation catheter into the coronary artery. The brachial artery guide catheter was developed to permit introduction of a single, multipurpose guide catheter which would allow intubation of either coronary ostium or of the saphenous vein graft ostium for the performance of single or multiple transluminal coronary angioplasties [3]. Patient selection and the brachial technique with its advantages and disadvantages are discussed.

Patient Selection

All patients undergoing transluminal coronary angioplasty in our series have had coronary atherosclerosis causing severe angina pectoris, or severe stenosis(es) producing significant myocardial ischemia documented by objective noninvasive studies, including stress testing and myocardial scintigraphy (when not clinically contraindicated) and by coronary cinearteriography. The patient's anatomy, i.e., the site of the stenosis(es), is the primary determinant of whether or not transluminal coronary angioplasty is attempted, and in fact influences the choice of guide catheter entry (brachial or femoral). Each patient agrees to an attempt at angioplasty with the proviso that immediate myocardial revascularization will be performed if necessary. Some patients have undergone coronary angioplasty being aware that the risk involved in surgical myocardial revascularization was prohibitive and that this would be attempted only in the event of a catastrophe.

Each patient is treated with an antiplatelet regimen of aspirin (10 grains) and dipyridamole (150 mg) for 1 or 2 days before, and indefinitely after the procedure. A calcium antagonist (nifedipine 40 mg daily or diltiazem 120 mg daily) is started the night before and continued for 1 week after angioplasty, or longer if clinically required.

The patient's clinical status is discussed with a cardiovascular surgeon who is aware of the patient's medical history and has reviewed the cinearteriograms. The surgical team is available if needed.

Technique for Brachial Angioplasty

In the standard manner, a cutdown is performed under local anesthesia in the right (or left) antecubital fossa. The brachial artery is isolated with an accompanying vein. A temporary pacing catheter is frequently placed into the main pulmonary artery. Heparin, 7000 units, is administered. An arteriotomy is made. Heparin, 3000 units, is then injected distally. The guide catheter, usually an 8.3-F, 90-cm multipurpose woven Dacron catheter with a Teflon lining (USCI, Billerica, Mass), is preloaded with an 0.035-in. Teflon-coated safety J-tip wire 145 cm long. Within the guide catheter is a 3-F lead catheter, which extends 10 cm beyond the guide catheter tip (Fig. 1). The guide catheter is introduced into the arteriotomy over the guidewire and the 3-F lead catheter, which facilitates the entry of the nontapered tip into the arteriotomy site. The catheter is then advanced through the artery over the guidewire to the aortic root. The guidewire and introducing lead catheter are removed. The catheter is connected to a pressure manifold. Advancement of the guiding catheter into the coronary ostium is achieved by modified Sones' maneuvers (Fig. 7a and b). Coronary angiography is performed in multiple oblique and craniocaudal views. The angiographic projection permitting the best discrete delineation of the stenosis against the surrounding vessel and separation of the major and/or minor vessels from one another is selected. The pacing catheter can be used as an intracardiac spatial reference point to help mark the stenosis.

The selection of the preshaped guide catheter depends upon the size and configuration of the aortic root, the spatial orientation of the coronary ostium, and the placement within the ascending aorta of the saphenous vein grafts. The guide catheters manufactured by USCI are of two types: an 8.3-F woven Dacron, Teflon-lined catheter and an 8- or 9-F, preshaped, polyethylene, Teflon-lined catheter (Fig. 1).

The woven Dacron guide catheters, which are used in the majority of cases, are a multipurpose type and can be used to intubate either coronary ostium. They are available in small, medium, and large, and are chosen according to aortic root size. They are manufactured both with side holes (for maintenance of coronary flow after ostial engagement) and without side holes (as are the preshaped polyethylene guide catheters). Additional models available include those with extended catheter tips to reach higher ostial origins, and modified Castillo catheters for engagement of a high left coronary ostium or supraselective entry of the circumflex artery. The malleable distal tip of the catheter (the attenuated portion of the Teflon) can extend 4–8 cm from the tip. This allows more catheter flexibility as well as tip softness. These two qualities enable safer intromission of the guiding catheter deep into the coronary (Figs. 2 and 3).

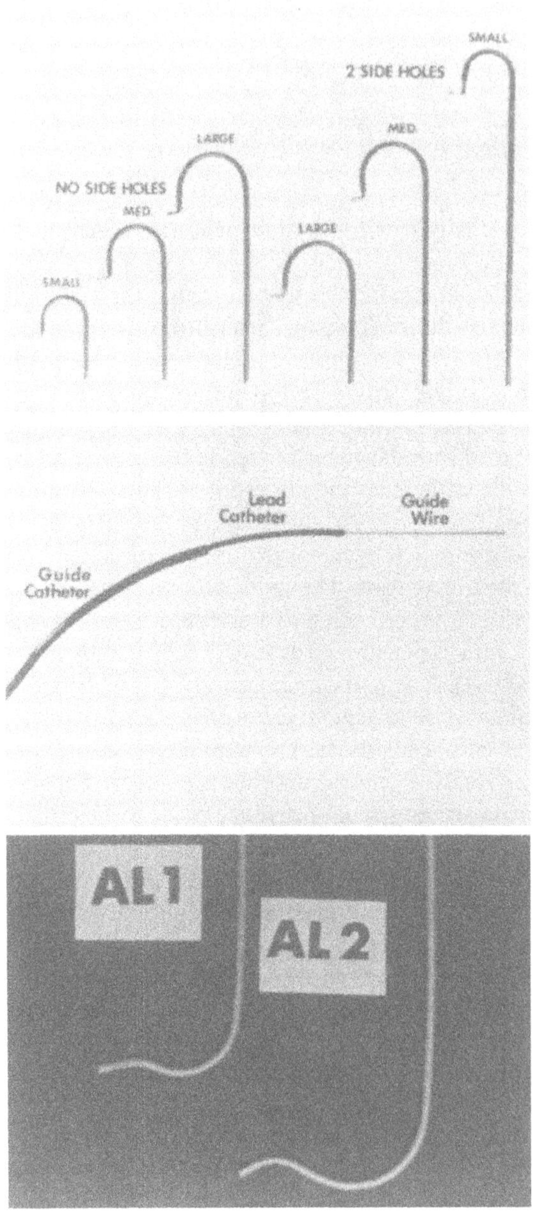

Fig. 1. The USCI Stertzer brachial guide catheters (*top*) are 90 cm long and 8.3 F in diameter and made of woven Dacron. The catheters are Teflon lined, with the Teflon attenuated for flexibility in the last 5 cm. Small, medium, and large sizes are available, being selected according to the aortic root size, and they are manufactured with and without side holes. The brachial guide catheter is introduced into the brachial arteriotomy over a guidewire and a 3-F lead catheter (*middle*), which facilitates entry of the nontapered tip into the arteriotomy site. The USCI AL1 and AL2 guide catheters (*bottom*) are 100 cm long and 8 or 9 F in diameter, made in polyethylene and lined with Teflon

The woven Dacron guide catheters with their soft distal end permit easy ostial engagement as well as supraselective catheter placement. Supraselective guide catheter advancement can be routinely achieved in the left anterior descending artery, the circumflex artery, or the ramus medianus of the left coronary with careful clockwise rotation of the catheter while it is engaged in the left main coronary artery. Intromission of the guide catheter into the left or right coronary artery

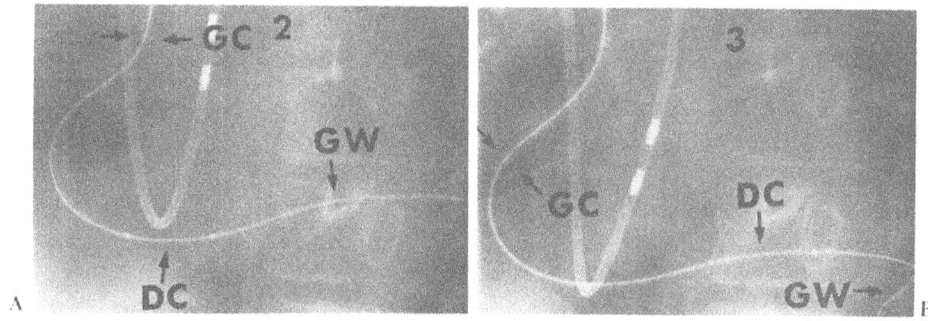

Fig. 2. A, B. Angiograms showed a severe stenosis which allowed the guidewire (*GW*) to cross (**A**), but not the dilatation catheter (*DC*); the guide catheter (*GC*) is at the right coronary ostium. Deep intromission of the guide catheter permitted the dilatation catheter (**B**) to cross the stenosis

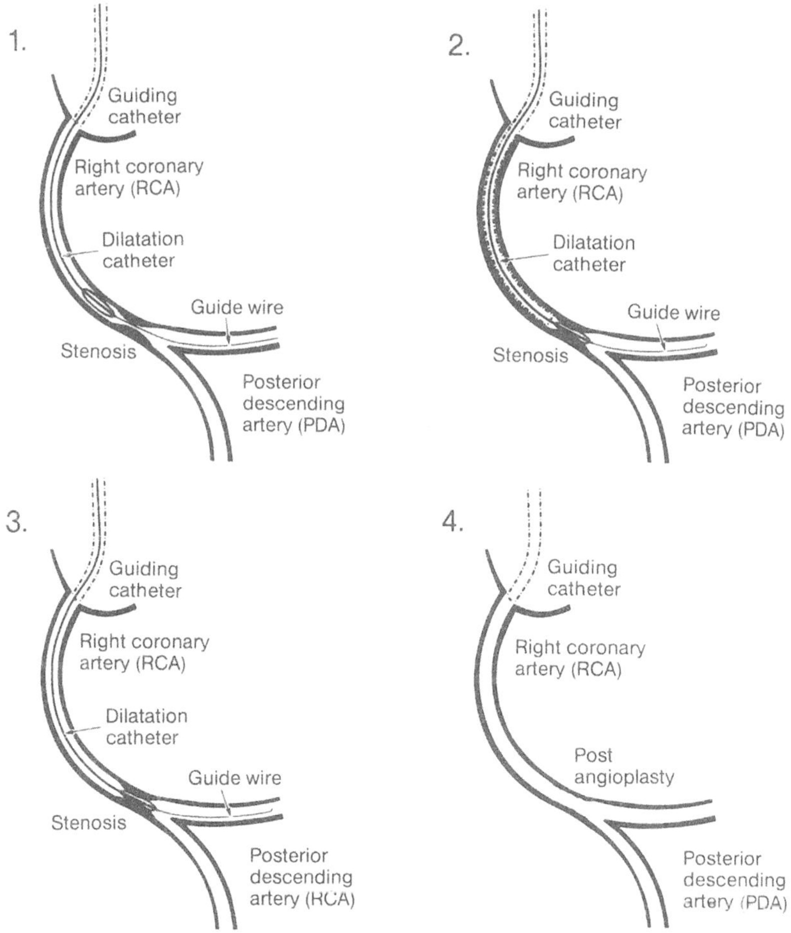

Fig. 3. Schematic of a severe stenosis which does not permit passage of the dilatation catheter (**1**). Deep intromission of the guide catheter gives sufficient support to the dilatation catheter (**2**) to allow it to traverse the stenosis. The guide catheter is withdrawn (**3**) with the dilatation catheter in place, which allows angioplasty to be carried out (**4**)

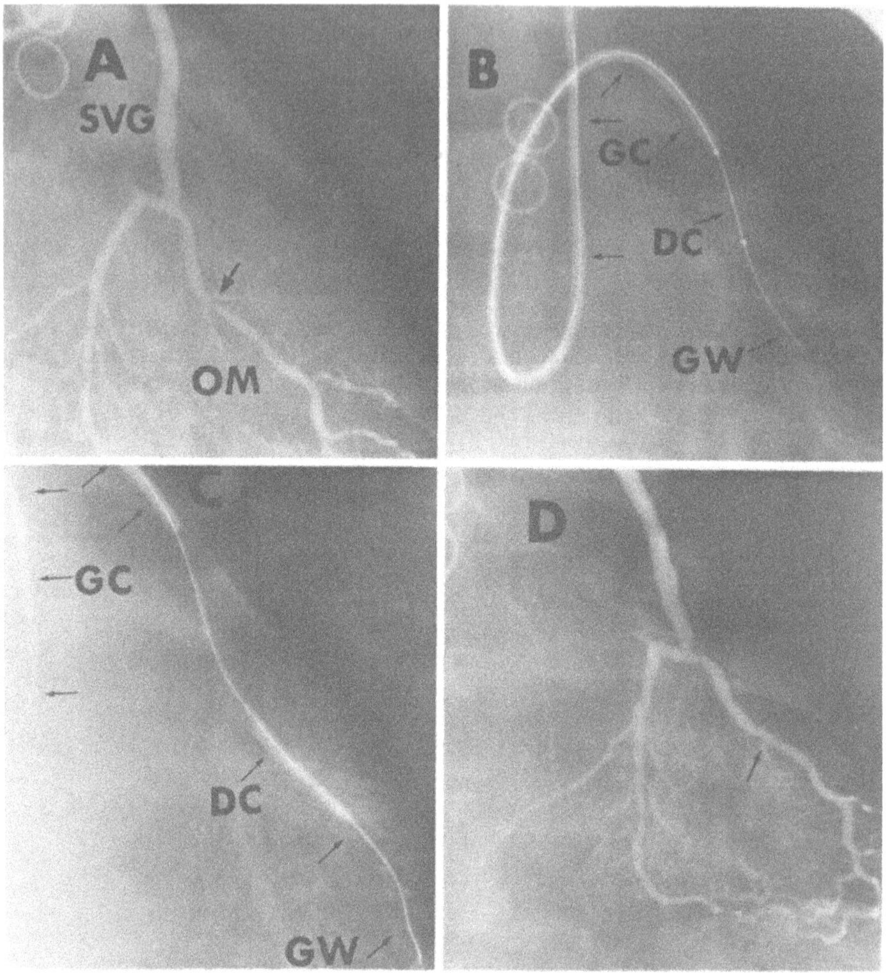

Fig. 4 A–D. Dilatation of an obtuse marginal (*OM*) stenosis which occurred (4 years after bypass surgery) distal to the anastomic site. The preangioplasty (**A**) angiogram shows the saphenous vein graft (*SVG*) and the stenosis, which did not permit passage of a low-profile dilatation catheter. Deep intromission of the guide catheter (*GC*) down the vein graft shaft after the guidewire (*GW*) had already traversed the stenosis (**B**) gave sufficient support to the dilatation catheter (*DC*) to permit the DC to cross the stenosis (**C**). The postangioplasty angiograms (**D**) show a successful result

with this catheter causes momentary coronary obstruction, but allows for rapid entry of the dilatation catheter into the coronary artery. Quick retraction of the guide catheter will enable the dilatation catheter to remain in the coronary artery with the guide catheter in position at the coronary orifice. This maneuver is ideal for tight midcoronary or distal coronary artery stenosis, in any major arterial trunk, or even in a native artery distal to a saphenous vein graft insertion (Fig. 4) which will not permit the dilatation catheter to cross the stenosis easily until sufficient support is provided for the dilatation catheter.

The polyethylene catheters are 100 cm in length, as against 90 cm for the woven Dacron catheters. The preshaped catheters have modified Amplatz shapes for the left coronary, and come in medium and large sizes. The 9-F catheter is similar to the 8-F catheter, but its body is more substantial, provides firmer support, and permits introduction of the larger dilatation catheters (i.e., the 3.7-mm, 4.2-mm, and 5.0-mm USCI dilatation catheters). These catheters can be used for cannulation of the left coronary ostium, while with the smaller size it is possible to cannulate the right coronary ostium. I do not utilize either of these guide catheters preferentially for normal coronary intubation. The tip is much firmer than those of the woven Dacron catheters, and its whip-like Amplatz catheter entry into the coronary ostium tip can lead to coronary dissection. These Amplatz catheters are preferentially utilized for intubation of saphenous vein graft ostium (Fig. 7). They can be maneuvered into place, remain relatively stable, and permit passage of a larger dilatation catheter. The vein graft ostium, which is firm and fibrotic, and not soft like the coronary ostium, is not easily dissected by these catheters. However, when necessary, the 8-F catheter is chosen preferentially for native coronary intubation, since it is less likely to occlude the coronary ostium and permits introduction of the USCI standard 3-mm steerable catheter as well as the Advanced Catheter Systems (ACS) catheter and the Meditech Corporation catheter. If a larger USCI dilatation catheter is required this will necessitate the use of the 9-F guide catheter.

After entry into the appropriate coronary ostium, the dilatation catheter is advanced into the arterial segment containing the stenosis. In the vast majority of cases, a steerable dilatation catheter is used. A Y connector (USCI) permits comparison of the guide catheter tip pressure and the dilatation catheter pressure. The steerable guidewire is advanced down the appropriate vessel under fluoroscopic control, with contrast injections achieved through both the dilatation catheter and the guide catheter to help localize the guidewire's position. The wire is advanced through and beyond the stenotic lesion. The dilatation catheter is then advanced under fluoroscopic control and with intracoronary pressure monitoring through and beyond the stenosis. The distal coronary pressure is recorded and the trans-stenotic gradient is calculated. The dilatation catheter is flushed with heparinized saline, and is centered across the lesion. The dilatation catheter is inflated to about 8 atm (range 5–12 atm). The appropriate pressure is developed by use of a hand-held, spring-loaded pump, the Dorros-Spring Pressurizer [4] (Cardiovascular Diagnostic Services, Inc., Milwaukee, Wis) (Fig. 5). The total inflation time varies between 50 and 90 s per dilatation. Three to six dilatations are usually necessary to abolish or significantly (i.e., to a mean of $\leqq 20$ mmHg) reduce the trans-stenotic gradient. This would satisfactorily complete the dilatation procedure.

When the distal gradient remains high although (a) inflation pressures are adequate and the balloon is fully expanded; (b) contrast injection via the guiding catheter shows that the stenosis is still severe; or (c) initially a small, low profile dilatation catheter has had to be utilized for partial opening of the lesion, either an exchange-wire technique is used to position a larger dilatation catheter without having to cross the dilated segment again with a guidewire or the lesion is recrossed with a very soft, flexible, and floppy guide. When the exchange wire technique

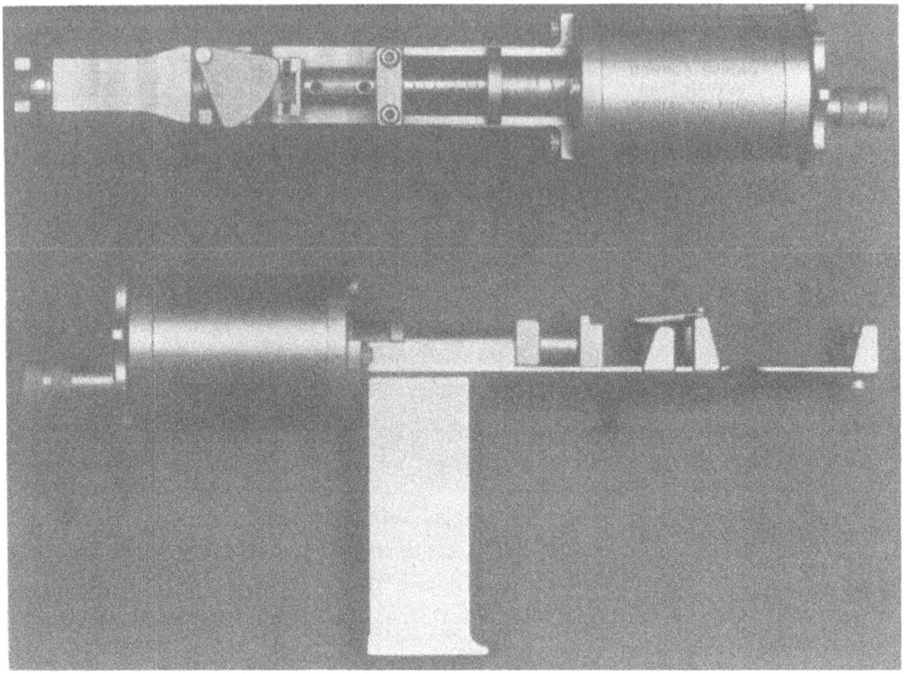

Fig. 5. The Dorros-Spring pressurizer is a hand-held and hand-operated angioplasty inflation device (U.S. patent # 4,429,724) (Cardiovascular Diagnostic Services, Inc., Milwaukee, WI 53202) which uses a calibrated spring to develop incremental and reproducible pressures in the distensible segment of the angioplasty catheter

is used the dilatation catheter is placed distal to the lesion and the steerable wire is removed. A 0.015-in. Teflon-coated 260-cm exchange wire is inserted and located distal to the lesion. The wire is kept in place under direct fluoroscopic visualization. The dilatation catheter is removed and then replaced with the selected dilatation catheter.

During the actual procedure, the success of the dilatation is assessed by the reduction in the mean trans-stenotic pressure gradient, achievement of full inflation of the dilatation balloon, and a satisfactory angiogram of the stenotic area following injection via the guide catheter with the dilatation catheter in place. After a satisfactory increase in the distal coronary pressure has been obtained, (i.e., less than 20 mmHg residual gradient) the dilatation catheter is removed under continuous pressure monitoring. Cinearteriography is performed, the guide catheter being used to record angiographic improvement.

The catheters are removed and the heparin is not reversed. The arteriotomy is repaired with fine suture material, either simple interrupted sutures, or a continuous interlocking suture being used. The patient is monitored and usually discharged within 24 h.

When multiple dilatations have been attempted, the plan has been to approach and dilate the stenosis considered critical initially and only to attempt the less severe stenosis(es) if this is successful. Thus, the initial guide catheter chosen will be the one that permits easy cannulation of the desired ostium. Once this dilatation is achieved the next lesion is attempted after waiting 10–15 min. Usually, the medium-sized multipurpose catheter, the workhorse of the guide catheters, permits successful cannulation of either coronary ostium with no necessity for catheter exchange. If a vein graft is then cannulated the modified Amplatz, polyethylene catheter is utilized to permit intubation and create a stable guide catheter position through which the dilatation catheter is introduced.

Results

The initial publication [3] describing the brachial artery method reported the results of a technique applied during the evolution of a guide catheter system. The authors' results were collated to provide an overall experience for analysis, since individual group analyses showed no statistical difference in their success rate. Each author preferentially chose the brachial method for the performance of angioplasty. In all, 300 angioplasties were performed, nearly 200 via the brachial and about 100 via the femoral artery approach. Analysis of these data indicated that successful angioplasty of the left anterior descending artery was equally effective with either technique, whereas successful angioplasty of the right coronary was significantly ($P<0.05$) more easily accomplished with the brachial artery technique. In addition, inability to enter the diseased coronary artery via the brachial approach was sometimes overcome by application of the femoral artery method (and vice versa).

In 1983, a comparison [5] of the brachial and femoral artery methods was published by the same authors, with the addition of one member who applied the femoral artery method exclusively. Thus, two authors utilized both techniques, while one author utilized the brachial, and one, the femoral method exclusively. The authors who utilized both methods preferred the brachial technique for angioplasty because this was their first choice for diagnostic coronary arteriography. The femoral artery method was initally chosen when there had been multiple brachial cutdowns, when the brachiocephalic system was known to be tortuous, or when the referring physician attending the procedure desired to learn the femoral technique. The brachial technique was preferentially chosen for right coronary artery stenoses and for saphenous vein grafts, since the brachial catheters were more maneuverable than the femoral catheters available. Their published data did not indicate the results that can presently be achieved with newer and more maneuverable guide catheters and the steerable dilatation catheters.

There were 901 angioplasty attempts, with 60% via the brachial and 40% via the femoral approach. There was no difference between the techniques in passing the dilatation catheter across the stenoses, regardless of the arterial segment attempted, or in successfully achieving dilatation. However, a comparison of the individual vessels dilated indicated that a stenosis of the left anterior descending artery was statistically more likely to be successfully crossed than a stenosis in the right or circumflex arteries or a saphenous vein graft.

These data helped mold the concept that interventional angiographers in relatively straightforward situations (remembering that the aforementioned data were collected at a time when relatively simple cases of proximal, concentric stenoses only were treated) should utilize the angiographic approach with which they are most familiar. However, refinement of the technique and the application in more difficult angioplasty cases has made it advantageous to use both techniques. These data showed, as anticipated, that if the dilatation catheter traversed the lesion the success of the dilatation did not depend upon how the dilatation catheter got there.

Experience, which cannot be verified by a controlled study, has taught me many things. Situations which were problematic though they initially appeared straightforward often required long and arduous procedures. However, these same formerly difficult situations are now recognized with relative ease because of this experience. The purpose of angioplasty is not to demonstrate the angiographers' prowess or persistence in the face of adversity, but rather to perform the technique smoothly, safely, and effectively so as to minimize patient discomfort, shorten the time needed for the procedure, and maximize success while minimizing complications. Thus, one technique may be preferentially used in certain situations to attain these goals.

Femoral or Brachial Technique?

The concept that the techniques are equally effective presupposes that the angiographer is equally skilled in the use of both methods, which is usually not the case when angiographers who generally use the femoral approach utilize the brachial technique. The brachial artery method requires knowledge of how to perform a cutdown, brachial artery identification and exposure, arteriotomy and its repair, and performance of the Sones' maneuvers or deliberate movements of multipurpose catheters.

A priori, coronary angioplasty should be performed in the most simple, safe, and successful manner possible, with the guide catheter technique chosen to be in keeping with this aim. One angiographer's attitude: "I can do any patient by one particular route," with no account taken of previously known or readily identifiable obstacles, is mentioned only to be condemned.

A brachial angiographer who is aware of problems found at previous catheterizations (a small brachial artery, superimposed brachial artery spasm, a tortuous brachiocephalic system, multiple prior brachial cutdowns, a high left coronary ostium, a difficult intubation of the left coronary artery, or an abnormal origin of the right innominate artery) should utilize the femoral method preferentially. Similarly the femoral angiographer should be aware of technical problems (severe iliofemoral disease, abdominal aortic aneurysm, tortuous abdominal/thoracic aorta, widened ascending aorta, difficult intubation of the coronary ostium, and aberrant ostial origins) that really indicate selection of the brachial approach from the first. However, the femoral angiographer who is not skilled in the brachial technique should not simply try to do it. Angioplasty is not a game,

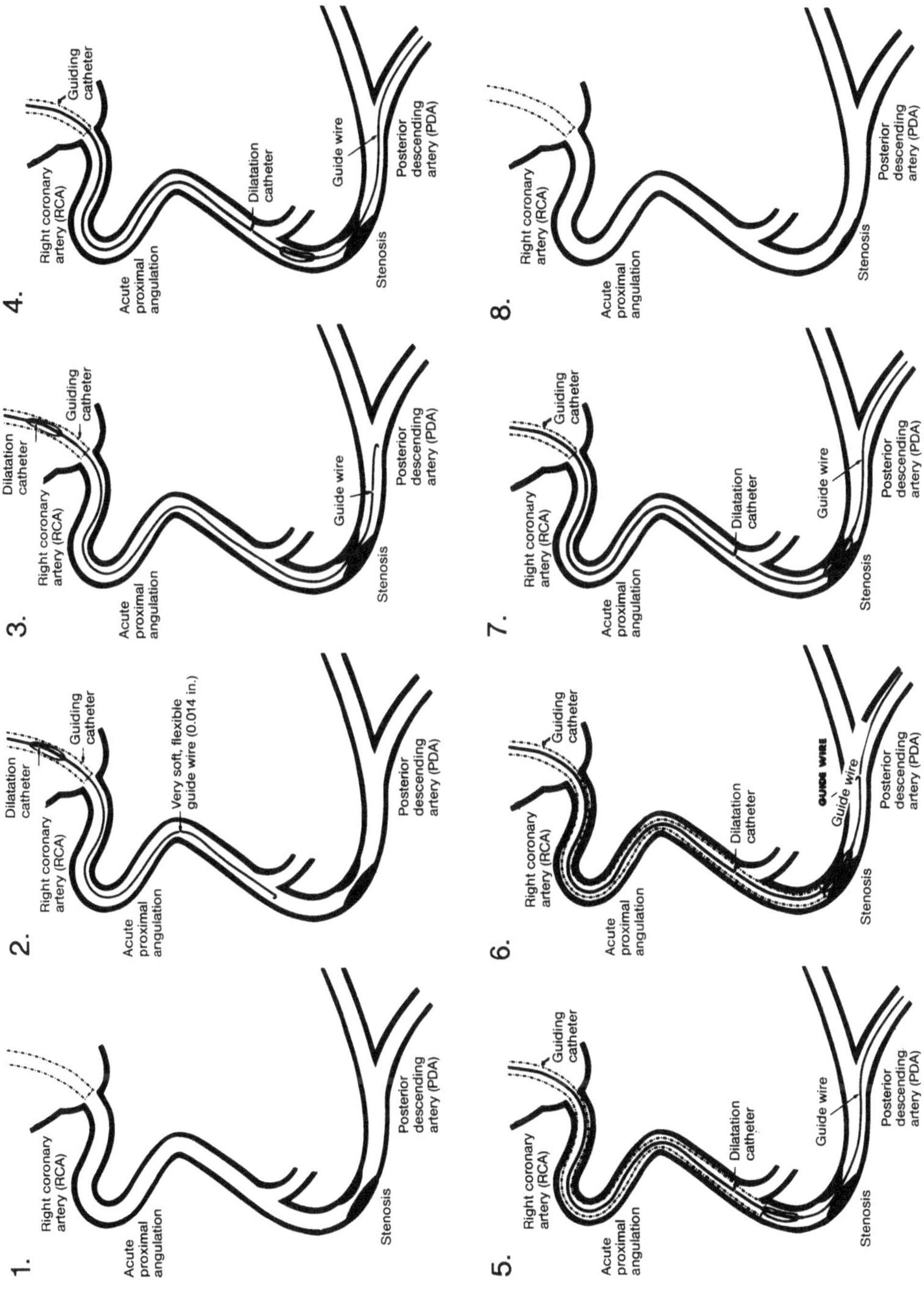

Fig. 6. Schematic showing how the problem of an acute proximal right coronary angulation can be overcome by using a soft, flexible guidewire, passage of the dilatation catheter, and then deep intromission of the guide catheter to traverse and successfully dilate a severe stenosis

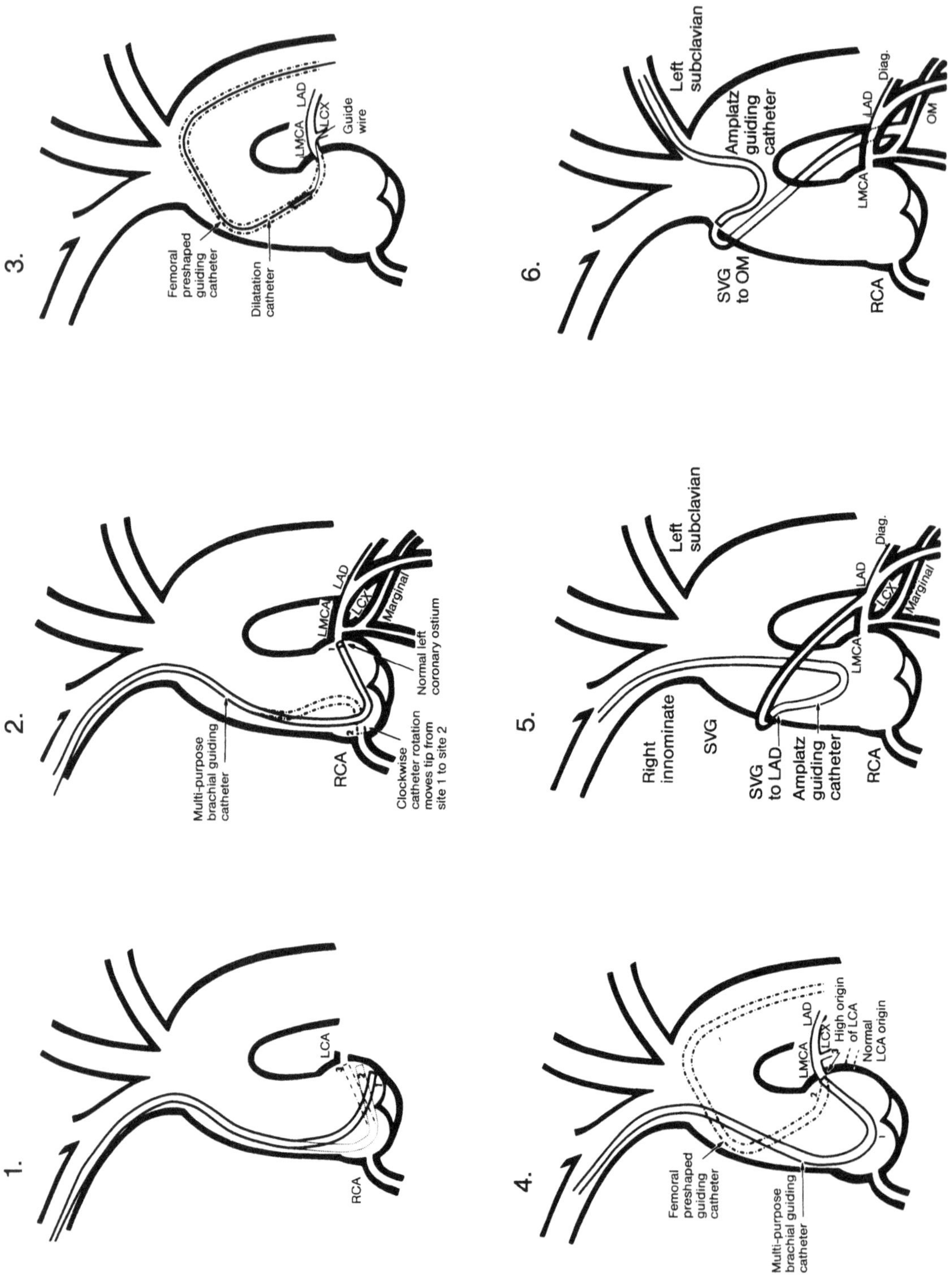

Fig. 7. This schematic shows different aspects of the brachial guide catheter. The careful placement and maneuvering of the guide catheter (**1**) permits easy entry into the left coronary ostium. Clockwise rotation of the guide catheter (**2**) will change the direction of the catheter tip and per-

and should not be looked at in this way. A skilled brachial angiographer familiar with the technique of angioplasty should be found to perform the intervention if the femoral angiographer is not well versed in the technique, and vice versa.

The brachial artery method is my first choice for the right coronary artery. The woven Dacron guide catheters are easy to manipulate, permit consistent ostial intubation, and have a soft, flexible tip that allows intromission deep into the coronary. The deep catheter penetration permits better support of the dilatation catheter, and thus enables it to traverse a severe stenosis. The acute angulation of the proximal right coronary arteries (Fig. 6) can easily be negotiated via the brachial approach; traversing the upward bend of the proximal coronary with a soft, flexible guidewire which enables the dilatation catheter to slide beyond the crook. Once the dilatation catheter is beyond it can act as a mandrel over which the guide catheter can be passed into the artery beyond the curve and provide for better dilatation catheter support.

When the right coronary stenosis is considered to be the critical stenosis and there is a less severe stenosis in the left anterior descending artery the multipurpose brachial guiding catheter can be used to cannulate the left coronary ostium after completion of the right coronary angioplasty.

The left anterior descending artery can be approached by either the brachial or the femoral technique without difficulty. However, certain situations will require preferential utilization of the femoral technique. When the left coronary artery has been difficult to intubate (Fig. 7) (especially when an extended-tip Sones or multipurpose catheter or an Amplatz catheter has been required), this indicates to me that intubation of the coronary will be more difficult with a guide catheter, and that even if intubation is achieved the guide catheter will not be stable. This potential problem can often be avoided by use of the femoral technique. The preshaped woven Dacron, Teflon-lined, Castillo and the polyeythylene, Teflon-lined Amplatz shaped guide catheters are difficult to use, especially the polyethylene catheters, which have stiffer tips than their multipurpose counterparts. In addition, introduction of these catheters into the coronary ostium is often achieved by a snapping movement which is beyond the angiographer's control. Rapid entry of this stiff-tipped catheter into a soft coronary ostium may lead to a left main coronary dissection. Most diagnostic angiographers prefer not to utilize the Amplatz catheter, for this reason. Moreover, the Amplatz catheter requires techniques which are exactly opposite to those automatically used with the Sones, multipurpose, or Judkins type catheters. For example, inadvertent withdrawal of

◄

mit intubation of the right coronary ostium. The steerable wire system is most maneuverable when used in a guidewire system with as few acute bends (**3**) as possible. The relatively smooth curvature of the preshaped femoral catheters minimizes the acute angulation usually encountered within the sinus of Valsalva when cannulating a high left coronary artery (*LCA*) origin (**1** in schema **4**). The right brachial approach utilizing an Amplatz shaped guiding catheter (**5**) can easily cannulate most vein grafts. However, a vein graft ostium originating high on the anterior surface of the ascending aorta, or originating on the posterior surface and leading to a saphenous vein graft (*SVG*) traversing the transverse sinus can easily be engaged via the left brachial approach (**6**). *LMCA*, left main coronary artery; *RCA*, right coronary artery; *LAD*, left anterior descending artery; *OM*, obtuse marginal artery; *DIAG*, diagonal branch; *LCX*, left circumflex artery the Amplatz-type catheter from the arm or leg does not cause disengagement of the catheter from the ostium but will only cause the stiff catheter tip to advance further into the coronary artery. Disengagement is accomplished by pushing the catheter in to release the tip from the ostium. Thus, I exercise caution when using these catheters. When it is known from previous brachial studies that coronary intubation will be difficult, or when there is great difficulty during an angioplasty procedure not only in intubating the coronary but also in establishing a stable guide catheter position, then the femoral artery technique is preferable.

Guide catheter stability is extremely important for the success of dilatation catheter entry into the coronary artery and for subsequent successful angioplasty. Inadequate guide catheter stability is a potential cause of multiple problems. A very high left coronary ostium which has been tenuously intubated (Fig. 7) with a large curved guide catheter can easily be disengaged as the dilatation catheter negotiates the last curve of the guide catheter, which tends to straighten the guide catheter and thereby disengage it from the ostium. In addition, the more severe angulation required to advance the guide catheter tip into the high coronary ostium often impedes the maneuverability of the steerable wire, which can also preclude the procedure's success.

The extreme brachial guide catheter curve within the sinus of Valsalva limits the maneuverability of the steerable wire, whose mobility in different directions is affected by the number and sharpness of bends and acute angulations within the guide catheter system as well as the dilatation catheter. Therefore, entry into an acutely angulated circumflex origin may be more difficult because of guide catheter bends which do not permit easy guidewire movement. Similarly, a tortuous left anterior descending artery with numerous diagonal branches and arterial curves may not be negotiable with the wire because of the sharpness of bends within the guide catheter system, which will significantly affect guide wire mobility. The preshaped femoral catheters (Fig. 7) are much easier to use and permit greater guidewire maneuverability in these situations, since the acute angulation of the brachial catheter lying deep within the sinus of Valsalva is not present. Another worrying problem is the likelihood of acute closure of the coronary artery, presumably by spasm, either initially or subsequent to the angioplasty procedure. Reinsertion of the dilatation catheter into the occluded arterial segment can often successfully reopen the occluded vessel [6]. However, a difficult intubation in a hemodynamically unstable patient does not provide an atmosphere conducive to success. Therefore, I always try to make sure that intubation of the coronary artery by the brachial method can be easily accomplished, that the guide catheter

Fig. 8 A–G. The anatomic configuration of the left main coronary, left anterior descending *(LAD)*, ramus and left circumflex *(LCX)* arteries can be best assessed using a pronounced (30°) caudal angulation in the anteroposterior projection. This projection will eliminate the foreshortening of the LAD in the LAO projection and the overlapping of the LCX origin with the LAD in the RAO projection: In (**A**) stenosis in the LAD is viewed in LAO. Caudal angulation separates the origin of the LCX (**B**) and facilitated entry into the LAD (**C**, after dilatation). Entry into a ramus stenosis is easy if the arteries' origins are spread out (**D**). The degree of angulation of the LAD, LCX and left main coronary arteries often determine how easy (**E**, **F**) or how difficult (**G**) the entry into an artery will be (for angiographic views see also Chap. 8, page 141)

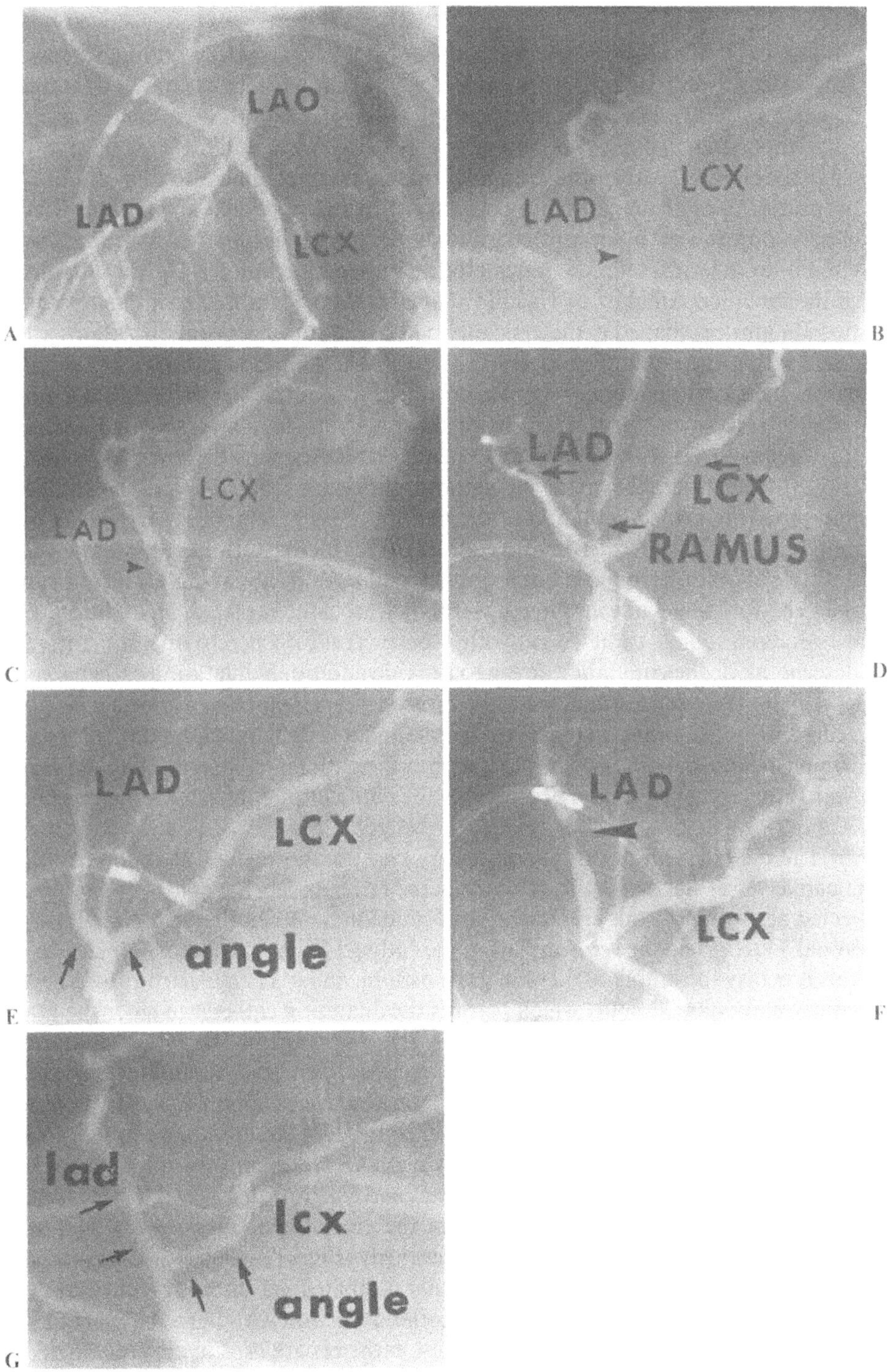
A
LAO
LAD
LCX
B
LCX
LAD
C
LCX
LAD
D
LAD
LCX
RAMUS
E
LAD
LCX
angle
F
LAD
LCX
G
lad
lcx
angle

is stable, and that if necessary intubation can be achieved under less than ideal circumstances. If this is not the case, then I immediately opt for the femoral technique.

The circumflex artery has been the most difficult artery within which to achieve consistent success with angioplasty, even with the steerable dilatation catheter systems. The anatomic configuration of an obtuse circumflex origin angulation (Fig. 8) did not permit easy guidewire entry, and if the guidewire did enter the circumflex the obtuse angulation was an impediment to dilatation. Appropriate views of the left main coronary with severe caudal angulation, which clearly show the left main coronary and the origins of the anterior descending and circumflex arteries, failed to elucidate the reasons for failure. The development of the modified Amplatz or Castillo shaped catheters and of the in-plane-modified Judkins preshaped catheters contributed to more successful dilatation of lesions within the circumflex artery. The steerable dilatation catheter has significantly increased the possibility of access, and as a result the success rate is now excellent. However, the steerable wire system is most maneuverable and successful when utilized with as few acute bends in the guidewire system as possible (Fig. 8). Therefore, the relatively smooth curvature from the Judkins catheter minimizes the acute angulation of the multipurpose brachial or Amplatz shaped guide catheter lying in the sinus of Valsalva. This factor must be considered when multiple dilatations in the left anterior descending and the circumflex arteries and the need for easy guidewire maneuverability are contemplated. In addition, the 8-F Judkins guide catheter can often be inserted deep into the left anterior descending or the circumflex artery to provide additional dilatation catheter support permitting severe stenoses to be crossed. This is not an easy or a safe procedure with the Amplatz shaped catheters, and it is certainly more difficult to accomplish with the brachial catheter within the circumflex artery. Thus, the femoral Judkins shaped guiding catheter is the catheter of choice for left circumflex lesions.

The patient with prior bypass surgery [7, 8] is approached as follows. When a native vessel stenosis is the one considered critical, then the guide catheter is selected according to the aforementioned guidelines. When the vein graft itself is initially attempted the 9-F Amplatz guide catheter (Fig. 7) is chosen, because with this it is easy to cannulate the vein graft ostium, and once in place it provides adequate stationary support which permits the dilatation catheter to enter the graft and even cross a severe stenosis. With the 9-F catheter the larger dilatation catheters (3.7- and 4.2-mm balloons) can be used. The brachial multipurpose 8.3-F catheter does not consistently provide the necessary support unless it is placed deep within the graft. The brachial method provides easier maneuverability and more catheter control than the femoral method, although this difference is not nearly as obvious as it has been in the past. A vein graft that was difficult to cannulate during diagnostic studies because the graft ostium was created high and anteriorly on the ascending aorta or posteriorly (Fig. 7) (with the graft traversing the transverse sinus), has often been easily intubated via the left brachial artery. The possibility of creating a vein graft ostial dissection with these Amplatz guide catheters is less of a worry than when these catheters are used in the native artery, since the site of aortic anastomosis has healed with formation of a fibrotic scar.

Finally, when a severe vein graft stenosis is accompanied by a severe, distal marginal stenosis, I use the femoral approach, initially utilizing the Amplatz catheter for the vein graft and a preshaped Judkins catheter for the circumflex artery.

Summary

The brachial artery method is an acceptable alternative to the femoral artery method for the performance of coronary angioplasty. The brachial technique differs from the femoral technique in that a multipurpose guide catheter is most often used, so that manipulation in the aortic root makes intubation of either coronary ostium possible. For the femoral method a preshaped guide catheter is used to intubate the ostium. Creation of the preshaped Castillo or modified Amplatz shapes permitted a preshaped catheter to be utilized via the brachial artery. However, the stiffer tips made them less desirable for use in the native coronary, though they were preferentially chosen for cannulation of saphenous vein grafts. There is no difference between the brachial and femoral artery methods in the ease with which the dilatation catheter can cross a stenosis in a simple angioplasty case (regardless of the arterial segment attempted), nor is there a difference in the achievement of successful dilatation once the stenosis has been crossed. However, accumulated experience of interventional angiography, better understanding of slight differences in coronary anatomy, newer guide catheters, and steerable dilatation catheters, has allowed the formulation of some guidelines: (a) The right coronary and saphenous vein graft stenoses are initially approached using the brachial method; (b) the left circumflex artery, either alone or in conjunction with a left anterior descending artery lesion, is preferentially approached via the femoral technique; and (c) an isolated stenosis of the left anterior descending artery can be approached with equal success by either technique. When multiple dilatations are contemplated the technique chosen will provide the easiest and safest access for attainment of successful dilatation of the stenosis considered critical. The additional lesions are approached, subsequently, with the same guide catheter technique or even with an alternative technique, or in another operative session. Clearly, the goal of the interventional angiographer is to perform the procedure in a simple, safe, and successful manner. The guide catheter which initiates the angioplasty procedure must accomplish coronary intubation simply, safely, and efficiently and be established in a stable position before the actual dilatation procedure takes place.

The complications encountered with the brachial technique are few, and are clearly related to the care expended on the brachial artery repair of a larger arteriotomy than is usually encountered during diagnostic angiography.

Presently angiographers contemplating the performance of coronary angioplasty procedures might elect to use both approaches. However, one word of caution: Angiographers who are unaccustomed to the brachial artery approach would be acting in the best interests of their patients if they refined their technique with the femoral approach to coronary angioplasty rather than performing brachial guide catheter manipulation as their initial experience with the Sones technique.

References

1. Zeitler E, Schoop W, Zahnow E (1971) The treatment of occlusive arterial disease by transluminal catheter angioplasty. Radiology 99:19–26
2. Gruentzig AR, Senning A, Siegenthaler WE (1979) Nonoperative dilatation of coronary artery stenosis, percutaneous transluminal coronary angioplasty. N Engl J Med 301:61
3. Dorros G, Stertzer SH, Bruno MS, Kaltenbach M, Myler RK, Spring DA (1982) The brachial artery method to transluminal coronary angioplasty. Cathet Cardiovasc Diagn 8:233
4. Spring DA, Dorros G (1982) The Dorros-Spring pressurizer as an inflation device for use in transluminal angioplasty procedures. Cathet Cardiovasc Diagn 8:209
5. Dorros G, Stertzer SH, Myler RK, Kaltenbach M, Spring DA (1983) Transluminal coronary angioplasty: comparison of brachial and femoral artery methods. Cathet Cardiovasc Diagn 9:547
6. Hollman J, Gruentzig AR, Douglas JS, King SB, Ischinger T, Meier B (1983) Acute occlusion after percutaneous transluminal coronary angioplasty – a new approach. Circulation 68:725
7. Douglas JS, Gruentzig AR, King SB, Hollman J, Ischinger T, Meier B, Craver JM, Jones EL, Waller JL, Bone DK, Guyton R (1983) Percutaneous transluminal coronary angioplasty in patients with prior coronary bypass surgery. J Am Coll Cardiol 2:745
8. Dorros G, Johnson WD, Tector AJ, Schmahl TM, Kalush SL, Janke L (1984) Percutaneous transluminal coronary angioplasty in patients with prior coronary artery bypass grafting. J Thorac Cardiovasc Surg 87:17

Chapter 10. Assessment of Results of Coronary Angioplasty

BERNHARD MEIER and THOMAS ISCHINGER

Assessment of the results of coronary angioplasty is a staged process. The laboratory assessment is followed by the inpatient assessment and finally by the long-term assessment. The laboratory and inpatient assessments combine to give the "primary result" of coronary angioplasty. Long-term assessment of patients after successful coronary angioplasty yields the "long-term result."

Assessment for Primary Result

The assessment for the primary result is based on hemodynamic and angiographic data. Functional parameters, electrocardiographic and enzymatic changes, and patients' symptoms are also considered.

Laboratory Assessment

Hemodynamic Assessment

The trans-stenotic pressure gradient is determined by subtracting the coronary pressure distal to the lesion from the aortic pressure. The distal coronary pressure is measured through the hole at the tip of the balloon catheter and the aortic pressure through the guide catheter in the coronary orifice. Two equicalibrated pressure transducers are used. The pressure tracings are checked for congruence at the beginning (Fig. 1) and at the end of the procedure. Efforts should be made to eliminate a "system-intrinsic" pressure gradient, which is commonly due to trapped air or leaks in the pressure lines. If an intrinsic gradient remains it needs to be accounted for when the trans-stenotic gradient is assessed.

Once the balloon is in place across the stenosis the initial gradient is recorded (Fig. 1). It may be significantly accentuated by the balloon catheter, which causes a further reduction in the lumen of the stenosed vessel. The smaller the difference between lumen diameter and balloon diameter the more the initial gradient will be overestimated. After each balloon inflation the pressure gradient is recorded again. About 30 s is allowed for the postocclusional hyperemia to settle [1]. The accentuation of the gradient after successful dilatation by the presence of the balloon catheter is usually less than 50% [2], because the ratio of the artery diameter to that of the deflated balloon diameter (about 1 mm) may be almost 3 to 1, except in small or tortuous artery segments.

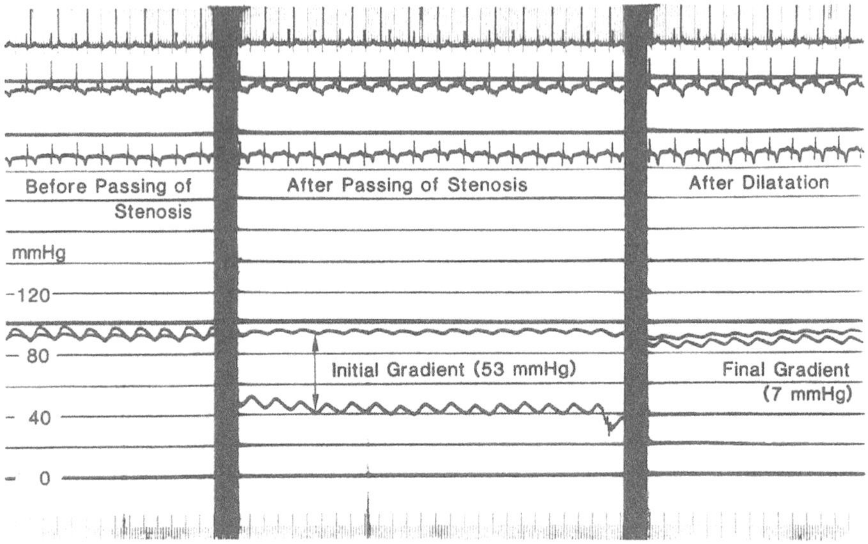

Fig. 1. Trans-stenotic pressure gradient during coronary angioplasty. Aortic and intracoronary pressures are practically identical before passing of the stenosis (*left*). After passing of the stenosis the coronary pressure drops and the initial trans-stenotic pressure gradient is apparent (*middle*). At completion of angioplasty the gradient is markedly reduced (*right*). Right coronary artery of a 62-year-old female patient

In the presence of a residual gradient of more than 20 mmHg repeat inflations should be carried out with increasing dilatation pressure and duration. If they fail to improve the residual pressure gradient intracoronary injection of vasodilators may be of use.

The average initial and final gradients in a large series of more than 1000 patients were 48 and 12 mmHg, respectively [3]. Residual pressure gradients are directly correlated with recurrence rate [4, 5].

The coronary occlusion pressure (distal pressure taken during balloon inflation) or the transocclusional pressure gradient (aortic pressure minus coronary occlusion pressure) may also be measured. Reliable measurements can only be obtained during inflation at 1–2 bar, because higher pressures within the balloon may compress the channel transmitting the distal pressure. The higher the coronary occlusion pressure the better the collateralization [6]. Collateral circulation is of great importance with reference to the risk of infarction in the event of acute or late coronary occlusion after angioplasty.

Assessment of the coronary flow reserve (coronary vasodilatory reserve) may serve as another hemodynamic parameter. Special electronic equipment is required for this technique, which is based on a comparison of contrast flow velocity in a coronary artery at rest and during artificially induced hyperemia [7]. It may be useful during followup catheterization when the trans-stenotic pressure gradient is not available.

Coronary vein flow measurements before, during, and after angioplasty showed that resting flow in the great cardiac vein will not increase after successful angioplasty of the left anterior descending coronary artery. Hyperemic flow, however, increases by 30%–90% [1,8].

Angiographic Assessment

It is important to base the angiographic assessment of coronary stenoses before and after angioplasty on several projections. Experienced angiographers may be able to estimate stenoses visually with sufficient accuracy for practical decisions. Acceptable consistency in the assessment of a stenosis can only be achieved by taking caliper measurements and using mean values of several views [9] or with sophisticated densitometric computerized methods [10]. Automated digital calipers (Fig. 2) provide an acceptable and practicable compromise for the assessment of stenoses. In the large series mentioned above where this instrument was employed, the mean initial and residual degrees of stenosis were 72% and 28%, respectively [3].

On the preangioplasty film attention should be paid not only to the severity of the stenosis but also to the other lesion characteristics. Eccentric stenoses and

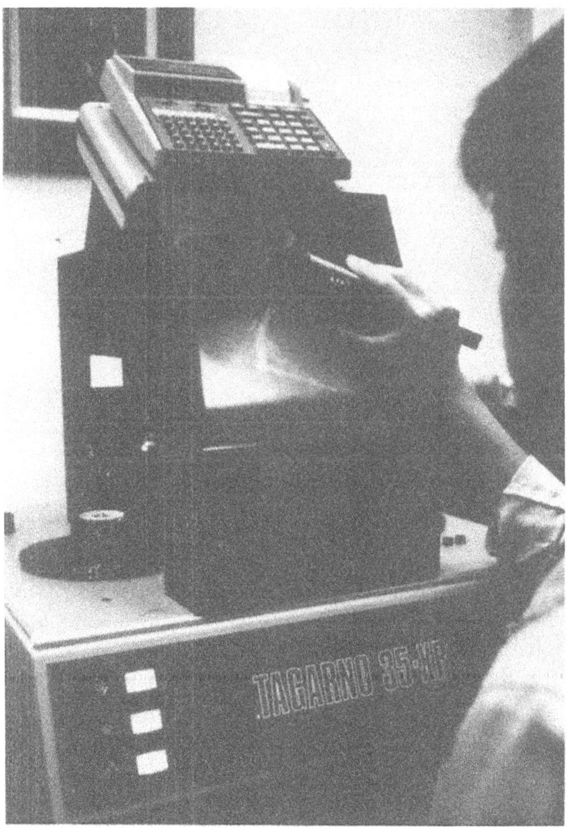

Fig. 2. Digital caliper used for assessment of coronary stenosis (A_2D cinemetric viewer and Prodical 1101 programmable digital caliper)

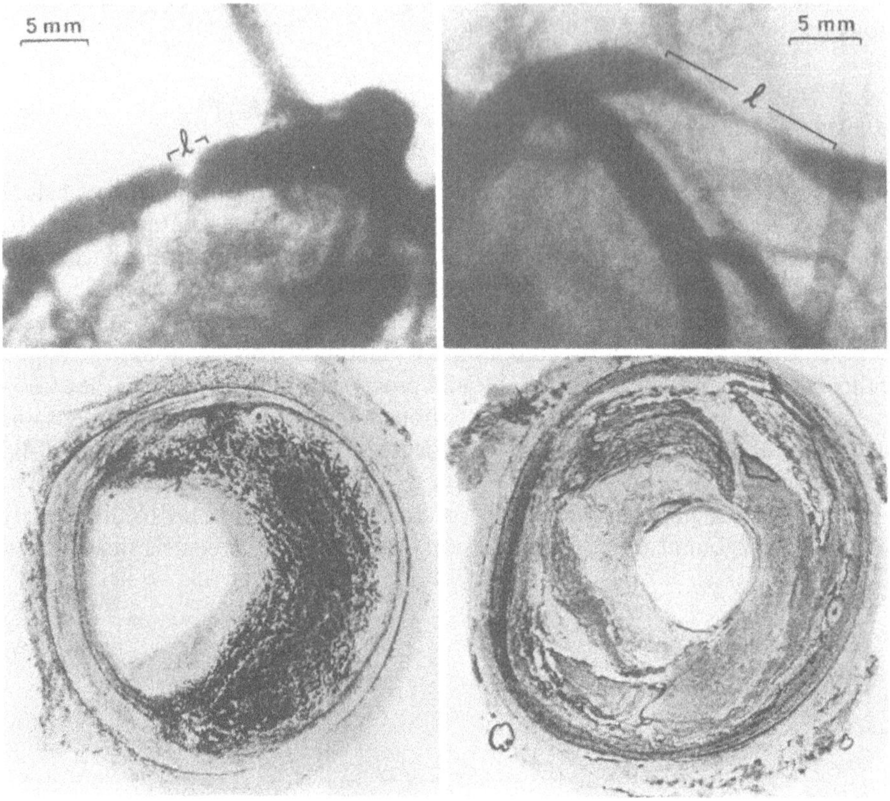

Fig. 3. *Left,* 2-mm-long eccentric stenosis. The residual lumen is confined to one half of the normal lumen (lateral projection). *Right,* 14-mm-long concentric stenosis (right anterior oblique projection). Both lesions are in left anterior descending coronary arteries. (Histologic pictures from Lossnitzer K, Pfennigsdorf G, Bräuer H. Myocardium, Vessels and Calcium, Knoll, Whippany, NJ, USA, 1983, with permission of the publisher)

long stenoses (Fig. 3), as well as stenoses in curves, have an increased incidence of acute complications during angioplasty [11, 12]. Thrombi, on the other hand, are easy to dilate but tend to recur immediately.

On the postangioplasty film an intimal flap can be seen in many instances [13]. It represents the main mechanism of angioplasty, i.e., splitting of the atheromatous plaque [14]. If the intimal flap is short and does not slow the flow or retain contrast material, it is not an ominous sign. More concern should be felt over long dissections that form a cul-de-sac with stagnation of contrast medium. They may harbinger an acute occlusion, which usually occurs within 12 h after the intervention. Prolonged heparinization and maximal vasodilatory therapy are advisable. Figure 4 shows that even with extremely large dissections there can be a favorable long-term result.

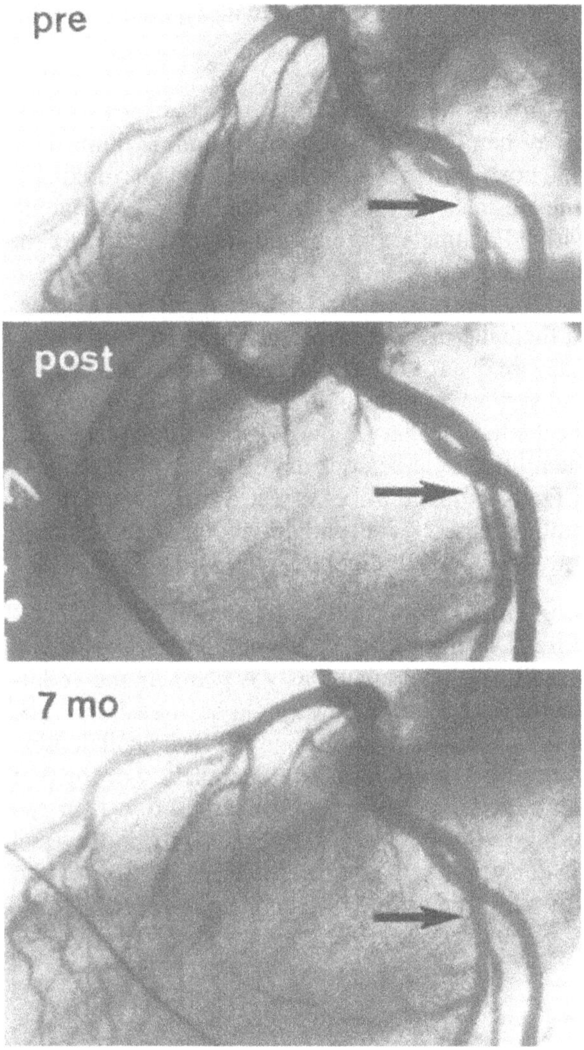

Fig. 4. Short- and long-term result of angioplasty of the circumflex coronary artery in a 57-year-old man. Immediately after angioplasty (*middle*) a long dissection is visible. Seven months later the artery appears normal. (Lateral projection)

When to Terminate the Intervention

It is often difficult to decide when to withdraw the balloon catheter system. It is not always possible to reinsert the balloon catheter properly should the final angiogram show an unsatisfactory result. An intimal dissection caused by angioplasty may direct the coronary guidewire into a false lumen. The necessity for recrossing an insufficiently dilated stenosis can be obviated by the following procedure.

1. After each balloon inflation 0.5–1 ml contrast medium is injected through the balloon catheter for observation of the runoff. This maneuver clears the tip of

the balloon catheter of blood, prevents clogging, and insures accurate pressure transmission. Moreover, the briskness of the runoff provides a qualitative hemodynamic information.
2. The trans-stenotic pressure gradient is recorded.
3. Contrast medium is injected through the guide catheter to check the aspect of the stenosis. Visualization may be poor. The contrast medium is thinned by the balloon in place in the stenosis. Furthermore, it cannot be delivered at a high flow rate owing to the obstacle of the balloon catheter in the guide catheter. Guide catheters with 9 F diameter or thin-wall guide catheters 8 F in diameter are advantageous for this purpose. A 5-ml, small-caliber glass syringe may also increase the amount of contrast medium delivered per unit of time. If a steerable system is used the balloon catheter can be retracted proximal to the stenosis leaving the guidewire distal to it. Simultaneous injection through both the guide catheter (5-ml syringe) and the balloon catheter (2-ml syringe) improves visualization of the dilated coronary segment without complete withdrawal of the dilatation system. It should be done in at least two projections.
4. Only if tests 1–3 prove satisfactory or cannot be corrected by further balloon inflations should the dilatation catheter be withdrawn from the guiding catheter to perform the control coronary angiogram.

After angioplasty an injection into the contralateral artery is of interest if collaterals had been present before. Disappearance of these collaterals reflects a good hemodynamic result. If multiple-vessel angioplasty is planned and collaterals are visible, the vessel receiving the collateral flow should be dilated first. The vessel providing the collateral flow should only be attempted if the collateralization is no longer visible or is reversed in direction after completion of the first dilatation. In case of a complication in the second vessel collateral flow from the first vessel can prevent a major infarction. In contrast, if angioplasty of the vessel providing the collateral flow is done first and complicated by an occlusion both myocardial regions will be simultaneously devoid of blood flow.

Inpatient Assessment

During the first 12 h after the intervention the patient is closely watched for myocardial damage caused by the intervention. Patient interrogation, electrocardiograms, telemetry (if available), and creatine phosphokinase determinations are used for this purpose. After mobilization and before discharge the functional result of balloon dilatation should be assessed.

Electrocardiogram and Creatine Phosphokinase

Two postinterventional electrocardiograms are usually sufficient. The first one should be done within a few hours after the procedure, while the second can be combined with the exercise test before discharge. Any chest pain not completely responding to vasodilators should prompt an additional electrocardiogram. Electrocardiographic signs of an ongoing infarction call for immediate action if they persist for more than 20 min. The choice between control angiography with an attempt to resolve the problem by repeat angioplasty [15] and/or by fibrinolysis [16] or immediate bypass surgery depends on the coronary situation found during initial angioplasty and on the logistics within the hospital. The appearance of new Q waves only indicates acute reintervention if they are coupled with continuing chest pain. Nevertheless, they should initiate a careful search for their cause. They may be due to a new conduction abnormality, which occurs in fewer than 1% of cases of coronary angioplasty [17]. In this case they are probably reversible and of little importance. More often such pains are due to myocardial necrosis that may have been clinically silent. In the majority of cases this means occlusion of the dilated vessel by dissection and/or thrombosis. Other causes, such as transient spasm of the dilated segment or side branch occlusion, are less frequent. Serial creatine phosphokinase levels add little to the assessment of coronary angioplasty [18]. They will rise slightly after the intervention, but stay within normal limits unless acute ischemia occurs. Such problems, however, are reflected in angiographic, hemodynamic, clinical, and electrocardiographic signs long before elevated creatine phosphokinase is found [1]. If myocardial infarction occurs creatine phosphokinase levels are helpful for estimation of the amount of damage.

Functional Assessment

From the viewpoint of the patient functional improvement is the most important benefit of angioplasty; a first functional assessment is made by the patient on walking in the hospital and climbing stairs the day after angioplasty.

An exercise test as a quantitative functional assessment should be performed in all cases, preferably before discharge from hospital. Unsatisfactory functional results should not be first noticed by the patient during a recreational or professional activity at a later stage; if detected while the patient is still in hospital they can be discussed and further therapy or a control angiography can be initiated.

Nuclear exercise studies can provide further information about the benefit in terms of coronary flow and cardiac function, especially if comparative values before and after angioplasty are available.

Bicycle ergometry after angiographically successful coronary angioplasty showed a marked increase in mean work capacity 2 days after the procedure [19]. Improvement of myocardial perfusion and cardiac function during exercise have also been documented by thallium-201 scan and nuclear assessment of the ejection fraction a few days after coronary angioplasty [20]. Thallium-201 perfusion defects during exercise disappeared after coronary angioplasty according to a report from another group [21], and nuclear ventriculography showed improvement of regional and global ejection fraction abnormalities during atrial pacing at rapid heart rates [22].

Primary Success and Failure

The National Heart, Lung, and Blood Institute Percutaneous Transluminal Coronary Angioplasty Registry proposed, as a simple definition of primary success, a reduction of the diameter narrowing by at least 20% of the normal artery diameter [23]. A reduction of at least 30% and a residual stenosis of less than 50% have also been proposed as criteria. These merely angiographic definitions of success were sufficient in the early days of coronary angioplasty, when inability to reach the stenosis was the most common reason for failure. Later, additional criteria for primary success were added.

A decrease of the pressure gradient to about 20 mmHg or less should be achieved. Higher residual pressure gradients signify a substantial residual obstruction of blood flow and predict a high chance of recurrence [4]. As mentioned earlier, small and tortuous vessels in which the residual pressure gradient will be artificially accentuated by the presence of the balloon catheter may be an exception.

It is not admissible to infer conclusions on the pressure gradient from the degree of stenosis. The correlation between degree of stenosis and pressure gradient is poor [24] owing to the influence of collateral circulation and to the inaccuracy of stenosis assessment.

The patient should be subjectively improved or at least unchanged if only mild symptoms were present. The postinterventional exercise test should give a normal result for the treated myocardial area, or at least a significantly improved result.

A coronary angioplasty that results in complications requiring heart surgery or cardiopulmonary bypass can hardly be called a success. An infarction of the part of the myocardium affected during the postinterventional hospitalization will destroy an initial angiographic and hemodynamic success, unless perhaps it is a small infarction caused by occlusion of a side branch considered negligible from the start.

With these more stringent criteria the primary success rates of around 90% that are currently reported when the technique is applied by experienced operators [25] already seem to be at the upper limit of the potential of coronary angioplasty.

For multiple-vessel angioplasty the definition of primary success is more complicated. The application of the above criteria to all lesions in which treatment is attempted reduces the primary success rate per patient drastically. It seems acceptable to restrict the global assessment of success or failure to the strategically important stenosis or stenoses i.e., those that would have been bypassed by the surgeon. Failure to improve lesions sufficiently in arteries too small or too severely diseased to be bypassed and lesions that have little bearing on the symptoms and the risk to the patient (e.g., infarcted areas) can be disregarded in estimating the overall result of an angioplasty procedure.

Assessment of Long-Term Results

The assessment of long-term results of coronary angioplasty is primarily based on functional tests. Angiographic controls are important in special situations. The long-term results after successful coronary angioplasty in the large followup series of Emory University [26] are displayed elsewhere (Chap. 11).

Functional Assessment

Patients are usually encouraged to be physically active after successful coronary angioplasty. Work can generally be resumed immediately after hospital discharge and should be recommended to both the patient and the primary care physician. A controlled exercise program with an exercise load adjusted for age and general health is ideal. Daily walks on a given circuit are an alternative. Even physical activity in a blue-collar job may suffice. A feeling of well-being, improved circulation, and, perhaps, deceleration of disease progression are possible benefits. The main purpose of exercise is monitoring for recurrence. Restenosis will be heralded earlier by functional limitation in the physically active than in the sedentary patient. Any recurrence or exacerbation of symptoms should prompt an exercise test. A drop in exercise capacity must lead to repeat coronary angiography and further treatment, be it coronary bypass surgery, repeat angioplasty, or modification of medical therapy.

Several studies have shown that exercise test performances of patients with angiographically documented recurrent stenoses dropped back to the pre-angioplasty levels [19, 27]. On the other hand, sustained normal exercise test performance in patients with abnormal exercise tests before angioplasty is a good predictor of sustained patency of the dilated vessel [27]. This can be further substantiated by nuclear exercise studies [21, 28, 29].

Exercise tests at 3, 6, and 12 months after coronary angioplasty seem appropriate in patients who have no symptoms during regular exercise. Afterwards a yearly test may be advisable, even though recurrences after angioplasty usually occur within the first 3 [30] to 8 months [26]. The patients may develop new coronary lesions.

Angiographic Assessment

Routine control coronary angiography was recommended during the initial evaluation of coronary angioplasty as a new mode of therapy. Although angiography can be partly replaced by functional tests, it still provides valuable prognostic information. In all patients with recurrent symptoms it should be performed without delay. In asymptomatic patients control angiography is most helpful several months after the procedure, when no further change of the dilated artery segment is likely.

Several definitions of angiographic recurrence have been proposed, such as a loss of more than 50% of the increase in luminal diameter achieved during angioplasty or a stenosis causing greater than 50% diameter reduction seen on followup angiogram. The diagnosis of long-term success or recurrence should not be based solely on an angiogram but derived from a synopsis of angiogram, functional tests, and subjective symptoms.

References

1. Rothman MT, Baim DS, Simpson JB, Harrison DC (1982) Coronary hemodynamics during percutaneous transluminal coronary angioplasty. Am J Cardiol 49:1615–1622
2. Leiboff R, Bren G, Katz R, Korkegi R, Ross A (1983) Determinants of transstenotic gradients observed during angioplasty: an experimental model. Am J Cardiol 52:1311–1317
3. Ischinger T, Gruentzig AR (1984) Perkutane transluminale Koronarangioplastie. In: Roskamm H (Hrsg) Handbuch der inneren Medizin, vol IX, 3. Springer, Berlin Heidelberg New York, S 1301–1317
4. Leimgruber P, Hollman J, Gruentzig AR, Meier B, Ischinger T, King SB III, Douglas JS Jr, Galan K (1984) Recurrent stenosis following successful percutaneous transluminal coronary angioplasty. Circulation
5. Holmes DR Jr, Vlietstra RE, Smith HC, Vetrovec GW, Kent KM, Cowley MJ, Faxon DP, Gruentzig AR, Kelsey SF, Detre KM, Van Raden MJ, Mock MB (1984) Restenosis after percutaneous transluminal coronary angioplasty (PTCA): a report from the PTCA Registry of the National Heart, Lung, and Blood Institute. Am J Cardiol 53:77C–81C
6. Meier B, Luethy P (1984) Coronary wedge pressure as predictor of recruitable collateral arteries. Circulation 70:II–266 (abstract)
7. O'Neill WW, Walton JA, Bates ER, Colfer HT, Aueron FM, LeFree MT, Pitt B, Vogel RA (1984) Criteria for successful coronary angioplasty as assessed by alterations in coronary vasodilatory reserve. J Am Coll Cardiol 3:1382–1390
8. Serruys PW, Wijns W, van den Brand M, Meij S, Slager C, Schuurbiers JCH, Hugenholtz PG, Brower RW (1984) Left ventricular performance, regional blood flow, wall motion, and lactate metabolism during transluminal angioplasty. Circulation 70:25–26
9. Meier B, Gruentzig AR, Goebel N, Pyle R, von Gosslar W, Schlumpf M (1983) Assessment of stenoses in coronary angioplasty. Inter- and intraobserver variability. Int J Cardiol 3:159–169
10. Nichols AB, Gabrieli CFO, Fenoglio JJ Jr, Esser PD (1984) Quantification of relative coronary arterial stenosis by cinevideodensitometric analysis of coronary arteriograms. Circulation 69:512–522
11. Ischinger T, Gruentzig AR, King S, Douglas J, Hollman J, Meier B, Galan K (1983) Coronary dissection and total coronary occlusion with percutaneous transluminal coronary angioplasty (PTCA): significance of initial angiographic morphology of coronary stenoses. Circulation 68:III–208 (abstract)
12. Meier B, Gruentzig AR, Hollman J, Ischinger T, Bradford JM (1983) Does length or eccentricity of coronary stenoses influence the outcome of transluminal dilatation? Circulation 67:497–499
13. Holmes DR Jr, Vlietstra RE, Mock MB, Reeder GS, Smith HC, Bove AA, Bresnahan JF, Piehler JM, Schaff HV, Orszulak TA (1983) Angiographic changes produced by percutaneous transluminal coronary angioplasty. Am J Cardiol 51:676–683
14. Block PC (1984) Mechanism of transluminal angioplasty. Am J Cardiol 53:69C–71C
15. Hollman J, Gruentzig AR, Douglas JS Jr, King SB III, Ischinger T, Meier B (1983) Acute occlusion after percutaneous transluminal coronary angioplasty – a new approach. Circulation 68:725–732

16. Ischinger T, Zack P, Aker U (1984) Acute coronary occlusion during balloon angioplasty due to intracoronary thrombus and coronary spasm: a reversible complication. Am Heart J 107:1271–1275
17. Dorros G, Cowley MJ, Simpson J, Bentivoglio LG, Block PC, Bourassa M, Detre K, Gosselin AJ, Gruentzig AR, Kelsey SF, Kent KM, Mock MB, Mullin SM, Myler RK, Passamani ER, Stertzer SH, Williams DO (1983) Percutaneous transluminal coronary angioplasty: report of complications from the National Heart, Lung, and Blood Institute PTCA Registry. Circulation 67:723–730
18. Berclaz S, Meier B, Barthélémy JC, Rutishauser W (1984) Changes in creating phosphokinase after coronary angioplasty. In: Meyer J, Erbel R, Rupprecht HJ (eds) Improvement of myocardial perfusion – thrombolysis, angioplasty, bypass surgery. Nijhoff, Boston
19. Meier B, Gruentzig AR, Siegenthaler WE, Schlumpf M (1983) Long-term exercise performance after percutaneous transluminal coronary angioplasty and coronary artery bypass grafting. Circulation 68:796–802
20. Kanemoto N, Hör G, Kober G, Maul FD, Klepzig H Jr, Standke R, Kaltenbach M (1983) Noninvasive assessment of left ventricular performance following transluminal coronary angioplasty. Int J Cardiol 3:281–292
21. Hirzel HO, Nuesch K, Gruentzig AR, Luetolf UM (1981) Short- and long-term changes in myocardial perfusion after percutaneous transluminal coronary angioplasty assessed by thallium-201 exercise scintigraphy. Circulation 63:1001–1007
22. Weiss AT, Gotsman MS, Shefer A, Halon DA, Lewis BS (1984) Improvement in regional ventricular function after percutaneous transluminal coronary angioplasty. Int J Cardiol 5:299–311
23. Mock MB, Kent KM, Bentivoglio LG, Block PC, Bourassa M, Cowley MJ, Detre K, Dorros G, Gosselin J, Gruentzig A, Myler RK, Simpson J, Stertzer SH, Williams DO, Mullin SM, Costa B, Mitchell H, and Participating Medical Centers (1982) The National Heart, Lung, and Blood Institute Percutaneous Transluminal Coronary Angioplasty Registry: the first 1116 cases. In: Kaltenbach M, Gruentzig A, Rentrop K, Bussmann WD (eds) Transluminal coronary angioplasty and intracoronary thrombolysis. Springer, Berlin Heidelberg New York, pp 11–19
24. Ganz P, Harrington DP, Gaspar J, Barry WH (1983) Phasic pressure gradients across coronary and renal artery stenoses in humans. Am Heart J 106:1399–1405
25. Meier B, Gruenzig AR (1984) Learning curve for percutaneous transluminal coronary angioplasty: skill, technology or patient selection. Am J Cardiol 53:65C–66C
26. Meier B, King SB III, Gruentzig AR, Douglas JS, Hollman J, Ischinger T, Galan K, Tankersley R (1984) Repeat coronary angioplasty. J Am Coll Cardiol 4:463–466
27. Scholl JM, Chaitman BR, David PR, Dupras G, Brévers G, Val PG, Crépeau J, Lespérance J, Bourassa MG (1982) Exercise electrocardiography and myocardial scintigraphy in the serial evaluation of the results of percutaneous transluminal coronary angioplasty. Circulation 66:380–389
28. Kent KM, Bonow RD, Rosing DR, Ewels CJ, Lipson LC, McIntosh CL, Bacharach S, Green M, Epstein SE (1982) Improved myocardial function during exercise after successful percutaneous transluminal coronary angioplasty. N Engl J Med 306:441–446
29. Sigwart U, Grbic M, Essinger A, Bishof-Delaloye A, Sadeghi H, Rivier JL (1982) Improvement of left ventricular function after percutaneous transluminal coronary angioplasty. Am J Cardiol 49:651–657
30. Kober G, Scherer D, Koch M, Dowinsky S, Kaltenbach M (1982) Transluminale koronare Angioplastie. Früh- und Langzeitergebnisse bei 250 Eingriffen. Herz Kreisl 6:309–318

Chapter 11. Outcome of Coronary Angioplasty

THOMAS ISCHINGER and BERNHARD MEIER

Early Results

Most of the overall experience of coronary angioplasty has been collected in patients with single-vessel coronary artery disease. More recently, the indications for coronary angioplasty have been extended to include multiple stenoses and multiple-vessel disease. The recent report from the NHLBI PTCA Registry analyzes the results recorded in 3079 patients enrolled by 105 centers [1]. The mixed data from the Registry include early and limited experience recorded in many contributing centers and may therefore reflect what a patient can realistically expect from coronary angioplasty.

The numbers of patients contributed by the individual centers varied widely. Only 18 centers contributed more than 50 cases, and 48 centers enrolled fewer than 10. During the first 3 years of the PTCA Registry 21% of the patients enrolled patients had multivessel disease, and in only 7% was there an attempt to treat multiple stenoses. During the final year of the PTCA Registry (10/81 until 9/82) enrollment was limited to patients with multivessel disease, who account for a total of 25% of the Registry patients. The data from the Registry show that in the majority of the selected patients PTCA can be performed successfully and with an acceptable risk. The primary success rates increased from 61% (combined Registry sites) to 85% (centers with experience of more than 100 cases). The major complications remained relatively stable throughout the Registry experience. Emergency coronary bypass surgery following failed PTCA was performed in 7% of the patients treated.

Increasing expertise in coronary angioplasty and the availability of steerable over-the-wire dilatation systems have now led to primary success rates in excess of 90% in specialized centers [3, 4]. The ability to reach and cross coronary stenoses has increased markedly with the use of low-profile and steerable dilatation catheters. In experienced hands, uncomplicated (technical) failures account for approximately 50% of failed procedures and are mostly due to the inability to cross the lesion with the balloon catheter. Insufficient engagement of the guide catheter in the coronary ostium or insufficient stenosis reduction by balloon dilatation are less frequent causes of failed angioplasty. The chance of successful stenosis dilatation has become similar with respect to the different segments of the coronary circulation, but proximal LAD stenoses are still associated with the highest primary success rates [4].

In most patients with single-vessel stenosis successful lesion dilatation – according to the common angiographic and coronary hemodynamic criteria (Meier and Ischinger, Chap. 10) – means correction of the entire myocardial ischemia

Table 1. Degree of revascularization following multiple-vessel PTCA in 135 patients. [7]

No. of vessels	No. of pts	Dil rate/pt	Patient success (functional)	Revascularization	
				Complete	Incomplete
1	22	2.1	20/22 (91%)	18 (90%)	2 (10%)
2	65	2.3	59/65 (91%)	28 (47%)	31 (53%)
3	48	2.7	38/48 (79%)	8 (21%)	30 (79%)

Dil, dilatation

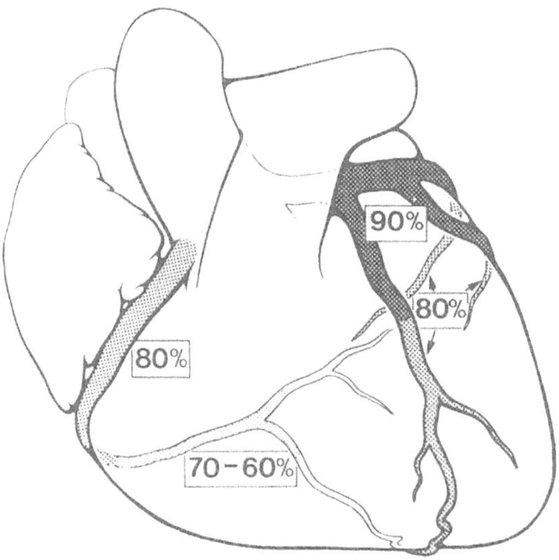

Fig. 1. Primary success of PTCA referred to stenosis location

and therefore clinical success for the patient. The situation is more complex in patients with multiple stenoses or multivessel disease.

Patients with more diffuse disease have less chance to achieve complete revascularization (Table 1). Incomplete revascularization most frequently results from non-attempted occluded vessels or non-attempted insignificant coronary lesions [7, 45]. However, successful dilatation of critical stenosis(es) may result in marked improvement of symptoms and clinical success for the patient, although revascularization is anatomically incomplete. In some of these patients the success of the PTCA procedure is to be determined by functional rather than angiographic results. Based on these less stringent criteria the PTCA success rates in patients with single-vessel stenosis and patients with multivessel disease are comparable [4–7]. Figure 1 shows the overall chance of primary success that currently should be expected in patients selected for coronary angioplasty [8].

Successful coronary angioplasty is usually associated with a significant reduction in coronary stenosis and an improvement in coronary flow, the latter being reflected in a reduction of the trans-stenotic pressure gradient. In the Emory series

Table 2. Rate of complications encountered with PTCA in a center with experienced staff. [4]

Complication	Rate (%)
Emergency coronary bypass operation	4
Myocardial infarction (Q wave)	2
Ventricular fibrillation (DC shock)	1.5
Surgical repair of femoral artery	0.5
Death	0.2

of 1500 patients coronary stenoses were reduced from a mean of 72% to one of 28% and the pressure gradient, from 48 mmHg to 12 mmHg [4]. The functional effectiveness of coronary angioplasty has been documented by electrocardiographic exercise stress testing in combination with thallium perfusion or radionuclear blood pool imaging [9–12].

Complication rates of coronary angioplasty have not improved so significantly as the primary success rates. Throughout the PTCA Registry experience complications have remained relatively stable and acceptably low, the major complications being myocardial infarction (5%), emergency coronary surgery (7%) and death (1%) [2]. Markedly lower complication rates are now achieved in centers with extensive experience (Table 2) [3, 4].

The typical complication of PTCA is coronary occlusion resulting from the "controlled injury" to the dilated vessel by mechanical dilatation: Occlusive plaque disruption or detachment, expanding intramural hematoma, spasm, and coronary thrombosis can occur and complicate the procedure. Coronary embolism and perforation or rupture of the coronary artery were the potential complications most feared at the inception of the technique, but turned out to be extremely rare (0.2%) [13–15]. With experience, use of over-the-wire dilatation systems, adequately sized balloons, and submaximal inflation pressure, coronary perforation or rupture are unlikely. Plaque disruption and splitting are frequent with successful stenosis dilatation and are part of the mechanism of action. Intimal dissection at the dilated site is considered a complication only when associated with major luminal obstruction, myocardial infarction, or myocardial ischemia calling for an emergency intervention.

Coronary dissection and coronary occlusion associated with myocardial ischemia are the most frequent events that precipitate the need of coronary bypass surgery to prevent myocardial infarction [16, 17]. However, the majority of myocardial infarctions associated with the performance of coronary angioplasty occur in patients undergoing emergency coronary bypass surgery. In most patients who are urgently operated on for evolving myocardial infarction following PTCA complete myocardial infarction will develop [18].

Other complications of coronary angioplasty are complications of cardiac catheterization, including ventricular fibrillation, bleeding from the puncture site and hematoma formation, and rare events such as pericardial tamponade due to perforation of the right ventricle by a pacemaker wire [4].

The mortality and the incidence of myocardial infarction associated with coronary angioplasty are similar to those associated with coronary bypass surgery in comparable patient subsets [19]. In women, PTCA is associated with a less favorable short-term outcome, notably a higher mortality, than in men [20].

However, the outcome of PTCA depends heavily on the types of cases attempted. As more high-risk patients are selected for coronary angioplasty and more complex procedures are performed, local vascular and myocardial ischemic complications are likely to increase. Investigator experience and the use of modified technical equipment may partially counterbalance this development.

Certain clinical and angiographic factors are associated with increased frequency of coronary vascular and myocardial ischemic complications [13]. Female sex, unstable angina, PTCA of the right coronary artery, multivessel disease, and "complicated" stenosis morphology were identified as involving an elevated rate of coronary vascular (coronary dissection and occlusion) and myocardial ischemic (prolonged angina, myocardial infarction) complications. Higher mortality is associated with PTCA in patients older than 60 years, patients with previous coronary bypass surgery, and patients with left main coronary artery disease [19]. In practice, only a combination of these factors – except for left main coronary artery disease, which we consider a relative contraindication in itself – may constitute a contraindication for PTCA.

Although steady improvement of the primary results is still being reported even from specialized centers with stable patient selection policies, the technique of coronary angioplasty seems to be approaching its final potential. A steady rate of coronary vascular complications is likely, because these are inherent in the mechanism of mechanical dilatation and cannot be predicted with certainty. Any further decline in complication rates, therefore, is likely to result from ways of preventing myocardial ischemia and myocardial infarction should coronary dissection occur.

Late Results

A persistent problem with PTCA has been the occurrence of restenosis after a successful procedure. Overall restenosis rates are reported to range from 20% to 50% [4, 21–27]. Recurrence rate can be as high as 50% in patients with variant angina (David, Chapter 18) and after dilatation of a venous graft at the aortic anastomosis site or the graft body [27]. Men seem to have a higher restenosis rate and to need additional revascularization procedures (repeat PTCA or bypass surgery) more frequently [20]. Recurrent stenoses usually occur within the first 6 months after successful PTCA (Fig. 2), but most frequently within the first 4 months; late recurrences are rare. Patients in whom the dilated vessel is shown to be patent on coronary angiography 6–8 months after PTCA have a high chance of continued success.

Anginal symptoms similar to those prior to angioplasty usually herald a recurrent stenosis. However, the recurrence of angina pectoris does not have a perfect correlation with angiographic evidence of recurrent stenoses. Not all symptom-

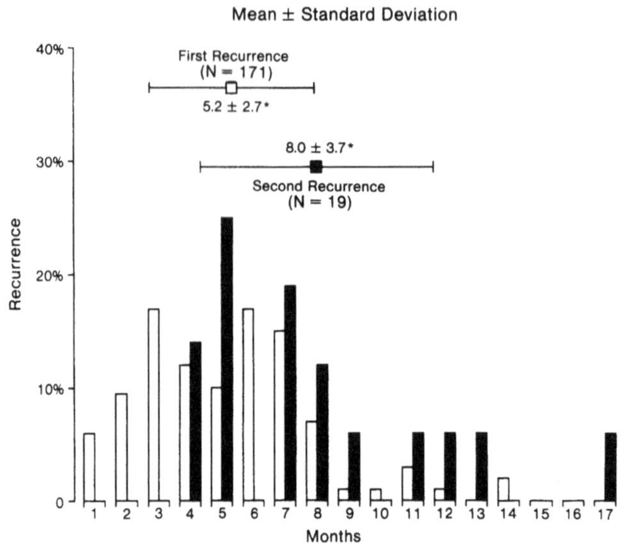

Fig. 2. Time of documentation of first and second recurrences in 514 consecutive patients with successful coronary angioplasty followed over more than 1 year. Percentages refer to the total number of recurrences

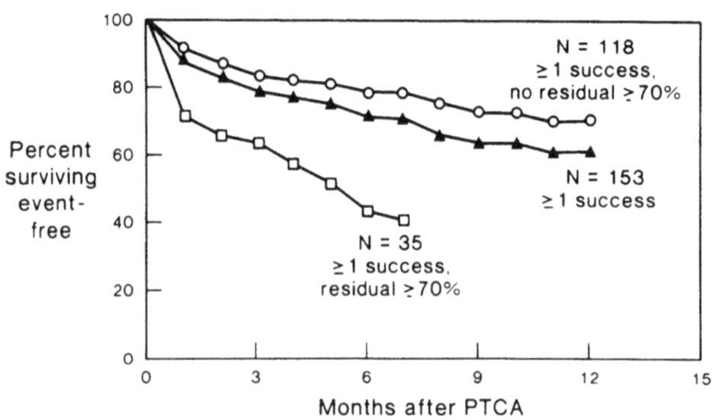

Fig. 3. Event-free survival after successful dilatation of at least one vessel (n = 153) and in subgroups: with complete revascularization (no residual stenosis, n = 118) and with incomplete revascularization (one or more residual stenoses ≧70%, n = 35). Cardiac events were angina pectoris, repeat PTCA, CAGB, myocardial infarction and cardiac death. The difference between the subgroups is significant ($p<0.001$) [45]

atic patients have recurrent stenoses, and the converse is also true. Progression of disease in a nondilated coronary segment or coronary spasm can also cause recurrent angina. On the other hand, over 10% of asymptomatic patients will have angiographic evidence of recurrent stenoses. Electrocardiographic exercise testing with thallium perfusion imaging appears to detect restenoses more reliably than symptomatic assessment alone. In practice, we follow our patients after PTCA with repeated exercise tests and perform coronary angiography only if myocardial ischemia recurs.

Table 3. Summary of reports on restenosis rate and associated drug regimen after PTCA

Group	Pts with followup *n*	Restenosis rate (%)	Drug regimen
Kaltenbach et al. [21]	333	16	Aspirin 1.5 g, verapamil 0.24–0.48 g
Scholl et al. [22]	45	24	Sulfinpyrazone 0.8 g
Kent et al. [11]	38	29	Aspirin 0.15 g, Persantine 0.15 g
Thornton et al. [24][a]	126	27	Aspirin 0.3 g
	122	36	Coumadin

[a] Randomized study

The comparison of restenosis rates from different centers is complicated by the lack of a common definition of recurrence [21]. The duration of followup after successful angioplasty is also important for a valid assessment of recurrence rates and should not be shorter than 6–12 months.

At present we have data on long-term results 4–7 years after successful coronary angioplasty, with Gruentzig's report on his initial patients providing the longest followup information [28]. Results from this report (31% restenosis rate), the Emory series (33% restenosis rate) [25], and the Registry patients (34% restenosis rate) [29] indicate that restenosis occurs in about one-third of patients in whom successful dilatation is achieved. However, using the same definition of recurrence, Kaltenbach [21] reports a significantly lower restenosis rate (16%).

The late clinical results recorded in the Registry patients [30] are in keeping with a relatively high angiographic recurrence rate: 72% of the patients remained improved at 1–4 years after successful angioplasty and did not need a further intervention. Approximately half the patients remained free of symptoms with no subsequent incidents after the initial dilatation.

With the object of preventing recurrent stenoses various drug regimens are used. Medical treatment before and after PTCA most commonly includes a combination of antiplatelet drugs with calcium antagonists and nitrates, which are continued for 6 months or longer after a successful procedure. Table 3 summarizes some of the published long-term results and the associated drug regimens. Except for the results of Kaltenbach [21], none of the different medical treatments post PTCA so far have shown to be associated with a significantly reduced recurrence rate. Anticoagulation with Coumadin after successful PTCA has not proved to be more effective than treatment with aspirin and is therefore not recommended [24].

Clinical or angiographic predictors of recurrent stenoses that are of practical value for patient selection and performance of PTCA have not yet been clearly identified [31] (Hollman, Chapter 12). There is, however, some evidence, that presence of residual stenosis post PTCA is associated with a higher restenosis rate [31, 32]. So, in practice, the best we can currently do to prevent restenosis is to strive for complete initial stenosis dilatation.

Again, most of the data available refer to patients with single-vessel disease. Recently, preliminary reports have shown similar restenosis rates and late functional results in patients after multivessel dilatation [7, 33, 34]. However, in patients with more extensive coronary artery disease incomplete revascularization

Table 4. Comparative results with multilesion coronary angioplasty

	n	Successfully dilated/total no. of lesions	% MVD	% Complications			Late complications			
				Urgent CABG	MI	Death	Mean follow-up (months)	Repeat PTCA	CABG	MI
Hartzler [35]	80	168/180 (91%)	NA	1%	1%	1%	6.9	4%	4%	NA
Vlietstra et al. [5]	100	72/100 (72%) [a]	100	6%	2%	0	> 6	NA	16%	NA
Cowley et al. [36]	72	179/195 (92%)	100	3%	4%	0	26	11%	19%	4%
Dorros et al. [37]	309	599/685 (87%)	64	4%	4%	1%	> 7	15%	6%	<1%
Vandormael et al. [34]	135	264/329 (80%)	84	4%	3%	0	> 6	9%	9%	2%

CABG, coronary artery bypass graft surgery; MI, myocardial infarction; MD, multivessel disease; NA, not available

[a] Patient success

is a more frequent result of angioplasty [35–37]. In incompletely revascularized patients residual myocardial ischemia requiring a second revascularization procedure is significantly more common than in patients with complete revascularization [7, 45] (Fig. 3).

The late mortality and late myocardial infarction rates during the first year of followup are low in patients with single-vessel disease (1% and 3%, respectively, according to the report from the PTCA Registry). Multivessel disease and left main coronary artery disease are associated with a higher rate of late complications [29]. Table 4 summarizes reports on early and late results for multilesion coronary angioplasty.

The improvement in cardiac functional status as a result of successful coronary angioplasty persists until restenosis occurs, as a number of studies using ex-

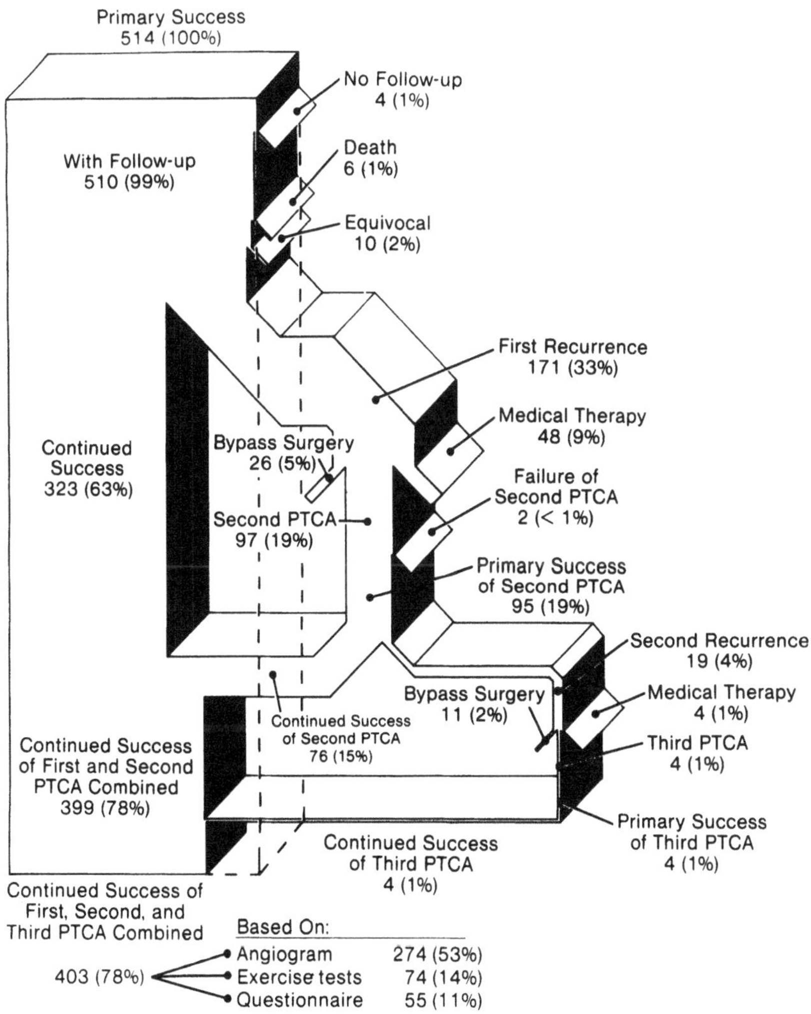

Fig. 4. Long-term results after successful coronary angioplasty (PTCA) in 514 consecutive patients followed over more than 1 year [25]. A favorable long-term result was attained with PTCA alone in 78% of patients

ercise testing and nuclear studies have demonstrated. For most patients with recurrent stenosis repeat coronary angioplasty can be performed with a higher chance of primary success (95%) and fewer complications than the initial angioplasty [25]. The recurrence rate after repeat angioplasty is 25%–30%, which is similar to that after the initial procedure. In view of this favorable prospect repeat PTCA seems to be performed less often than it might be: 50%–60% of patients with restenosis undergo repeat PTCA [25, 30], and the rest of these patients are treated medically or by coronary bypass surgery. Third angioplasties have been performed with a similar success rate in a few patients, but the data available do not permit a definitive judgement about the therapeutic value of a third angioplasty for coronary restenosis at the same site. We tend to recommend coronary bypass surgery in patients with a second recurrence, and in patients with recurrent stenosis against a background of progressive multivessel disease.

Repeat coronary angioplasty for restenosis in patients with initially successful angioplasty can substantially increase their chance of long-term success, which may reach almost 80% including second and third angioplasties. Repeat PTCA should therefore be considered an integral component of PTCA therapy. The long-term result that can be expected after successful PTCA is shown in Fig. 4, which provides details of the outcome in 514 consecutive patients with primarily successful PTCA at Emory University in Atlanta, Ga. USA [4, 25].

In the 7 years it has been in clinical use coronary angioplasty has proved to be effective in a substantial number of patients in need of myocardial revascularization. If it is assumed that up to 30% of patients with symptomatic coronary artery disease are suitable for coronary angioplasty, more than 20% of patients with coronary artery disease may experience long-term benefit from coronary angioplasty if its current potential is utilized.

Learning Curve for Coronary Angioplasty

Proficiency in the performance of coronary angioplasty requires practical skill, appropriate technical equipment, and experience in patient selection. Primary success rates therefore correlate with the "learning curve" of the angioplasty operators and increase with improvements in catheter technology and associated equipment.

The learning curve for coronary angioplasty is reflected by changes in success rate, complications, and case selection criteria with growing number of patients treated by a given operator. The learning curve per se is based on skill but cannot be separated from the influence of improving technology.

Skill and Experience of Operator

Manual dexterity is essential for adequate performance of coronary angioplasty. However, experience plays a part in the choice of catheters and X-ray projections, in the development of maneuvers to overcome difficulties, in the knowledge of when to abort a procedure, and in the management of complications.

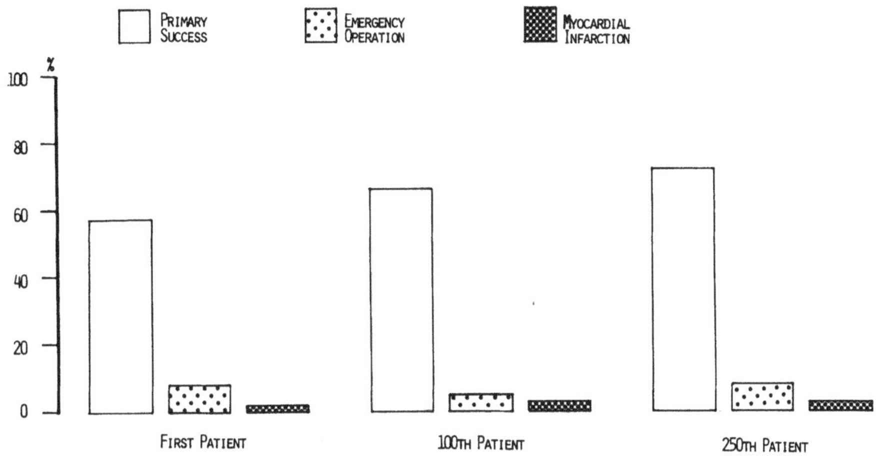

Fig. 5. Chances of primary success, emergency operation, and myocardial infarction for the 1st, the 10th, and the 250th patient of a given operator performing coronary angioplasty. Calculations are based on data collected before 1982 by the National Heart, Lung, and Blood Institute Percutaneous Transluminal Coronary Angioplasty Registry [33]

Table 5. Primary success achieved by Gruentzig and coworkers

	Patients per year	Primary success (%)	Emergency operation (%)
1978	30	63	17
1979	58	79	9
1980	103	87	3
1981	368	88	6
1982	678	91	3
1983	1234	94	2

The data from the National Heart, Lung, and Blood Institute's PTCA Registry show that the primary success rate rises with increasing number of cases treated by the same operator (Fig. 5) [38]. In that particular survey the incidence of complications did not decline correspondingly. The figures were obtained before the advent of steerable angioplasty catheters. Therefore, little change is achieved by technological advances. Table 5 demonstrates the steady increase in primary success rate over time in the results of Gruentzig and coworkers [39]. Reduction of inadvertent injury to the artery owing to improved skill and material was not the most important factor in the reduced need for emergency operation. More importantly, obstructions caused by the dilatation process itself were reopened by repeat dilatation or intracoronary injections of spasmolytic or fibrinolytic agents with increasing frequency, thus obviating the need for emergency surgery.

Furthermore, the indications for emergency surgery were restricted to signs of acute ischemia after failed angioplasty. Patients who had vessel occlusion following angioplasty and in whom ischemia was precluded by collateral circulation were treated by elective surgery or received conservative treatment.

Extensive experience at a center contributes to the quality of coronary angioplasty; not only the experience of the main operators is important in this regard, but also that of their assistants and of the technicians and the nursing staff.

Repeated exposure of the cardiosurgical team to emergencies after failed angioplasty results in a more expert and expeditious handling of these patients, which may limit infarct size or even prevent casualties.

The impact of experience on patient selection is ambiguous. On the one hand, growing experience boosts self-confidence and results in more permissive acceptance policies. On the other hand, possible pitfalls are recognized and unsuitable patients are excluded from the start. Figure 6 shows that patients with multiple-vessel disease gain ground compared with patients with single-vessel disease at the beginning of an angioplasty practice. After the first 200 patients this effect is again reversed. At this stage of experience, operators may realize that single-vessel disease is indeed the optimal indication for coronary angioplasty. As their reputation is established, they are able to apply more restrictive selection criteria and still stay busy. The curves for multiple-vessel disease and multiple lesions in which treatment is attempted draw together with growing experience (Fig. 5). This indicates that expert operators strive for complete revascularization if they accept a patient with multiple-vessel disease.

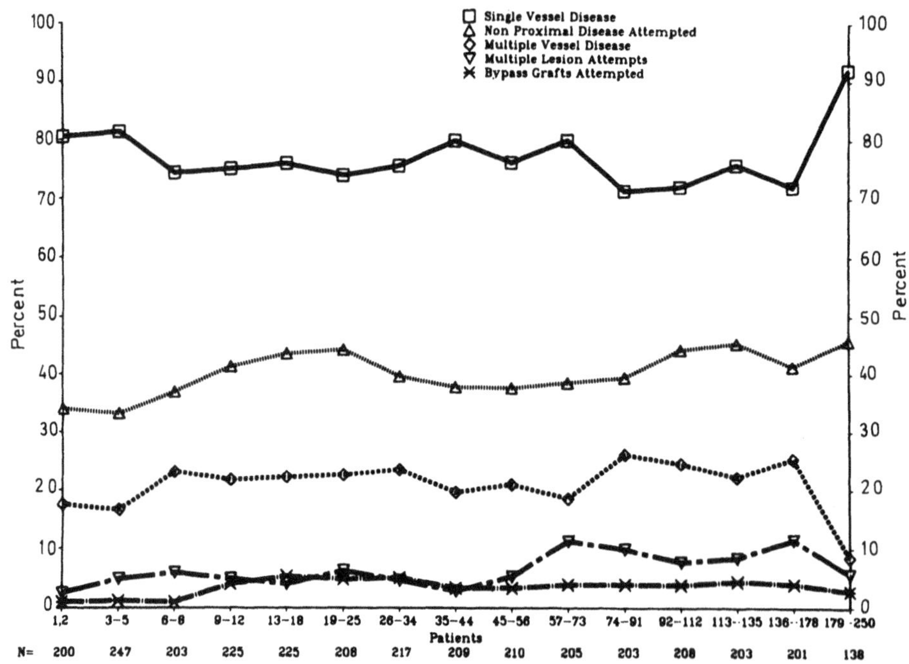

Fig. 6. Change with increasing investigator experience in acceptance of single- and multiple-vessel disease for coronary angioplasty and in attempts to treat lesions in nonproximal locations, lesions in bypass grafts, and multiple lesions. The corresponding chronological case numbers of 105 different centers are grouped together on the *abscissa*. After an initial increment in multiple-vessel disease during early experience single-vessel disease gains ground again beyond the first 200 patients. Distal lesions increase steadily with operator experience. [35]

Technology

The introduction of the steerable guidewire system for coronary angioplasty [40, 41] had a conspicuous influence on both results and patient selection. With the standard system, even in experienced hands, about 10% of the stenoses selected for angioplasty could not be reached [42]. With the current steerable system this proportion has dropped to less than 1%. A group of operators who had just changed from the standard to the steerable system reported an increase in primary success rate from 80% to 94% within 100 patients [43]. Apparently, after only a small number of patients they were familiar with the steerable system and able to gain the full benefit of its advantages. The same group reported a reduced incidence of complications with the steerable system. Yet, the most typical complication of angioplasty is an obstructive dissection caused by the actual dilatation. Its incidence is more dependent on the impact of the expanding balloon on the diseased vessel segment than on negotiation of the lesion. Nonetheless, recrossing of a stenosis for correction of an angiographically unsatisfactory result is safer with the steerable, i.e., over-the-wire catheter system, provided that the guidewire has been left in place during the control injection.

The steerable system also allowed for an expansion of indications for coronary angioplasty. Today more distal, difficult, complex, and multiple lesions are attempted.

Inability to pass a stenosis with the balloon once it has been passed by the steerable guidewire accounted for roughly 50% of the failures in the early use of the steerable system [42]. This problem has been largely overcome by low-profile balloons with an outer diameter of less than 1 mm in the deflated state and by improved guide catheters, which provide better support than the earlier ones. Custom shaping of guide catheters with hot air may also be helpful. Subtle and concerted manipulation of guide catheter, balloon catheter, and guidewire, is a necessary skill if the full benefit of these technological advances is to be enjoyed.

The higher pressure tolerance of the new generations of dilatation balloons has not significantly improved the primary success rate [44]. This is because stenoses resistant to the 7–10 bar attained by older balloons are extremely rare. The use of higher pressures, however, has resulted in a lower residual pressure gradient, indicating a better hemodynamic result.

High-resolution television systems and continuously displayed still frames for reference during advancement of the balloon catheter are considered an additional tremendous support by operators who have these facilities available.

Learning Curve and Long-Term Results

The effect of operator experience and technological advances on the long-term result is obscured by more important factors such as the healing process of the disrupted plaque, the coronary vasomotion, and the natural course of coronary artery disease. Some evidence has been presented to show that a good short-term result of coronary angioplasty (low residual pressure gradient and degree of stenosis) is correlated with a lower recurrence rate [27]. However, it has not yet been shown that these short-term indicators of success improve with increasing experience of the operator.

Eventually there will be a learning curve for long-term management of patients after coronary angioplasty, as investigators collect experience in what medications to use during followup and when and how to reexamine patients in whom the primary result of coronary angioplasty is good.

Socioeconomic Aspects

B. Meier

Return to Work After Coronary Angioplasty

Much like coronary artery bypass surgery, coronary angioplasty is a rather poor means of vocational rehabilitation.

In a study in Geneva [46] in patients who worked right up to the intervention or stopped working shortly before because of their heart problem, only 81% of patients with successful angioplasty returned to work. In a comparable group of patients with coronary artery bypass surgery, 87% resumed work. Hence, both interventions resulted in a similar net loss to the work force. If only the patients that resumed work at a level equal to or higher than that before the intervention are counted the result is even more sobering: 43% after angioplasty and 49% after bypass surgery. The more medication the patients received the lower was their return-to-work rate. The poor correlation between the number of drugs and residual anginal pain demonstrated that overprotection by physicians played a role in failure to return to work. The results are comparable to those of a multicenter study in the United States of America [2].

A study in Frankfurt revealed a return-to-work rate of about 90% both in patients with successful angioplasty and in those with failed angioplasty and subsequent bypass surgery [48].

Return-to-work rates are dependent on local economic situations and types of employment. A self-employed white-collar worker is more likely to return to work than a blue-collar worker supported by an excellent disability insurance system. This is exemplified by a very high return-to-work rate after coronary angioplasty in a study of patients of a highly reputable private hospital in the United States. It was 98%, irrespective of the outcome of angioplasty [49].

Cost and Economic Impact of Coronary Angioplasty

Coronary angioplasty reduces medical expenses in the United States, where medicine relies largely on private institutions and coronary artery bypass surgery facilities are abundant and not fully booked. The early experience of the Mayo

Clinic with coronary angioplasty and the assumption that 15% of the candidates for bypass surgery are also candidates for angioplasty were used as the basis of an estimate of the contemporary annual savings in the United States [50]. The total expenditure for bypass surgery per year was put at $ 2 billion. The corresponding expenditures for the 15% of bypass operations replaceable by angioplasty is thus $ 300 million. Expenditure for angioplasty was found to be 15% less than that for bypass surgery. Annual savings of $ 45 million were concluded. This figure is already adjusted for the charges for standby of a surgical team during angioplasty (a service free of charge in many other institutions), the charges for surgery after failed or complicated angioplasty (27% of the patients in that particular study), the charges for bypass surgery for recurrence after successful angioplasty (11%), and the charges for repeat angioplasty (8%). It was speculated that an increase of their primary success rate from 70% to 95% and a reduction of their recurrence rate from 33% to 20% would more than double the savings.

An American multicenter study on patients with single-vessel disease reported an average hospital bill for angioplasty of $ 5000, versus $ 15000 for bypass surgery. An average saving of $ 7000 per angioplasty procedure was calculated, accounting for primary failures but not for recurrences [51]. Considering a recurrence rate of about 30% after angioplasty and repeat angioplasty in about 20% (some followed by second recurrence), the chance that treatment by angioplasty will prove adequate on a long-term basis is about 80% [52, 25]. The 20% needing bypass surgery in the later course mean a further decrease in the savings.

The same calculations cannot be applied to the situation in other western countries with nationalized or seminationalized medical services, where many candidates for coronary angioplasty would not be readily accepted for elective bypass surgery because of insufficient operating facilities. The cost of all sophisticated interventions is heavily subsidized from taxes. Surgical waiting lists are shortened by coronary angioplasty, but the length of a waiting list has little impact on hospital cost. Therefore, coronary angioplasty increases actual medical cost in these countries (including many western European countries) and financial considerations are not in its favor.

Economic benefits can be expected from patients in whom bypass surgery is successfully replaced by angioplasty and who return to work. This is not because they would not return to work after bypass surgery but because they return to work earlier, i.e., after a few weeks instead of a few months [46, 48]. The sick leave after angioplasty is bound to become shorter as the confidence of primary care physicians in this new therapy grows.

Reflections and calculations on return-to-work rates and expenditure are interesting but should not be overemphasized. Putting people back to work and saving money should not be the primary incentives in the treatment of coronary artery disease.

References

1. Detre KM, Myler RK, Kelsey SF, van Raden M, To T, Mitchell H (1984) Baseline characteristics of patients in the national heart, lung and blood institute PTCA registry. Am J Cardiol 53:7 C
2. Mock MB (1984) Acute and chronic outcome of percutaneous transluminal coronary angioplasty. Am J Cardiol 53:67 C
3. Gruentzig AR, Meier B (1983) Percutaneous transluminal coronary angioplasty. The first five years and the future. Int J Cardiol 2:319
4. Ischinger T, Gruentzig AR (1984) Perkutane transluminale Koronarangioplastie. In: Roskamm H (Hrsg) Handbuch der Inneren Medizin IX/3. Springer, Berlin Heidelberg New York
5. Vlietstra RE, Holmes DR, Reeder GS, Mock MB, Smith HC, Bove AA, Bresnahan JF, Piehler JM (1983) Balloon angioplasty in multivessel coronary artery disease. Mayo Clin Proc 58:563
6. Ischinger T, Zack P, Russ T, Aker U, Kennedy H (1984) Percutaneous transluminal coronary angioplasty (PTCA): is the widening of indication justified? An updated experience. Eur Heart J 5(I):73
7. Vandormael MG, Chaitman BR, Ischinger T, Aker UT, Harber M, Hernandez J, Deligonul U, Kennedy HL (1985) Immediate and short-term benefit of multilesion coronary angioplasty: influence of degree of revascularization. J Am Coll Cardiol (in press)
8. Ischinger T, Aker U, Kennedy H (1984) Percutaneous transluminal coronary angioplasty (PTCA): current status and indications. Cardiovasc Rev Rep 5:782
9. Rosing DR, van Raden M, Mincemoyer RM, Bonow RO, Bourassa MG, David PR, Ewels CJ, Detre KM, Kent KM (1984) Exercise, electrocardiographic and functional responses after percutaneous transluminal coronary angioplasty. Am J Cardiol 53:36 C
10. Hirzel HO, Nuesch K, Gruentzig AR, Luetolf UM (1981) Short and long-term changes in myocardial perfusion after percutaneous transluminal coronary angioplasty assessed by thallium 201 exercise scintigraphy. Circulation 63:1001
11. Kent KM, Bonow RO, Rosing DR, Ewels CJ, Lipson LC, McIntosh CL, Bacharach S, Green M, Epstein SE (1982) Improved myocardial functions during exercise after successful PTCA. N Engl J Med 306:441
12. Meier B, Gruentzig AR, Siegenthaler WE, Schlumpf M (1983) Long term exercise performance after percutaneous transluminal coronary angioplasty and coronary artery bypass grafting. Circulation 68:796
13. Cowley MJ, Dorros G, Kelsey SF, van Raden M, Detre KM (1984) Acute coronary events associated with percutaneous transluminal coronary angioplasty. Am J Cardiol 53:12 C
14. Kimbiris D, Iskandrian AS, Goel I, Bemis C, Gehl L, Owens J, Segal B (1982) Transluminal coronary angioplasty complicated by coronary artery perforation. Cathet Cardiovasc Diagn 8:481
15. Saffitz J, Rose T, Oaks J, Roberts W (1983) Coronary arterial rupture during coronary angioplasty. Am J Cardiol 51:902
16. Ischinger T, Gruentzig AR, Meier B, Galan K (to be published) Coronary dissection and total coronary occlusion with percutaneous transluminal coronary angioplasty (PTCA): significance of initial angiographic morphology of coronary stenoses. Circulation
17. Cowley MJ, Dorros G, Kelsey SF, van Raden M, Detre KM (1984) Emergency coronary bypass surgery after coronary angioplasty: The National Heart, Lung and Blood Institute's Percutaneous Transluminal Coronary Angioplasty Registry experience. Am J Cardiol 53:22 C
18. Murphy DA, Craver JM, Jones EL, Gruentzig AR, King SB, Hatcher CR (1982) Surgical revascularization following successful percutaneous transluminal coronary angioplasty. J Thorac Cardiovasc Surg 84:342
19. Dorros G, Cowley MJ, Janke L, Kelsey S, Mullin SM, van Raden M (1984) In hospital mortality rate in the National Heart Lung and Blood Institute Percutaneous Transluminal Coronary Angioplasty Registry. Am J Cardiol 53:17 C

20. Cowley MJ, Mullin SM, Kelsey SF, Kent KM, Gruentzig AR, Detre KM, Passamani E (1985) Sex differences in early and long-term results of coronary angioplasty in the NHLBI PTCA Registry. Circulation 71:90
21. Kaltenbach M, Kober G, Scherer D, Vallbracht C (1984) Rezidivhäufigkeit nach erfolgreicher Ballondilatation von Kranzarterienstenosen. Z Kardiol 73(2):161
22. Scholl JM, Chaitman PR, David PR, Dupras G, Brevers G, Val PC, Crepeau J, Lesperance J, Bourassa MG (1982) Exercise electrocardiography and myocardial scintigraphy in the serial evaluation of the results of percutaneous transluminal coronary angioplasty. Circulation 66:380
23. Ischinger T, Gruentzig AR, Hollman J, King SB, Douglas J, Meier B, Bradford J, Tankersley R (1983) Should coronary arteries with less than 60% diameter stenosis be treated by angioplasty? Circulation 68:148
24. Thornton MA, Gruentzig AR, Hollman J, King SB, Douglas J (1984) Coumadin and aspirin in prevention of recurrence after transluminal coronary angioplasty. Circulation 69:721
25. Meier B, King SB, Gruentzig AR, Douglas J, Hollman J, Ischinger T, Galan K, Tankersley R (1984) Repeat coronary angioplasty. J Am Coll Cardiol 4:463–466
26. Jutzky KR, Berte LE, Alderman EL, Ratts J, Simpson JB (1982) Coronary restenosis rates in consecutive patient series one year post successful angioplasty. Circulation 66(II):331
27. Douglas J, Gruentzig AR, King SB, Hollman J, Ischinger T (1983) Percutaneous transluminal coronary angioplasty in patients with prior coronary bypass surgery. J Am Coll Cardiol 2:745
28. Gruentzig AR, Schlumpf M, Siegenthaler W (1984) Long term results after coronary angioplasty. Circulation 70(II):323
29. Holmes DR, Vlietstra RE, Smith HC, Vetrovec GW, Kent KM (1984) Restenosis after percutaneous transluminal coronary angioplasty (PTCA): a report from the PTCA Registry of the National Heart, Lung and Blood Institute. Am J Cardiol 53:77 C
30. Kent KM, Bentivoglio LG, Block PC, Bourassa MG, Cowley MJ, Dorros G, Detre KM (1984) Long term efficacy of percutaneous transluminal coronary angioplasty (PTCA): report from the National Heart, Lung and Blood Institute PTCA Registry. Am J Cardiol 53:27 C
31. Hollman J, Gruentzig AR, King SB, Douglas J (1984) Percutaneous transluminal coronary angioplasty. In: Hurst JW (ed) Essay on the heart. McGraw-Hill, New York, pp 297–315
32. Schmitz HJ, Meyer J, Kiesslich T, Effert S (1982) Greater initial dilatation gives better later angiographic results in percutaneous transluminal coronary angioplasty (PTCA). Circulation 66(I):123
33. Hall DP, Gruentzig AR (1984) Recurrence rate after double vessel dilatation. Circulation 70(II):107
34. Vandormael M, Ischinger T, Russ T, Aker U, Chaitman BR, Kennedy H (1984) Complex coronary angioplasty – immediate and six months functional results. Circulation 70(II):322
35. Hartzler GO (1983) Percutaneous transluminal coronary angioplasty in multivessel disease. Cathet Cardiovasc Diagn 9:537–541
36. Cowley MJ, Vetrovec GW, Lewis SA, Hirsh PD, Wolfgang TC (1984) Coronary angioplasty (PTCA) of multiple vessels: acute and long term results. Circulation [Suppl II] 70:II–322 (abstract)
37. Dorros G, Stertzer SH, Cowley MJ, Myler RK (1984) Complex coronary angioplasty: multiple coronary dilatations. Am J Cardiol 53:126C–130C
38. Gruentzig AR, Hollman J (1982) Improved primary success rate in transluminal coronary angioplasty using a steerable guidance system. Circulation [Suppl II] 66:II–330 (abstract)
39. Simpson JB, Baim DS, Robert EW, Harrison DC (1982) A new catheter system for coronary angioplasty. Am J Cardiol 49:1216–1222
40. Kelsey SF, Mullin SM, Detre KM, Mitchell M, Cowley MJ, Gruentzig AR, Kent KM (1984) Effect of investigator experience on percutaneous transluminal coronary angioplasty. Am J Cardiol 53:56C–64C
41. Meier B, Gruentzig A (1984) Resultate der transluminalen Koronardilatation. Dtsch Med Wochenschr 109:675–677
42. Meier B, Gruentzig AR (1984) Learning curve for percutaneous transluminal coronary angioplasty: skill, technology or patient selection. Am J Cardiol 53:65C–66C

43. Von Essen R, Merx W, Bertram B, Schmitz HJ, Braun C, Effert S (1984) Koronargefäßdilatation mit Hilfe steuerbarer Ballonkatheter – Erfahrungen mit den ersten 100 Dilatationen bei stabiler und instabiler Angina pectoris. Dtsch Med Wochenschr 109:651–655
44. Meier B, Gruentzig AR, King SB III, Douglas JS, Hollman J, Ischinger T, Galan K (1984) Higher balloon dilatation pressure in coronary angioplasty. Am Heart J 107:619–622
45. Mabin TA, Holmes DR, Smith HC, Vlietstra RE et al. (1985) Follow up clinical results in patients undergoing percutaneous transluminal coronary angioplasty. Circulation 71:754
46. Meier B, Chaves V, von Segesser L, Faidutti B, Rutishauser W (1984) Return to work after coronary angioplasty in comparison to coronary bypass surgery. In: Walter PJ (ed) Return to work after coronary bypass surgery. Psychosocial and economic aspects. Springer, Berlin Heidelberg New York Tokyo
47. Holmes DR Jr, van Raden MJ, Reeder GS, Vlietstra RE, Jang GC, Kent KM, Vetrovec GW, Cowley MJ, Dorros G, Kelsey SF, Detre KM, Mock MB (1984) Return to work after coronary angioplasty: a report from the national heart, lung, and blood institute percutaneous transluminal coronary angioplasty registry. Am J Cardiol 53:48C–51C
48. Vallbracht C, Kaltenbach M (1984) Return to work after coronary angioplasty. In: Walter PJ (ed) Return to work after coronary bypass surgery. Psychosocial and economic aspects. Springer, Berlin Heidelberg New York Tokyo
49. Holmes DR Jr, Vlietstra RE, Mock MB, Smith HC, Dorros G, Cowley MJ, Kent KM, Hammes LN, Janke L, Elveback LR, Vetrovec GW (1983) Employment and recreation patterns in patients treated by percutaneous transluminal coronary angioplasty: a multicenter study. Am J Cardiol 52:710–713
50. Reeder GS, Krishan I, Nobrega FT, Naessens J, Kelly M, Christianson JB, McAfee MK (1984) Is percutaneous coronary angioplasty less expensive than bypass surgery? N Engl J Med 311:1157–1162
51. Jang GC, Block PC, Cowley MJ, Gruentzig AR, Dorros G, Holmes DR Jr, Kent KM, Leatherman LL, Myler RK, Sjolander SME, Stertzer SH, Vetrovec GW, Willis WH Jr, Williams DO (1984) Relative cost of coronary angioplasty and bypass surgery in a one-vessel disease model. Am J Cardiol 53:52C–55C
52. Williams DO, Gruentzig AR, Kent KM, Detre KM, Kelsey SF, To T (1984) Efficacy of repeat percutaneous transluminal coronary angioplasty for coronary restenosis. Am J Cardiol 53:32C–35C

Chapter 12. The Problem of Restenosis

JAY HOLLMAN and THOMAS ISCHINGER

Recurrent stenosis following successful PTCA remains the most serious barrier to wider application of this technique. Solution of the problem is in its infancy. A reliable means of preventing recurrence will probably also increase our understanding of the atherosclerotic process. If recurrent stenosis can be prevented, it may be possible to slow down the progression of atherosclerosis by the same interventions.

Recurrence: The Clinical Interventionist's Perspective

There are at least four patterns of recurrence (see Table 1). The first is the acute occlusion syndrome, which occurs in about 2% of patients who have an otherwise unremarkable angioplasty [1]. Acute occlusion occurs within hours of the PTCA procedure. While there is controversy about the cause of acute occlusion [2, 3], hypotension, large intimal tears, and poor initial PTCA results predispose to acute occlusion. The use of intravenous heparin and nitrates help prevent acute occlusion. The mechanism may be multiple, but coronary artery spasm and/or hemorrhage into an atherosclerotic plaque are the most likely mechanisms. This is more usually considered a complication of PTCA and will not be considered further.

Coronary artery spasm occurring during hemodynamically insignificant disease is a second reason for recurrent symptoms. The onset is in the first 2 months after angioplasty. The symptoms are usually resting angina and early morning angina. Prompt relief with nitroglycerin is the rule. Angina on exertion is not usually present. These patients frequently progress to recurrent stenosis [4, 5]. While this may represent an intermediate step in recurrence, it is only present in

Table 1. Types of recurrences after PTCA

Recurrence type	Time from PTCA to onset or time of presentation	Frequency
Acute occlusion	<24 hours	2%
Variant angina	1 day to $1^1/_2$ months	1%
Thrombotic	1 day to 1 month	< 1%
Intimal hyperplasia	1 month to 9 months	25%

While most recurrences are of the intimal hyperplasia type, other types of recurrence should be considered when the clinical picture is unusual

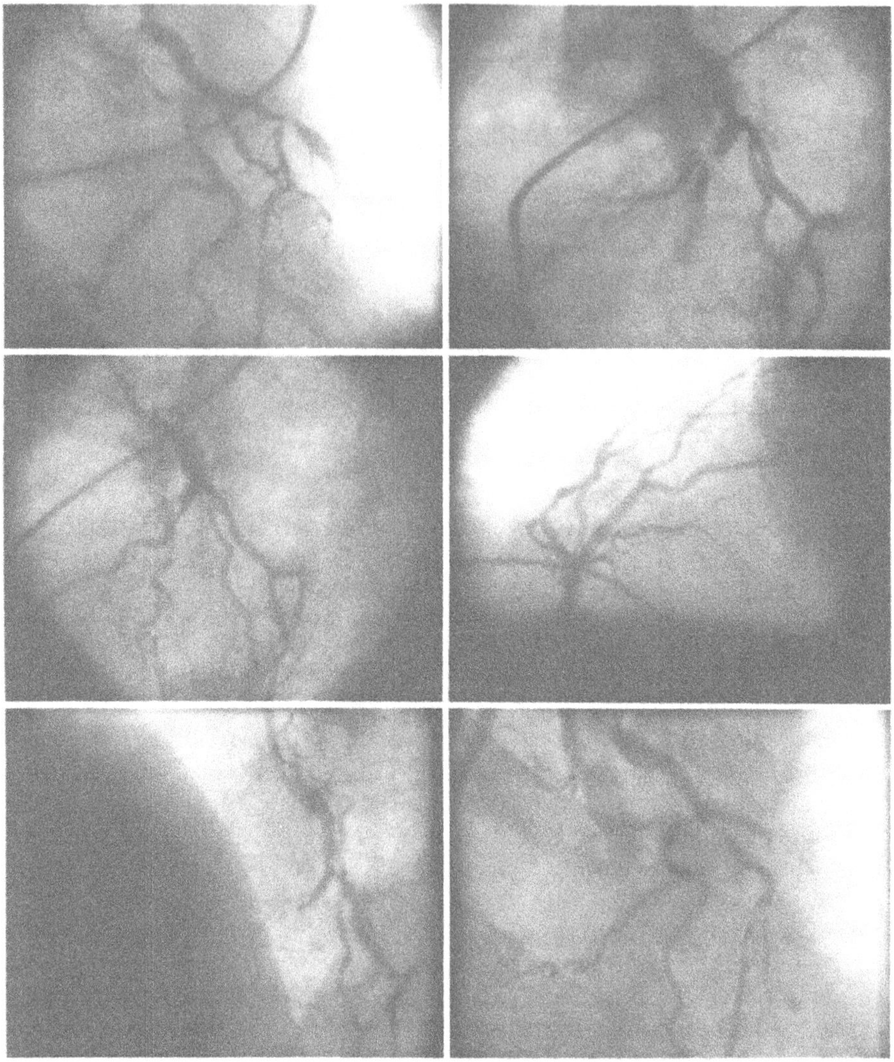

a b c d e f

Fig. 1 a–f. PTCA followed by thrombotic occlusion. Severe obstruction on the proximal left anterior descending artery at the first septal perforator is seen in the RAO projection (**a**) and the LAO cranial projection (**b**). Postangioplasty angiograms demonstrate a satisfactory result in LAO cranial (**c**) and 30° cranial projections (**d**). One week later, the patient experienced an acute myocardial infarction. Cardiac catheterization done within days of the infarction demonstrated occlusion at the site of PTCA (**e** LAO cranial, **f** RAO). Other patients presenting as this patient did have been successfully treated with streptokinase

a small number of patients who develop recurrent stenosis. This coronary spasm at the site of PTCA is probably responsible for many of the early deaths which occur in the first 30 days after angioplasty.

Thrombotic occlusion is a rare cause of recurrent stenosis, but can and does occur (see Fig. 1). Because this type of occlusion is so sudden, acute myocardial

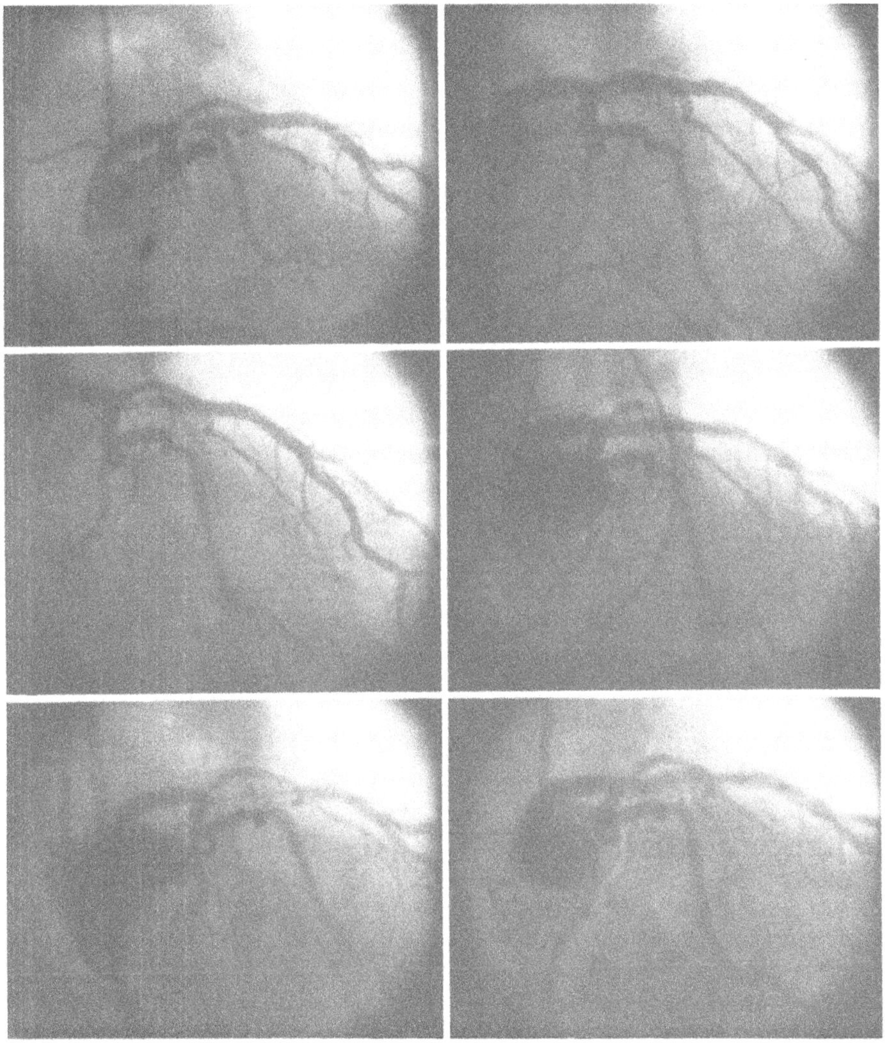

Fig. 2 a–f. Patient with two types of recurrence: Original de novo stenosis **a** before and **b** after PTCA; **c** First recurrence; **d** result of second PTCA. Note that the first recurrence is short and about the same length as the original stenosis, while second recurrence (**e**) is longer, extending over the entire length of balloon injury; **f** result of the third angioplasty

infarction may result. Only 4 patients in the Cleveland Clinic series of over 1000 angioplasty patients have had documented thrombotic occlusion.

The most usual recurrence pattern is for a patient to remain symptom-free until 1½ to 5 months after PTCA. At this time, the patient develops exertional angina relieved by rest. Patients who have a more active life-style usually present earlier and sedentary patients present with postprandial angina or angina on minimal exertion. This type of recurrence is seen in about 25% of patients.

Recurrent lesions by definition occur at the site of angioplasty. Angiographers have observed several features: The new stenosis is usually more concentric than the original stenosis; it can be shorter or longer than the original one but it does not extend beyond the area of previous balloon injury (see Fig. 2). It can be more severe or less severe than the original stenosis. Symptoms are generally present when the lesion has recurred according to angiographic criteria, but sometimes the lesion can be quite severe though there are no symptoms, while at other times recurrent symptoms of angina are experienced in the absence of recurrent stenosis. In the NHLBI Registry, 56% of patients with definite or probable angina had recurrent stenosis, while 14% of patients with no symptoms were found to have recurrent stenosis on followup angiography [6]. The most promising aspect of recurrence is that if it is going to occur, it usually occurs within the first 6–8 months. If angiography at 6 months documents good healing there will almost certainly be no recurrence at the site of angioplasty. This is probably related to the biologic effects of balloon injury. Grunwald and Haudenschild [7], using a rat aorta model have shown that the stimulus to in vitro smooth muscle proliferation following in vivo balloon injury is maximal at 7 days after injury and is no longer present at 21 days after balloon injury. Thus, balloon injury's stimulus to the development of recurrence (which probably occurs as a result of smooth muscle proliferation) is limited to a finite time period following angioplasty.

Mechanism and Pathology of Recurrence

The pathology of recurrence is still not completely defined for all subgroups.

Pathology

Coronary spasm-type occlusion has been documented in one patient dying 64 days after apparently successful PTCA (Fig. 3) [4]. While myofibroblastic (smooth muscle) proliferation was documented, the disorderly pattern was of such a kind that it could not account for the coronary artery spasm. The spasm was probably due to smooth muscle cells present in the muscular media. Coronary artery spasm at the site of PTCA will probably not occur if the lesion is old and the muscular media is completely destroyed by the atherosclerotic process.

The most common form of recurrent stenosis is that of intimal hyperplasia [8, 9]. This intimal growth has been identified as early as 5 days after PTCA. By 17 days after PTCA a proliferation several layers thick can be identified (Fig. 4). At 5 months, the hyperplastic growth may have nearly closed the lumen (Fig. 5). This intimal hyperplasia is similar to the early changes observed throughout vein grafts, particularly at the graft-arterial junction [10, 11]. Clearly, vein-graft anastomoses and vessels with balloon injuries must heal by forming a new lining endothelium. Intimal hyperplasia is probably an extension of the normal healing process.

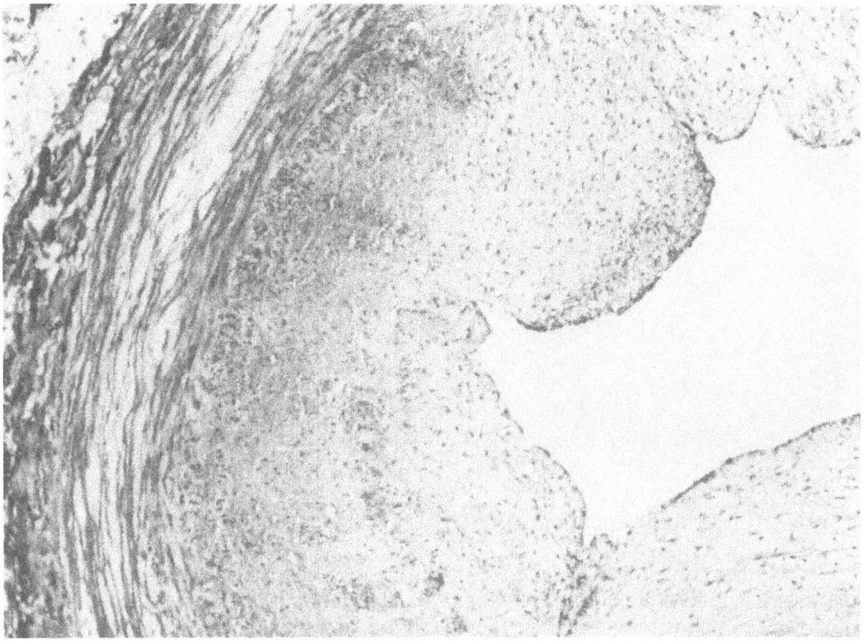

Fig. 3. An artery at 64 days after angioplasty. Note the inner cellular layer and the outer layer, which contains fully developed smooth muscle cells with cholesterol clefts

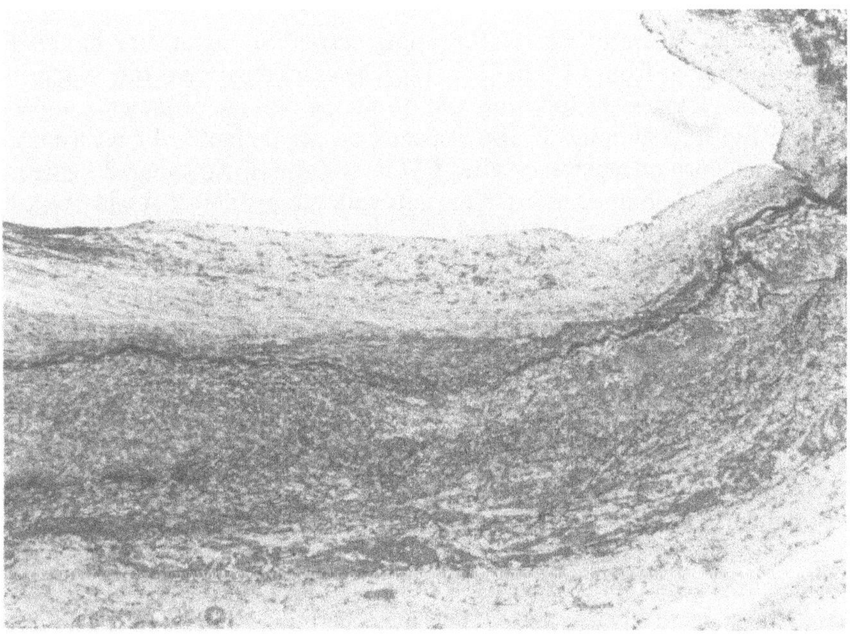

Fig. 4. This patient died 17 days after apparently unremarkable PTCA of a right coronary artery. The lumen is well preserved. The inner layer, as in Fig. 3, is relatively cellular without development of definitive smooth muscle elements

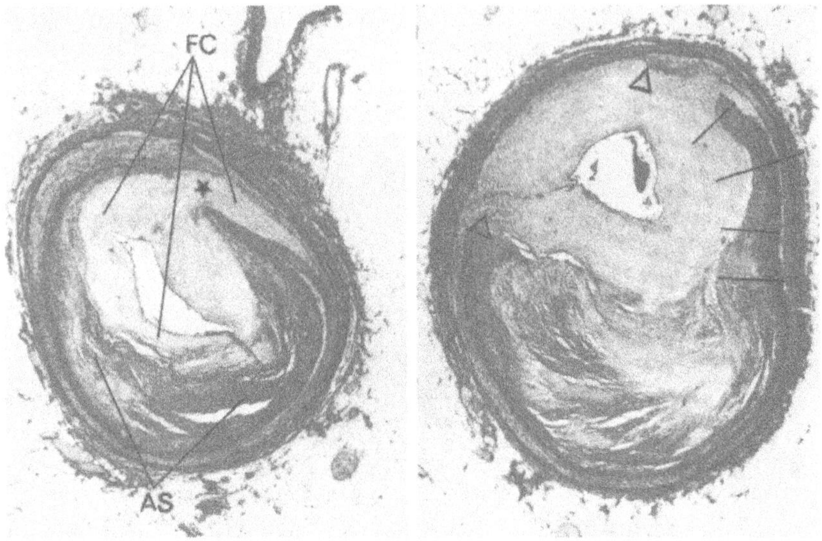

Fig. 5. Fibrocellular proliferation in a patient who had progressed to full, angiographically visible recurrence at 5 months after PTCA. Note the clear demarcation between the fibrocellular proliferation (*FC*), which is responsible for the recurrence, and the atherosclerotic plaque (*AS*). (Essed et al. [8])

Clinical Factors

The incidence of recurrent stenosis following successful angioplasty has been variously reported as from 13% to 47% [12]. The exact recurrence rate is dependent upon completeness of followup and on the percentage of patients undergoing followup angiography. It also depends on the definition of recurrence. Thus, the incidence of recurrence after PTCA is not easily compared between series and centers. About one-third of patients with successful PTCA will develop recurrent stenosis in the first 6–8 months.

Of the clinical variables, male sex, short duration of symptoms, and diabetes are likely to be found in patients with recurrence. The greater likelihood of recurrence in male than in female patients is in contrast to the data observed in bypass surgery [14, 15]; bypass graft patency is higher in men than women. This makes for interesting complementary roles of bypass surgery and PTCA. The reason for the higher recurrence rates in males is unclear: While speculation about hormonal influences on intimal hyperplasia may be of interest, no data are available to resolve this issue. A more plausible explanation is that at the time of angioplasty, in most patients in both the NHLBI Registry and in the Emory series dilatation was performed with a 3 mm balloon. This was the largest balloon available at the time. Since males tend to have larger arteries than females, many male arteries could have been relatively undersized. This hypothesis is supported by the finding in the Emory series that lesions of the left anterior descending artery were more likely to recur than right coronary or circumflex artery lesions. Again as a general rule, the left anterior descending artery tends to be the largest one. Further exploration of this hypothesis is possible now that balloon catheters are available in a variety of sizes.

Shorter duration of symptoms was more likely to be associated with recurrent stenosis in the NHLBI Registry. A similar trend was also seen in the Emory series, although no statistically significant difference was recorded. A correlation between duration of symptoms and age of the atherosclerotic lesion implies that recurrence is more likely in younger, active lesions. This is consistent with data from human aorta smooth muscle cultures: Cells from fatty streaks show proliferation, manifested by increased thymidine uptake, while smooth muscle cells from fully developed plaques do not [16]. Diabetes mellitus is the only risk factor that appears to be associated with a higher incidence of recurrence. With larger series other risk factors may become apparent.

Severe lesions recurred more often in the NHLBI Registry, but not in the Emory series. This may be related to experience. The Emory series of over 600 followup angiograms represents later experience than that of the NHLBI Registry, which contains a similar number of patients but is based on the early experience of a number of centers. Perhaps with more experience pre-PTCA lesion severity might no longer correlate with recurrence.

A variety of procedural variables have been published in abstract form to correlate with recurrent stenosis [17]. However, few are of any practical value. What appears to be consistent is that the better the initial result, the less likely a recurrence is. Efforts should be made to achieve a residual pressure gradient less than 20 mmHg. The results recorded in the two largest series indicate that residual gradients of greater than 20 mmHg are associated with an elevated incidence of recurrent stenosis [13]. No other procedural variables have been shown to be so consistently linked with recurrence. Unfortunately, the recent use of lower profile balloons and softer lumen catheters makes the measurement of distal arterial pressure more difficult and less accurate. The polyethylene balloon does not fold around the shaft as well as the polyvinylchloride balloon, which makes the comparison of gradients more difficult. Softer catheters tend to collapse their lumen when sharp bends are negotiated. In the practical situation the aim of a low residual gradient should still be pursued, but the limitations of the particular balloon system must be understood.

The presence of an intimal tear or nonocclusive dissection was associated with a lower recurrence rate in the Montreal Heart Institute series [17]. No statistical difference was found in the Emory series. However, the recurrence rate was lower in patients who had an intimal tear after PTCA associated with a residual gradient of less than 15 mmHg. On the other hand, the restenosis rate was considerably higher if the residual pressure gradient was more than 15 mmHg, regardless of whether a dissection was present or not [18].

Faxon et al. [12], using the New Zealand white rabbit model, have shown that extensive intimal hyperplasia occurs 4 weeks after angioplasty. This model also shows more thrombosis with organization. Thrombosis is seen in the clefts of the intimal splits following balloon angioplasty in human coronaries [9, 13]. Whether these thrombi are the stimulus to intimal hyperplasia or not is not definitely known. However, the artery must heal by forming a new endothelium. Recurrent stenosis probably represents intimal proliferation beyond that necessary for healing.

While the Emory series showed a higher incidence of recurrence among left anterior descending artery lesions, the NHLBI series did not. As previously mentioned, this difference might be due to relative undersizing of left anterior descending artery lesions. Dilatation of atherosclerotic graft body stenosis is associated with a higher incidence of recurrence. Distal anastomotic lesions that occur within 1 year after bypass surgery are easily handled by PTCA and the recurrence rate appears to be relatively low (about 20%) [19]. The difference in recurrence is probably not a function of balloon sizing only, but also of the underlying disease. The late atherosclerotic disease seen in vein grafts is pathologically different [10, 11]. The recurrence rate in late graft body dilatation is almost 50%.

Drug Therapy to Prevent Recurrence

The use of anticoagulants and antiplatelet agents in coronary angioplasty is based upon experience in peripheral angioplasty, where the use of these agents was associated with a lower incidence of recurrent stenosis. There are no randomized data to show the superiority of any form of drug therapy following successful PTCA.

Aspirin has been shown to be at least as effective as Coumadin in the treatment of patients with recurrent stenosis [20]. Overall, this study showed a trend for a lower incidence of recurrent stenosis among aspirin-treated patients, but the difference was not statistically significant ($P = 0.1$). However, when only patients who had had symptoms for longer than 3 months were considered, aspirin proved to be significantly more successful than Coumadin in the prevention of recurrent stenosis ($P = <0.05$).

Faxon et al., using the hypercholesteremic rabbit model, have shown that lower recurrence rates can be achieved with either sulfinpyrazone or aspirin and dipyridamole than are recorded in control animals [21]. Moreover, in this animal model, Faxon has shown that organized thrombus may account for some of the recurrences in the rabbit model [22]. However, in most cases intimal hyperplasia accounted for the majority of recurrences. What it is important to learn from these models, however, is that either thrombosis and/or platelet factors, which probably coat the freshly damaged angioplasty surface [23], can play a role in the development of recurrence. Platelet growth factor – although its local effect is almost impossible to measure – may be important in the development of the current stenosis. In the rabbit animal model, however, balloon injury induces smooth muscle cell proliferation independently of serum factors [7]. Thus, even if serum factors are controlled by antiplatelet or anticoagulant medication recurrence may still be a complication.

Drugs active against coronary artery spasm have been advocated as agents that may lessen the likelihood of recurrence [4]. Evidence for this is based on clinical data suggesting that lesions demonstrating spasm either before or after PTCA have a high incidence of recurrence [5]. Obviously, spasm can be only a symptom of a recurrent lesion. Drugs that prevent spasm may prevent symptoms and not the recurrence. However, it is important to prevent spasm after PTCA, since this may prevent some cases of the unusual but serious complications of sudden death and myocardial infarction observed in the first few months after PTCA.

Recurrent Stenosis – A Practical Clinical Approach

Certainly there is nothing in the clinical data amassed so far that gives definite direction in patient selection, except perhaps that old vein grafts should not undergo PTCA. The risk of embolism during late graft dilatation is real, and the high recurrence rate makes the presence of old vein grafts a relative contraindication. The fact that PTCA is better in women and coronary bypass grafting better in men might suggest that bypass grafting should be performed in men and PTCA, in women. Fortunately, repeat PTCA is safer (i.e., less likely to be associated with complications) and more likely to be initially successful [24]. The primary success rate for repeat PTCA at the Cleveland Clinic was greater than 99%; emergency surgery was needed in one case).

This high primary success and low complication rate are due in part to patient selection – patients with recurrence have already undergone successful dilatation. A second factor, the underlying pathology, is also important. Recurrent stenosis represents intimal hyperplasia without large areas of cholesterol plaques that might rupture and hemorrhage. Recurrent lesions are not associated with thrombosis.

For these reasons, a second PTCA is generally recommended for patients experiencing recurrent stenosis. The recurrence rate following the second PTCA is about the same (25%–30%), but recurrence tends to be 1–3 months later than after the original PTCA. (It may, however, occur even earlier than the first time.) Because the second recurrence can be later, a follow-up catheterization is usually undertaken 1 year after a second PTCA. A second recurrence is still sufficiently unusual for formulation of any fixed rules to be possible. More recently, third PTCAs have been undertaken, particularly if the interval between recurrences has been lengthening. If the biology of the lesion is limited by the number of times the smooth muscle cells (or myofibrocytes) can replicate this approach is logical. Nonmalignant cells in culture will only replicate a finite number of times. If PTCA is repeated enough times the capacity of the lesion for proliferation will eventually be exceeded, and the lumen will remain large.

The risk of recurrence must be explained to the patient when informed consent is given for the intervention. If the patient is completely revascularized with PTCA an active exercise program is indicated. This will give an early warning if recurrent symptoms are developing. Once symptoms recur, prompt repeat catheterization and repeat PTCA should be undertaken. It is our practice to perform this in the same session.

Recurrent Stenosis in Patients with Mild Stenosis

The problem of PTCA in lesions causing narrowing by less than 60% of the diameter is a difficult one. While the majority of such patients will have a satisfactory long-term result with PTCA, some will have recurrent stenosis. In these circumstances the recurrence is frequently more severe than the original stenosis [25] (Fig. 6). For this reason, it is necessary to be sure of the indications before performing PTCA in patients with mild stenosis.

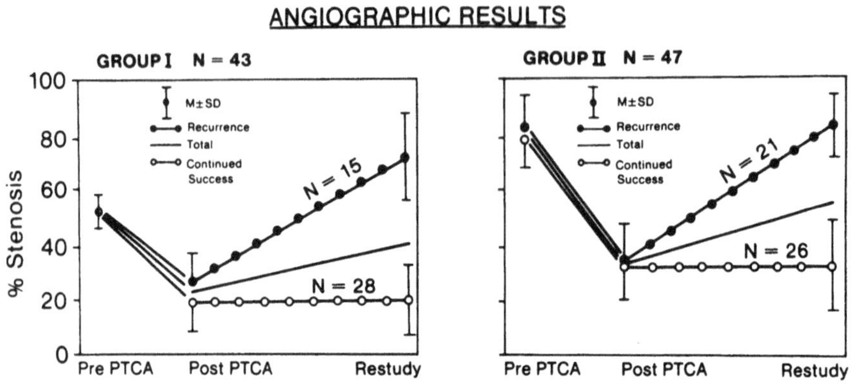

Fig. 6. This figure contrasts the results in patients with mild stenosis (group I) and severe stenosis (group II). While the majority of patients in both groups experienced good long-term results, the patients with mild stenosis who experienced recurrence had a lesion that was more severe on average than their original stenosis. (Ischinger et al. [25])

PTCA and Bypass Surgery

All revascularization procedures have a recurrence rate. At present the recurrence rate after PTCA appears to be higher than that following bypass surgery. In bypass surgery, earlier experience was associated with a lower graft patency [26]. It remains to be seen whether or not PTCA will show an improvement in recurrence rate with increased experience. Even if the recurrence rate in single-vessel disease does not show improvement, near-equal results to those of bypass surgery can be obtained with PTCA if repeat procedures are allowed for. In multivessel disease longer followup is needed to determine the relative value of PTCA and coronary artery bypass surgery.

Indications for Future Research

It is important to ascertain whether or not there are certain procedural changes that will change the recurrence rate. Is the size of the balloon relative to the size of the distal artery important? As in bypass surgery [27, 28], will PTCA of small arteries or of arteries with low flows be found to be associated with a higher recurrence rate? Drug therapy also needs to be resolved. Cheseboro et al. [29] have reopened this issue of antiplatelet therapy following aortocoronary bypass grafting with a well-controlled study of aspirin and dipyridamole versus placebo. Are antiplatelet drugs useful after PTCA, and if so, which combination is most effective? Calcium channel blockers are also frequently used. What is the value of these agents? Do they decrease symptoms? Do they prevent recurrence? Montreal Heart Institute recently reported their data on a randomized trial of diltiazem [30]. They found no effect of diltiazem in the prevention of recurrence; however, only 92 patients were randomized. Type II errors, i.e., real but small differences between subgroups, are missed when the sample size is so small. Large study groups of at least 500 patients or more will be necessary to detect a real difference of 10% with 95% certainty when the recurrence rate is 25%–35%. Thus, studies such as these must be well funded and carefully planned by large centers or carried out as multicenter trials.

An understanding of the real biology of recurrent stenosis may yield exciting new insights into what causes atherosclerosis to develop. This information may be the most helpful gain from the study of recurrence.

Acknowledgement. The authors would like to thank Paula LaManna for her expert technical assistance in the preparation of this manuscript.

References

1. Hollman J, Gruentzig AR, King S, Douglas J, Ishinger T, Meier B (1983) Acute occlusion following percutaneous transluminal coronary angioplasty – a new approach. Circulation 68:725
2. Schoffer J, Krebber HJ, Bleifeld W, Mathey DG (1982) Acute coronary artery occlusion during percutaneous transluminal coronary angioplasty: reopening by intracoronary streptokinase before emergency coronary artery surgery to prevent myocardial infarction. Circulation 66:1325
3. Ischinger T, Zack P, Aker U (1984) Acute coronary occlusion during balloon angioplasty due to intracoronary thrombosis and coronary spasm: a reversible complication. Am Heart J 107:1271–1275
4. Hollman J, Austin GE, Gruentzig AR, Douglas JS Jr, King SB III (1983) Coronary artery spasm at the site of angioplasty in the first two months after successful percutaneous transluminal coronary angioplasty. J Am Coll Cardiol 2:1039–1045
5. David PR, Waters DD, Scholl JM, Crepeau J, Szlachcic J, Lesperance J, Hudon G, Bourassa MG (1982) Percutaneous transluminal coronary angioplasty in patients with variant angina. Circulation 66:695–702
6. Holmes DR, Vlietstra RE, Smith HC et al. (1984) Restenosis after percutaneous transluminal coronary angioplasty (PTCA): a report from the PTCA registry of the National Heart, Lung, and Blood Institute. Am J Cardiol 53:77C–81C
7. Grunwald J, Handenschild CC (1984) Intimal injury in vivo activates vascular muscle cell migration and explant outgrowth in vitro. Arteriosclerosis 4:183–188
8. Essed CE, Van den Brand M, Becker AE (1983) Transluminal coronary angioplasty and early restenosis. Fibrocellular occlusion after wall laceration. Br Heart J 49:393–396
9. Austin GE, Ratliff NB, Hollman J, Tabei S, Phillips DF (to be published) Myofibroblastic intimal proliferation as an explanation for recurrent coronary artery stenosis following percutaneous transluminal coronary angioplasty. J Am Coll Cardiol
10. Bulkley BH, Hutchin GM (1977) Accelerated atherosclerosis: a morphologic study of 97 saphenous vein coronary artery bypass grafts. Circulation 55:163–169
11. Smith SH, Geer JC (1983) Morphology of saphenous vein-coronary artery bypass grafts. Arch Pathol Lab Med 107:13–18
12. Hollman J, Gruentzig AR, King SB III, Douglas JS Jr (1984) Percutaneous transluminal coronary angioplasty. In: Hurst JW (ed) Essay on the heart. McGraw-Hill, New York, pp 297–315
13. Hollman J, Gruentzig AR, Meier B, Ischinger T, King SB III, Douglas JS Jr, Galan K (to be published) Recurrent stenosis following successful percutaneous transluminal coronary angioplasty. Circulation
14. Loop FD, Golding LR, MacMillian JP, Cosgrove DM, Lytle BW, Sheldon WC (1983) Coronary artery surgery in women compared with men: analysis of risks and long-term result. J Am Coll Cardiol 1:383–390

15. Douglas JS Jr, King SB III, Jones EL, Craver JM, Bradford JM, Hatcher CR (1981) Reduced efficacy of coronary bypass surgery in women. Circulation [Suppl II]:11–16
16. Orekhov AN, Kosykh VA, Repin VN, Smirnov VN (1983) Cell proliferation in normal and atherosclerotic human aorta. Lab Invest 48:749–754
17. David PR, Rankin J, Moise A, Dangoisse V, Val PG, Bourassa MG (1984) Can patient selection and optimization of technique reduce the rate of restenosis after percutaneous transluminal coronary angioplasty? J Am Coll Cardiol 3:470 (abstract)
18. Leimgruber PP, Roubin GS, Rice CR, Tate JM, Gruentzig AR (1984) Influence of intimal dissection after coronary angioplasty (PTCA) on restenosis rate. Circulation 70(II):174
19. Douglas JS Jr, Gruentzig AR, King SB III, Hollman J, Ischinger T, Meier B, Craver JM, Jones EL, Waller JL, Bone DK, Guyton R (1983) Percutaneous transluminal coronary angioplasty in patients with prior coronary bypass surgery. J Am Coll Cardiol 2:745
20. Thornton MA, Gruentzig AR, Hollman J, King SB III, Douglas JS Jr (1984) Coumadin and aspirin in the prevention of recurrence after transluminal coronary angioplasty: a randomized study. Circulation 69:721–727
21. Faxon DP, Sanborn TA, Handenschild CC, Ryan TJ (1984) Effect of antiplatelet therapy on restenosis after experimental angioplasty. Am J Cardiol 53:72C–76C
22. Faxon DP, Sanborn TA, Weber VJ, Handenschild C, Gottsman SB, McGovern WA, Ryan TJ (1984) Restenosis following transluminal angioplasty in experimental atherosclerosis. Atherosclerosis 4:189–195
23. Pasternak RC, Baughman KL, Fallon JT, Block PC (1980) Scanning electron microscopy after coronary transluminal angioplasty of normal canine coronary arteries. Am J Cardiol 45:591
24. Williams DO, Gruentzig AR, Kent KM, Detre KM, Kelsey SF, To T (1984) Efficacy of repeat percutaneous transluminal coronary angioplasty for coronary restenosis. Am J Cardiol 53:32C–35C
25. Ischinger T, Gruentzig AR, Hollman J, King SB III, Douglas J, Bradford J (1983) Should coronary arteries with less than 60% diameter stenosis be treated with angioplasty? Circulation 68:148–154
26. Campeau L, Enjalbert M, Lesperance J, Vaislic C, Grondin CM, Bourassa MG (1983) Atherosclerosis and late closure of aortocoronary saphenous vein grafts: sequential angiographic studies at two weeks, one year, five to seven years, and 10 to 12 years after surgery. Circulation [Suppl II] 68:1–7
27. Walker JA, Friedberg HD, Flemma RJ et al. (1977) Determinants of angiographic patency of aortocoronary vein bypass grafts. Circulation [Suppl II] 11–18
28. Roth JA, Cukingnan RA, Braun BG (1979) Factors influencing patency of saphenous vein grafts. Ann Thorac Surg 28:176–183
29. Cheseboro JH, Fuster V, Elveback LR (1984) Effect of dipyridamole and aspirin on late vein graft patency after coronary bypass operations. N Engl J Med 310:209–214
30. Corcos T, David PR, Renkin J, Dangoisse V, Guiteras P, Rapold H, Bourassa MG (1984) A randomized trial of diltiazem for prevention of restenosis after percutaneous transluminal coronary angioplasty (PTCA). Circulation 70(II):175

Chapter 13. Complications Associated with PTCA

GERALD DORROS, and MICHAEL COWLEY

Introduction

Percutaneous transluminal coronary angioplasty (PTCA) has proven to be a safe and effective treatment of selected patients with coronary artery occlusive disease. Initially, PTCA was used to treat proximal, isolated coronary stenosis in patients with single-vessel disease [1]. Subsequently, the technique of PTCA has been used as an investigative technique in patients with more complex coronary artery disease (e.g., when there is a history of prior bypass surgery, multivessel coronary disease, disease in geriatric patients, and disease necessitating multiple dilatations). In March 1979, the United States National Heart, Lung, and Blood Institute (NHLBI) established an international registry of PTCA patients. The purpose of the registry was to accumulate baseline and followup data to facilitate evaluation of the safety, effectiveness, and long-term outcome of this technique. In 1981, the initial report of the NHLBI PTCA Registry [2] discussed coronary angioplasty in general, and a subsequent communication in 1983 [3] concerned the complications occurring in the first 1500 patients enrolled in the Registry. The complication report was subsequently modified by reports [4–6] analyzing the complications which occurred in the 3079 patients from 105 contributing centers enrolled in the PTCA Registry. This communication will summarize the NHLBI PTCA Registry complications data, with particular emphasis on analysis of the acute coronary vascular and ischemic events, the inpatient mortality, and the patients who underwent emergency bypass surgery. The January through August 1984, Milwaukee coronary angioplasty experience provides information that contrasts with the PTCA Registry data collected between 1978 and 1982, and perhaps some insight into how the problems associated with the procedure have changed.

Methods

The NHLBI PTCA Registry and the methods of data collection and data analysis techniques have been described elsewhere [4–6]. The patients included all those who underwent angioplasty under the initial protocols and excluded patients covered by special protocols, e.g., in combination with streptokinase, or patients in cardiogenic shock. The definitions of complications were taken from the PTCA Manual of Operations [3]:

"Angina was classified using the Canadian Heart Association criteria. Prolonged angina was defined as chest pain persisting longer than usual, or angina unrelieved promptly with sublingual or intravenous nitroglycerine. A myocardial infarction was diagnosed when two of the following three criteria occurred: (1) prolonged chest pain, (2) electrocardiographic evidence of myocardial infarction (Minnesota code), or (3) creatine kinase or creatine kinase-MB elevation more than three times normal values. Intimal tear was defined by the presence of angiographically evident intimal damage producing either an intraluminal filling defect, extraluminal extravasation of contrast material, linear luminal density or luminal staining. Intimal tear was considered a complication of PTCA when it caused major luminal obstruction, was associated with coronary occlusion, myocardial infarction, or deterioration of coronary flow resulting in emergency bypass surgery, or resulted in termination of the procedure before completion. Coronary artery spasm was defined as transient vasoconstriction resulting in myocardial ischemia. Hypotension was defined as a decrease in systolic pressure >30 mmHg lasting more than 30 min and requiring therapy. Acute coronary events include coronary vascular and myocardial ischemic events. Coronary vascular events were coronary dissection, occlusion, spasm, embolism, perforation, and rupture. Myocardial ischemic events include myocardial infarction and prolonged angina." [4].

The patient mortality was evaluated in a more detailed manner: "Data were collected by each investigator who participated in the NHLBI Registry and were submitted to the data coordinating center. The baseline form contained detailed information about the patient's medical history and specific data about the PTCA procedure, including a section pertaining to complications. When a patient died during the hospitalization for PTCA, a detailed narrative summary of the patient's hospitalization was submitted in addition to the baseline form. These summaries were then distributed for review to all members of the Registry Steering Committee and were submitted to an independent committee of experts (not participating in the Registry) for review and comment." [5)

Mortality rates by baseline characteristics of the patients and characteristics of the lesions attempted were calculated to discover risk factors for mortality. Chi-square tests, a univariate analysis, and a stepwise multivariable regression were used to determine factors significantly associated with mortality.

"Emergency surgery was defined as the need for urgent operation due to complications during or after PTCA. Surgery after PTCA was classified as emergency or elective by the physician performing the procedure at each institution. The baseline records of patients reported as having emergency surgery were reviewed by one of us to determine the indication for surgery in each patient. The primary complication was defined for this analysis as either the only complication reported or the probable cause of any associated complications when multiple complications were recorded. A hierarchichal system was used to determine the probable cause with multiple complications: dissection, spasm, occlusion and prolonged angina, that is, if dissection and occlusion were both reported, dissection was considered to represent the probable cause of occlusion and was classified as the primary complication." [6]

Table 1. Characteristics of the patient population

1. No. of patients	3079	
a) Males	2374	77%
b) Females	705	23%
2. Age (mean, years)	53.5	
3. Prior myocardial infarction	770	25%
4. Elderly (65 years and older)	370	12%
5. Prior bypass surgery	277	9%
6. Angina		
a) Unstable	2063	67%
b) Class III (CHC)	1139	37%
c) Class IV (CHC)	801	26%
7. Extent of coronary disease		
a) Single vessel	2386	77.5%
b) Multivessel	693	22.5%
c) Left main	77	2.5%
8. Lesion size ≧90% diameter stenosis	1078	35%
9. Multiple angioplasty attempts	246	8%
10. Vessels attempted		
a) LAD	1992	63%
b) RCA	820	26%
c) LCX	223	7%
d) SVG	116	4%

CHC, Canadian Heart Classification for severity of angina; LAD, left anterior descending coronary artery; RCA, right coronary artery; LCX, left circumflex coronary artery; SVG, saphenous vein bypass graft

Clinical Characteristics

The baseline clinical characteristics of the patients are shown in Table 1, which includes data which have been shown to be relevant to the procedure.

Results

Complications were encountered in 652 patients (21%) and a total of 1180 complications were reported during hospitalization. The types and frequencies of complications are listed in Table 2. The acute coronary vascular or ischemic events with which we are concerned occurred in 418 patients, with a total of 830 incidents reported. The most frequent complications encountered were prolonged angina, myocardial infarction, coronary occlusion, coronary dissection, and coronary spasm. Acute coronary events occurred more frequently, utilizing a univariate analysis, in women ($P<0.01$), in patients with unstable angina ($P<0.01$), with initial lesion severity ≧90% diameter stenosis ($P<0.01$), with eccentric lesions ($P<0.05$), with lesions of nondiscrete morphologic aspects ($P<0.01$), and with tubular lesions ($P<0.01$). According to multivariate analysis, increased frequency was associated with unstable angina ($P<0.001$), more severe stenosis ($P<0.01$), lesions of nondiscrete morphologic aspects ($P<0.01$), and tubular lesions ($P<0.05$).

Table 2. Complications of PTCA in 652 patients

Complications	Episodes
A. Acute coronary events (418 pts, 830 events)	
1. Prolonged angina	236 (20.0%)
2. Myocardial infarction	170 (14.4%)
3. Coronary occlusion	151 (12.8%)
4. Coronary dissection	135 (11.4%)
5. Coronary spasm	130 (11.0%)
6. Coronary embolism	5
7. Coronary perforation	2
8. Coronary rupture	1
B. Noncoronary events (234 pts)	
1. Ventricular fibrillation	57
2. Hypotension	47
3. Bradycardia	43
4. Hospital death	29
5. Ventricular tachycardia	23
6. Vascular problems	22
7. Excessive blood loss	17
8. Other[a]	110
Total	1178

[a] Conduction defects, central nervous system events, minor arrhythmias, coronary branch injury, pulmonary embolism, allergic reactions, pulmonary edema, respiratory arrest, febrile episode, transient hypotension, nausea, minor bleeding, impending infarction

Major complications were seen in 289 patients (9.4%) and included nonfatal myocardial infarction ($n=154$; 5.0%), emergency coronary bypass surgery without death or infarction ($n=106$; 3.4%), and death in hospital ($n=29$; 0.9%). Major complications (nonfatal myocardial infarction, emergency coronary bypass surgery, or death) occurred in 197 of the 323 patients (62%) who had acute coronary vascular incidents. These accounted for 68% of all major complications.

Acute Coronary Events

Myocardial Infarction

There were 170 myocardial infarctions (5.5%), and 110 (65%) of these were classified as definite; 67 infarctions (39%) occurred in the catheterization laboratory, 85 (50%) within 24 h after PTCA, and 18 (11%) between 24 h and 1 week after PTCA. Myocardial infarction occurred in 90 of 202 patients (45%) who underwent emergency bypass surgery, in 21 of 583 patients (3.6%) who had elective bypass surgery, and in 59 of 2294 patients (2.6%) who did not undergo bypass surgery.

In 16 patients (9.4%) myocardial infarction was fatal: 7 patients had the infarction in the catheterization laboratory; 6 patients, within 24 h of PTCA; and 3 patients, between 24 h and 1 week after PTCA. Fatal myocardial infarction occurred in 7 patients (6.4%) who had emergency surgery and in 4 patients who did not undergo surgery. Two deaths related to an acute myocardial infarction occurred within the catheterization laboratory.

The primary complications associated with the occurrence of a myocardial infarction were coronary dissection in 58 patients (34%), coronary occlusion in 36 patients (21%), prolonged angina in 24 patients (14%), and coronary spasm in 9 patients (5.3%).

Coronary Dissection

A coronary dissection or intimal tear (remote or distal from the lesion) was present in 397 patients (12.9%) undergoing PTCA. Coronary artery dissection was a complication of PTCA in 135 of the 397 patients (34%) with 60 patients having an associated occlusion. A major complication occurred in 120 of the 397 coronary dissection patients (30%): nonfatal infarction in 60 patients (15%), emergency bypass surgery in 92 patients (23%), and death in 6 patients (1.5%). No major adverse effect was encountered in the 277 patients (70%) with a tear or dissection. PTCA was successful in 218 of the 397 patients (51%), and in 218 of the 277 patients (79%) who did not have any adverse side effects.

Univariate and multivariate analysis showed that an intimal tear or coronary dissection was more likely to occur in women ($P<0.001$), in patients undergoing right coronary artery PTCA ($P<0.001$), in patients with multivessel disease ($P<0.01$), with eccentric lesions ($P<0.01$), and with nondiscrete lesions ($P<0.05$).

Coronary Occlusion

Coronary occlusion was reported in 151 patients (4.9%) after PTCA. A major complication occurred in 122 of these patients (81%): 62 (41%) had a myocardial infarction, 108 (72%) required emergency surgery, and 8 (5.3%) suffered death in hospital. However, 29 patients who had a coronary occlusion did not suffer a major complication, with only 15 patients subsequently undergoing elective surgery. Univariate analysis showed that predictors of coronary occlusion included onset of angina within 6 months ($P<0.05$), eccentric lesions ($P<0.01$), lesion severity >90% ($P<0.05$), and tubular or nondiscrete lesions ($P<0.01$).

Coronary Spasm

Coronary spasm occurred in 130 patients (4.2%) and was associated with a major complication in 41 of the 130 patients (32%): 16 (12%) had a nonfatal myocardial infarction, 31 (24%) required emergency bypass surgery, and 4 (3%) died in hospital. No adverse side effects occurred in 89 patients (68%). PTCA was successful in 51 of these 130 patients (39%). Isolated coronary spasm (i.e., not associated with either dissection or occlusion) occurred in 101 patients (78%) and was associated with a major complication in 18 patients (18%): 8 (8%) had a nonfatal myocardial infarction, 11 (11%) required emergency bypass surgery, and 2 (2%) died.

Analysis showed that spasm was more likely to occur with noncalcified lesions ($P<0.01$) and at a younger age ($P<0.05$).

Prolonged Angina

Prolonged angina was the most frequent complication reported, with 236 episodes occurring in 211 patients (6.8%): 18 episodes occurred in the catheterization laboratory. Prolonged angina was associated with major complications in 114 of 211 patients (54%): 57 (27%) had nonfatal myocardial infarctions, 90 (43%) required emergency bypass surgery, and 11 (5%) died. No major complications occurred in 97 patients (40%) with prolonged angina. PTCA was successful in 46 of the prolonged angina patients (22%). Prolonged angina not initially associated with a myocardial infarction or occlusion occurred in 115 patients, 96 of whom had a dissection or coronary spasm, and was associated with or resulted in a major complication in 40 patients (35%): 21 of these patients (18%) had a nonfatal myocardial infarction, 29 (25%) required emergency surgery, and 6 (5%) died. PTCA was successful in 37 of these 115 patients (32%).

Analysis (univariate) showed that prolonged angina was more likely to occur in the presence of unstable angina ($P<0.01$) or class IV angina ($P<0.01$), in the absence of previous myocardial infarction ($P<0.01$), with lesion severity >90% ($P<0.01$), and with lesion eccentricity ($P<0.05$).

Table 3. Predictors of coronary vascular and ischemic incidents. [3]

Variable	Complication	*P* Value
1. Clinical		
a) Younger age	a) Coronary spasm	<0.05
b) Female sex	b) Dissection	<0.05
c) No previous myocardial infarction	c) Prolonged angina	<0.05
d) Unstable angina	d) Any coronary incident	<0.01
	Coronary vascular incident	<0.05
	Prolonged angina	<0.05
	Myocardial infarction	<0.05
2. Angiographic		
a) Right coronary attempt	a) Dissection	<0.05
b) Greater lesion severity	b) Any coronary incident	<0.01
c) Eccentric lesion	c) Dissection	<0.01
	Coronary occlusion	<0.01
d) Nondiscrete lesion	d) Any coronary incident	<0.01
	Coronary vascular incident	<0.01
	Coronary occlusion	<0.01
e) Tubular lesion	e) Coronary vascular incident	<0.01
	Any coronary incident	<0.05
	Coronary occlusion	<0.05

Table 3 lists the clinical and angiographic predictors of coronary vascular and ischemic events.

Inpatient Mortality

The baseline characteristics of the 29 patients who died during hospitalization for PTCA are shown in Table 4 [4]. Twenty-nine patients (16 males and 13 females) died during the stay in hospital during which coronary angioplasty was attempted. Nineteen deaths (0.6%) were considered to be related to the PTCA procedure. Eighteen patients (0.8%) with single-vessel disease died, including 2 of 80 patients (2.5%) with prior bypass surgery (Table 5). Eight patients (1.0%) with multivessel disease died, including 3 of 162 patients (2.5%) with prior bypass surgery. Twenty patients without prior bypass surgery died (0.7%): 16 had single-vessel disease, 4 had multivessel disease, and 1 had left main coronary artery disease. Eight patients had prior bypass surgery (2.9%): 2 had single-vessel disease, 4 had multivessel disease, and 2 had left main coronary disease.

The complications encountered in each case are listed in Table 6 [4]. The incidence of complications occurring in the mortality group did not differ from the group of Registry patients who experienced at least one complication, except for the increased incidence of ventricular tachycardia, ventricular fibrillation, and prolonged hypotension among the patients who died. Analysis of the 29 inpatient deaths revealed that 19 were related (attributable) to PTCA, and 10 were not. The related problems included coronary occlusion (partial/total), acute myocardial infarction, coronary spasm, omission of anticoagulation, guiding catheter dissection of the left main coronary artery, emergency coronary artery bypass surgery in an unstable patient, and persistent hypotension after calcium antagonist administration. The unrelated problems included disseminated intravascular coagulopathy after successful bypass surgery, complications of coronary bypass surgery including technically difficult repeat elective surgery, postoperative vein graft occlusion, intestinal obstruction sepsis after bypass surgery, and perioperative myocardial infarction.

Clinical characteristics that had a demonstrable effect upon the mortality rates included gender (female, 1.8% mortality; male, 0.7% mortality), patient age (patients >60 years, 1.7% mortality; patients <60 years 0.7% mortality), and duration of angina (mortality rate increased from 0.5% when angina had been present for less than 6 months to 1.7% when angina had been present for over 1 year).

A stratified analysis of the extent of coronary artery disease, i.e., looking at single-vessel, multivessel, and left main coronary artery disease, showed that only the presence of left main coronary artery disease was a significant risk factor ($P<0.01$) (Table 5) [4]. In addition, prior bypass surgery significantly increased the mortality rate within each group, and is a statistically significant risk factor.

The mortality rate differed with the site of the lesion for which treatment was attempted. However, only a trend could be observed, in that the mortality rates in patients with circumflex or left main artery lesions were higher at 2.2% and 2.3%, respectively, than the 0.8% for the left anterior descending and right cor-

Table 4. In-hospital mortality by baseline characteristics. [4]

	Patients who died ($n=29$)	Registry (%) ($n=3079$)
1. Patients		
a) Male*	55% (16)	77% (2374)
b) Female	45% (13)	23% (705)
2. Average age (years)	58.5	53.5
3. Anginal classification		
a) Class 0	3.4% (1)	5.6%
b) Class I	0 (0)	3.8%
c) Class II	24.1% (7)	27.7%
d) Class III	41.4% (12)	37.1%
e) Class IV	31.0% (9)	25.8%
4. Previous myocardial infarction	34.5% (10)	25.0%
5. Overall mortality	0.9% (29/3079)[a]	
a) Related to PTCA	0.6% (19/3079)	
b) Probably not related to PTCA	0.3% (10/3079)	
6. Clinical characteristics		
a) Gender*		
I) Male	0.7 (16/2374)	
II) Female	1.8% (13/ 705)	
b) Age*		
I) ≧60 years	1.7% (14/ 814)	
II) <60 years	0.7% (15/2265)	
c) Duration of angina**		
I) <6 months	0.5% (9/1701)	
II) 6–12 months	1.1% (6/ 504)	
III) ≧12 months	1.7% (1/ 135)	
IV) Unknown	0.7% (1/ 135)	
d) Previous CABG*		
I) Yes	2.9% (8/ 278)	
II) No	0.8% (21/2801)	
e) Previous CABG and graft attempt		
I) Previous CABG and native artery attempt	3.0% (5/ 169)	
II) Previous CABG and graft attempt	2.8% (3/ 109)	
f) Previous myocardial infarction		
I) Yes	1.3% (10/ 768)	
II) No	0.8% (19/2311)	
g) Vessel disease (≧50% stenosis)		
I) Single	0.8% (18/2233)	
II) Multiple	1.0% (8/ 768)	
III) Left main*	3.8% (3/ 78)	
h) Time since first episode of chest pain**		
I) < 6 months	0.5% (9/1701)	
II) ≦12 months but >6 months	1.1% (6/ 504)	
III) >12 months	1.7% (13/ 749)	
IV) Unknown or no chest pain	0.7% (1/ 135)	

* $P<0.01$
** $P<0.05$
[a] Number of mortality group out of total number of this group within the Registry
PTCA, percutaneous transluminal coronary angioplasty; CABG, coronary artery bypass graft surgery

Table 5. In-hospital mortality rate and its relation to coronary disease. [4]

	Mortality group ($n=29$)	Registry ($n=3079$)
1. Extent of coronary artery disease		
a) Single	62.1% (189)	72.5%
b) Multiple	27.6% (8)	25.0%
c) Left main*	10.3% (3)	2.5%
2. Previous coronary bypass graft surgery	27.6% (8)	9.0%
3. Vessel distribution of single lesion attempts*		
a) LAD	53.6% (15)	64.2%
b) RCA	17.9% (5)	25.0%
c) LCX	14.3% (4)	6.0%
d) SVG	10.7% (3)	3.5%
e) LMCA	3.6% (1)	1.3%
4. Patients with multiple lesion attempts	3.4% (1)	7.6%
5. Extent of coronary artery disease[b]		
a) Single	0.8% (18/2231)[a]	
I) Without previous CABG	0.7% (16/2151)	
II) With previous CABG	2.5% (2/ 80)	
b) Multivessel	1.0% (8/ 768)	
I) Without previous CABG	0.7% (4/ 607)	
II) With previous CABG	2.5% (4/ 162)	
c) Left main*	3.8% (3/ 78)	
I) Without previous CABG	2.4% (1/ 42)	
II) With previous CABG	5.6% (2/ 36)	
6. Mortality rate according to vessel attempted		
a) LAD	0.8% (15/1953)	
b) RCA	0.8% (6/ 792)	
c) LCX	2.2% (4/ 181)	
d) LMCA	2.3% (1/ 44)	
e) SVG**	2.8% (3/ 109)	
7. Mortality rate according to lesion severity		
a) ≧90% diameter stenosis	0.9% (16/1721)	
b) <90% diameter stenosis	1.0% (13/1358)	

* $P<0.01$; ** $P<0.05$
[a] Number of mortality group out of total number of this group within the Registry
[b] Within each disease category previous CABG is a significant risk factor
CABG, coronary atery bypass graft surgery; LAD, left anterior descending coronary artery; RCA, right coronary artery; LCX, left circumflex coronary artery; LMCA, left main coronary artery; SVG, saphenous vein bypass graft

onary artery lesions. Only with an attempt at dilating a saphenous vein graft lesion was the mortality rate significantly increased ($P<0.05$) compared with that for other sites attempted.

The presence of left main coronary disease was a significant risk factor; however, the dilatation of a left main lesion is not a statistically significant risk factor, although a trend was present. Thus, whenever left main coronary artery disease is present the risk of dying is increased regardless of the site dilated.

Factors found to have no influence upon the inpatient mortality rates included lesion severity, history of diabetes, history of elevated cholesterol levels, unstable angina pectoris, Canadian Heart Association anginal classification, le-

Table 6. In-hospital mortality: complications. [4]

	Mortality group	Registry[a]	Registry
	($n=29$)	($n=652$)	($n=3079$)
1. Occurring in laboratory			
a) Prolonged angina	11 (38.0%)	(27.6%)	211 (6.8%)
b) Coronary occlusion	8 (27.6%)	(21.8%)	151 (4.9%)
c) Ventricular tachycardia or fibrillation	11 (38.0%)	(9.0%)	72 (2.9%)
d) Prolonged hypotension	10 (34.0%)	(5.5%)	46 (1.5%)
e) Coronary dissection	6 (24.1%)	(19.2%)	135 (4.1%)
f) Coronary spasm	4 (13.8%)	(19.8%)	130 (4.2%)
g) Myocardial infarction	16 (55.0%)		170 (6.0%)
2. CABG			
a) Emergency bypass surgery	13 (44.8%)	–	202 (6.4%)
b) Elective bypass surgery	11 (37.9%)	–	583 (1.9%)

[a] Registry patients who had at least one complication

Table 7. In-hospital complications in 202 patients undergoing emergency coronary artery bypass surgery. [5]

Complication	No.
1. Coronary occlusion	108
2. Coronary dissection	93
3. Prolonged angina	92
4. Myocardial infarction	90
5. Coronary spasm	31
6. Hypotension	19
7. Ventricular fibrillation	17
8. Bradycardia	13
9. Death	13
10. Other	27
Total	503

sion calcifications, previous myocardial infarction, and geometric or morphologic aspects of the lesion.

One or more complications of PTCA or of bypass surgery preceded each death. Clearly, the mortality rates were higher when associated with certain complications, affecting 16 of 170 myocardial infarction patients (9.4%), 10 of 46 patients with prolonged hypotension (21.7%), and 11 of 72 patients with ventricular tachycardia or fibrillation (15.3%). The mortality rate was 6.4% for patients undergoing emergency bypass surgery, as against 1.9% for patients undergoing elective bypass surgery.

Factors that were predictive of the occurrence of death were lesion location, age, sex, time since onset of chest pain, previous bypass surgery, and number of vessels diseased. Older age, particularly in men, and female gender had adverse effects on survival. The history of prior bypass surgery, the longer the time since the first onset of chest pain, and the presence of left main coronary artery disease were additional independent risk factors. A multivariate analysis differed from the univariate analysis since it confirmed only that female gender was significantly associated with PTCA-related deaths.

Emergency Coronary Bypass Surgery After PTCA

Emergency coronary bypass surgery was performed in 202 of the 3079 patients (6.6%) who underwent attempts at dilatation of 216 lesions. Twelve patients (5.9%) underwent multiple dilatations. Initial angiographic success was achieved in 57 lesions (26%) in 52 patients (26%). Angioplasty was unsuccessful in 178 patients (88%): the lesion could not be reached or crossed in 117 patients and could not be dilated once crossed in 61 patients. In all, 503 complications were reported in these 202 patients (Table 7) [5]. Emergency bypass surgery was performed within 24 h in 200 patients (99%).

The indications for emergency surgery based upon the primary complication are listed in Table 8 [5], with the most frequent problem being coronary dissection in 93 patients (46%). A major complication occurred in 96 patients (47%) who underwent emergency surgery: 90 patients had a myocardial infarction (45%), (Table 9), 83 being nonfatal (41%) and 7 fatal infarctions (3.5%). Thirteen patients (6.4%) died after emergency bypass surgery.

A coronary occlusion was present in 108 patients (53%) who underwent emergency bypass surgery, and was the primary complication in 41 of these patients. Patients who suffered a coronary occlusion and underwent emergency bypass surgery still had significant major complications: 49 of the 108 (45%) had a myocardial infarction, and 6 of the 108 (5.6%) died. Forty-nine patients with an acute coronary occlusion developed myocardial infarction: 32 (65%) of these infarcts occurred immediately (i.e., in the catheterization laboratory), 12 (25%) within 24 h of PTCA, and 5 (10%) between 24 h and 1 week of PTCA.

A coronary dissection was the primary complication occurring in 93 patients who underwent emergency bypass surgery after PTCA. The coronary dissection was not associated with coronary occlusion or coronary spasm in 33 patients (35%), and was associated with occlusion in 51 (55%), with spasm in 5 (5%), and spasm and occlusion in 4 (4%). Nonfatal infarction occurred in 33 patients (36%)

Table 8. Indications for emergency surgery. [5]

Primary complication	No.	%
1. Dissection	93	46
2. Occlusion	41	20
3. Prolonged angina	28	14
4. Coronary spasm	22	11
5. Myocardial infarction	10	5
6. Other	8	4
Total	202	100

and death in 5 patients (5.4%). No major postoperative problems occurred in 54 patients (59%).

Thirteen patients who required emergency surgery died in hospital. The most frequent primary complications in these patients were coronary dissection, coronary occlusion, and myocardial infarction.

The clinical hospital discharge status was reported in 175 of the 202 patients (87%), including the 13 inpatient deaths. Of these, 154 were clinically improved, 5 were unchanged, and 3 were worse.

Univariate analysis of baseline characteristics revealed an increase in the frequency of emergency surgery with eccentric lesions ($P<0.01$), nondiscrete lesions ($P<0.01$), and severe lesions (>90% stenosis) ($P<0.05$). Multivariate analysis showed that lesion eccentricity was the only predictor ($P<0.001$) of increased frequency of emergency bypass surgery. Clinical profiles are shown in Table 10.

Certain procedural difficulties, e.g., inability to pass the stenosis ($P<0.001$) and inability to dilate the lesion once traversed ($P<0.001$) were associated with an increased likelihood of emergency surgery. An additional factor that influenced the frequency of emergency surgery was investigator experience: the probability of emergency bypass surgery was 7% for an operator's first case, and 4% for his/her 150th case.

Discussion

The NHLBI PTCA Registry is the largest source of published data concerning coronary angioplasty. The statistics were provided by more than 100 centers and provide a broad-based view of the angioplasty procedure, even though the majority of interventions were performed in approximately 15 centers (or by 15 investigators). The PTCA Registry data provide insight into the coronary angioplasty procedure: the selection of patients, the determinants of a successful procedure, and the factors associated with the development of complications. Review of the Registry data enables an investigator to acquire a fundamental knowledge of the coronary angioplasty procedure, avoid certain pitfalls and, thereby, without having to reproduce the past, maximize the number of successes and minimize the incidence of complications. These data must always be viewed with reference to the fact that they represent the very earliest experience with angioplasty, and do not represent the current incidence of success or of complications with the technique in the hands of experienced operators in 1984. Clearly, the experienced operator using present-day angioplasty equipment including the low-profiled steerable dilatation catheters and improved fluoroscopic imaging, and with much more experience, has made tremendous strides not only in successful performance of the coronary angioplasty procedure and lowering of the complication rates, but also in achieving these results in difficult and complex cases which would have never even been considered for coronary angioplasty during the time of PTCA Registry data collection.

Table 11 shows the Milwaukee coronary angioplasty experience during the first 8 months of 1984. The data represent all cases who underwent coronary

Table 9. Electrocardiographic criteria for infarction with emergency surgery. [5]

Classification of Infarction	No.	%
1. Definite (Q wave)	52	58
2. Definite (ST wave)	9	10
3. Probable (Q or ST wave)	15	17
4. None of the above	10	11
5. Unknown	4	4
Total	90	100

angioplasty (author G. D.), and includes patients in cardiogenic shock, with advanced renal insufficiency, impending myocardial infarction, and severe chronic obstructive lung disease, and patients who were not considered candidates for myocardial revascularization. The patient baseline characteristics, dilatation data, and incidences of complications are presented. Coronary angioplasty is a dynamic procedure, which has been in a constant state of flux since its inception; comparison of these data should remain circumspect. But perhaps the Milwaukee coronary angioplasty experience, when compared with the PTCA Registry experience, can provide some insight into an evolving technique. Despite the more varied patient sample within the Milwaukee series undergoing angioplasty, the incidence of major complications was low: zero mortality, a 1.3% incidence of emergency surgery, and a 3.1% occurrence of a myocardial infarction. The three patients with subendocardial infarction developed it secondary to coronary embolization of atherosclerotic material in old (≧4 years) saphenous vein grafts which underwent dilatation. All patients had angiographically successful dilatation and were discharged from the hospital clinically improved. Thus, the overall incidence of significant major complications was low: 1.3% incidence of emergency surgery, and 1.8% occurrence of transmural myocardial infarction. One patient suffered a transmural infarction despite emergency surgery. In addition, whereas the incidence of complications occurring in the Registry's patient was 21%, the 1984 Milwaukee experience indicated that only 13% of patients experienced any complication, no matter how minor.

The PTCA Registry data indicate that the development of acute coronary events (vascular and ischemic) will be associated with a major complication (myocardial infarction, death, or emergency surgery) in approximately 60% of these patients. The frequency of major complications occurring with any specific event varied, but was quite high with the occurrence of a coronary occlusion (81%) and coronary dissection (89%). The probable reason for the absence of a major complication in nearly 20% of the coronary occlusion patients is that only a small branch vessel was occluded or significant collaterals were present. The term coronary dissection is difficult to define, since angiographic evidence of intimal disruption or intimal tear is present in a sizable proportion of patients undergoing angioplasty. Nearly two-thirds of these dissection patients had no problems associated with this angiographic finding and underwent angiographically successful dilatations. The distinction between a coronary dissection indicating a complication and an intimal tear as an angiographic finding is perhaps arbitrary, and in fact it may only be possible to differentiate them on the basis of the functional outcome. Thus, further analysis of the angiographic changes occurring with angioplasty appears justified and necessary.

Coronary spasm and prolonged angina were associated with a lower incidence of major complications, and a successful outcome was recorded in 51% and 32% of cases, respectively.

The incidence and nature of development of myocardial infarction is extremely interesting. The majority of patients had their myocardial infarction within the first 24 h after angioplasty. The mortality rate within this group was high (6.4%) and should be noted. These data have modified our attitude towards the use of emergency bypass surgery, with its own high mortality (6.4%), and the preferential use of intra-aortic balloon counterpulsation. Although the degree of success achieved with percutaneous intra-aortic balloon pump counterpulsation to attain hemodynamic stabilization and amelioration of myocardial ischemia remains to be validated in these circumstances, this nevertheless remains our primary mode of therapy, rather than indiscriminate performance of bypass surgery. However, acute occlusion of a major vessel is usually considered to warrant emergency surgery, unless concomitant medical problems would prohibitively increase the risks this surgery involves.

Certain patient characteristics were associated with an increased occurrence of acute coronary ischemic incidents, and especially unstable angina or severe ste-

Table 10. Clinical profiles of patients undergoing emergency surgery and of the total population. [5]

	Emergency surgery %	Total group %
1. Age (years)	54	54
2. Men	77	77
3. Angina class III or IV	64	63
4. Unstable angina	42	40
5. Symptom duration		
a) <6 months	64	58
b) 6–12 months	18	17
c) >12 months	18	25
6. Single-vessel disease	77	75
7. Multivessel disease	23	24
8. Left main disease	0	1
9. Previous bypass	5	9
10. PTCA vessel		
a) LAD	69	64
b) RCA	26	26
c) LCX	3	6
d) SVG	2	4

PTCA, percutaneous transluminal coronary angioplasty; LAD, left anterior descending coronary artery; LCX, left circumflex coronary artery; RCA, right coronary artery; SVG, saphenous vein bypass graft noses. There was an increased frequency of prolonged angina and of subsequent development of myocardial infarction in unstable angina patients. This association is not surprising. The angiographic features associated with an increased incidence of coronary events were tubular, nondiscrete, and eccentric lesions. These angiographic features are probably no longer so significant now that the steerable dilatation catheters are used exclusively. However, these factors were significant during the time of data collection, since only nonsteerable equipment was available. The lesion eccentricity and the diffuse nature of the stenosis were real obstacles, which can now be overcome with appropriate fluoroscopic visualization, isolation of the lesion, use of the kissing balloon technique when indicated, and careful guidewire manipulation.

The experience of the interventional angiographer can never be overlooked or dismissed. The incidence of acute coronary ischemic and vascular events [4], total complications [3], and emergency bypass surgery [6] were inversely related to investigator experience. Table 11 makes this point clearly despite the complexity of the cases treated. These Milwaukee patients, when compared with those of the Registry, had more extensive coronary disease, a higher incidence of prior bypass surgery, and a higher incidence of documented prior myocardial infarction. Nevertheless, 95% of the lesions attempted were successfully dilated, 87% of the patients experienced no complication (major or minor) during the procedure, and the major complications encountered included a 1.8% incidence of transmural myocardial infarction and required emergency surgery in 1.3% of cases. Thus, investigator experience and technological advances have enabled coronary angioplasty to be performed with a gratifying success rate and a low complication rate.

Early in the experience of coronary angioplasty, emergency surgery was something that was utilized whenever a significant complication occurred. Many factors led to this approach: (a) patients were primarily those with single-vessel disease, most often involving the left anterior descending artery, and with a significant amount of myocardium in jeopardy; (b) emergency surgery, performed immediately, could prevent the evolution of a myocardial infarction; (c) since a problem had been created, something must be done to solve that problem; and (d) the investigators' limited knowledge forced them to think along those lines. Clearly, the compromise of coronary blood flow by occlusion of a single vessel in the absence of contralateral collaterals will produce myocardial ischemia and will jeopardize myocardial tissue. Thus, the occurrence of an acute ischemic coronary incident as a result of compromise of coronary blood flow could lead to the performance of emergency surgery as a technique to overcome this problem. However, analysis of the inpatient mortality showed (a) that emergency surgery was associated with significant mortality, and (b) that nearly half the patients still evolved a myocardial infarction. Thus, the decision to perform emergency surgery must not be taken lightly. At present we attempt hemodynamic stabilization by means of drugs and intra-aortic balloon pump counterpulsation in the hope of partially ameliorating the ischemic syndrome, after which repeat angiography is performed to determine whether there is partial or complete occlusion. An attempt at repeat angioplasty to open the compromised vessel is then made, which is usually successful in more than two-thirds of cases, obviating the need for emer-

Table 11. Milwaukee experience with coronary angioplasty (January through August 1984)

	No.	(%)
I. Patient baseline characteristics		
1. Cases	226	
2. Patients	210	
a) Male	152	(72)
b) Female	58	(28)
3. Angina class III	44	(19)
4. Angina class IV	39	(17)
5. Successful cases	214	(95)
a) Single-vessel disease	100/104	(96)
b) Multivessel disease	114/122	(93)
6. Prior bypass surgery	53	(23)
7. Prior myocardial infarction	91	(40)
8. Impending infarction	15	(6.6)
9. Prior stroke	4	(1.8)
10. Severe renal disease	7	(3.9)
11. Severe obstructive lung disease	4	(1.8)
II. Dilatation data		
1. Attempted dilatation	338	
2. Success/lesion attempts	321/338	(95)
3. Mean degree of stenosis		
a) Before	84%	
b) After	17%	
4. Mean trans-stenotic gradient		
a) Before	38 mmHg	
b) After	7 mmHg	
5. Kissing balloon technique	5 cases	
6. Lesions attempted per case		
a) 1 only	62%	
b) 2	28%	
c) 3	6%	
d) 4	3%	
e) 5	1%	
III. Complications		
1. Cases with no complications	196	(87)
2. Deaths	0	
3. Emergency surgery	3	(1.3)
4. Myocardial infarction	7	(3.1)
a) Transmural	4	(1.8)
b) Subendocardial[a]	3	(1.3)
5. Ventricular tachycardia/fibrillation	4	(1.8)
6. Prolonged hypotension	4	(1.8)
7. Coronary dissection/occlusion	6	(2.7)
8. Coronary spasm	10	(4.4)
9. Coronary embolization	3	(1.3)
10. Prolonged angina	10	(4.4)
11. Stroke	0	–

[a] All three occurred secondary to embolization of atherosclerotic material in old saphenous vein grafts. All three patients were clinically improved at discharge, and PTCA was angiographically and clinically successful in each

gency surgery in these. As more complex anatomic cases underwent attempts at angioplasty (single or multiple dilatation attempts), and as individuals underwent angioplasty despite anticipated prohibitively high surgical morbidity and mortality rates, the realization dawned that perhaps medical (nonoperative) management of many acute ischemic coronary events could be safely performed and would involve lower morbidity and mortality despite the evolution of a myocardial infarction. Therefore, most acute ischemic coronary incidents related to angioplasty are now managed vigorously and nonoperatively. However, certain anatomic situations in which the proximal occlusion of a major vessel (the left anterior descending artery or right coronary artery) in a patient who has not had earlier bypass surgery will be managed by immediate insertion of the percutaneous intra-aortic balloon pump, hemodynamic stabilization, angiographic visualization, and an attempt to reopen the partial/total occlusion which, if unsuccessful may be followed by the performance of emergency bypass surgery. If the time taken for all these procedures, from the onset of the problem until achievement of cardiopulmonary bypass, is less than 2–3 h emergency surgery is performed. If the time goes beyond 3 h the patient is managed with drug treatment. Therefore, the relatively low incidence of emergency surgery, coupled with a fairly stable myocardial infarction rate, is in part an expression of this philosophical approach.

Prolonged hypotension and prolonged angina are treated with plasma expanders, medication (nitrites, calcium antagonists), hypertensive agents, and even intra-aortic balloon pump counterpulsation. The problem of intracoronary embolization seems more significant now than in the past. The intracoronary, or more accurately the intrasaphenous vein graft embolization of atherosclerosis and thrombotic material following angioplasty occurs in about 15% of these vein graft dilatations. Management of these patients includes the standard treatment for a subendocardial infarction as well as empirical utilization of heparin and occasionally intracoronary streptokinase. These patients will have a rise in the creatine kinase level and transient electrocardiographic changes.

All those of our patients who had this problem were clinically improved despite the occurrence of embolization, and were considered successful angioplasty cases.

The incidence of fatal complications reported in the PTCA Registry was not insignificant. Factors that adversely affected mortality were female gender, prior bypass surgery, presence of left main coronary artery disease, attempted dilatation of a vein graft stenosis, increasing duration of angina, and age over 60 years, especially in men. Clearly, the omission of anticoagulation can be avoided. Emergency surgery in a hemodynamically unstable patient is a situation that one hopes to avoid, but this is not always possible. Replacement of the original Teflon guide catheters by softer and more maneuverable guide catheter systems and the introduction of steerable dilatation catheter systems are important methodological improvements that have made the procedure safer and more successful.

Investigator experience, in conjunction with technological developments and improvements in methodology, has enabled great strides to be made in coronary angioplasty, dramatically increasing the success rate while simultaneously reducing the incidence of associated complications. However, as the boundaries of coronary angioplasty are expanded, despite investigator experience, methodological improvements, and technological advances, complications will continue to occur. By its very nature, this therapeutic procedure does not permit control of all the variables, so that problems are inevitable. The purpose of any review is to create an awareness of features and facts that will permit progress. There is no reason to repeat the past. Clearly, awareness of angioplasty's history so far, together with an investigator's experience, insight, and courage will allow angioplasty to play an increasingly significant role in the treatment of patients with coronary artery occlusive disease.

References

1. Gruentzig AR, Senning A, Siegenthaler WE (1979) Nonoperative dilatation of coronary artery stenosis. Percutaneous transluminal coronary angioplasty. N Engl J Med 301:61–68
2. Kent KM, Bentivoglio LG, Block PC, Cowley MJ, Dorros G, Gosselin AJ, Gruentzig A, Myler RK, Simpson J, Stertzer SH, Williams DO, Fisher L, Gillespie MJ, Mullin SM, Mock MB (1981) Percutaneous transluminal coronary angioplasty: report from the NHLBI registry. Am J Cardiol 47:2100–2020
3. Dorros G, Cowley MJ, Simpson J, Bentivoglio LG, Block PC, Bourassa M, Detre K, Gosselin AJ, Gruentzig AR, Kelsey SF, Kent KM, Mock MB, Mullin SM, Myler RK, Passamani ER, Stertzer SH, Williams DO (1983) Percutaneous transluminal coronary angioplasty: report of complications from the national heart, lung and blood institute PTCA registry. Circulation 67:723–730
4. Cowley MJ, Dorros G, Kelsey SF, Van Raden M, Detre KM (1984) Acute coronary events associated with percutaneous transluminal coronary angioplasty. Am J Cardiol 53:12C–16C
5. Dorros G, Cowley MJ, Janke L, Kelsey SF, Mullin SM, Van Raden M (1984) In-hospital mortality rate in the National Heart, Lung and Blood Institute Percutaneous Transluminal Coronary Angioplasty Registry. Am J Cardiol 53:17C–21C
6. Cowley MJ, Dorros G, Kelsey SF, Van Raden M, Detre KM (1984) Emergency coronary bypass surgery after coronary angioplasty: the national heart, lung and blood institute's percutaneous transluminal coronary angioplasty registry experience. Am J Cardiol 53:22C–26C

Chapter 14. The Role of the Cardiothoracic Surgeon in PTCA

George C. Kaiser, Lawrence R. McBride, and Thomas Ischinger

Introduction

The role of the cardiothoracic surgeon is to support the invasive cardiologist when PTCA is performed, a reversal of the relationship which they usually enjoy in the management of patients with ischemic heart disease. It is necessary to have surgical expertise available to manage PTCA complications should they occur. The most frequent indication for emergency surgical intervention is myocardial ischemia.

The acuteness of the signs and symptoms associated with PTCA failure will dictate the intensity of surgical involvement and the timing of operative intervention. In patients without unstable symptoms and with lesions that remain unsuccessfully dilated, or in those with restenoses after a successful PTCA, coronary artery bypass grafting (CABG) may be performed electively. Since these patients clinically have chronic stable angina pectoris, their preoperative and postoperative management is essentially the same as that of patients undergoing elective CABG without prior PTCA. The role of the surgeon in the management of these patients is to perform the elective CABG. The techniques required are standardized. No further attention will be paid to surgical management of this group in this discussion.

In contrast, those patients developing clinical signs and symptoms of myocardial ischemia associated with or following PTCA should be considered as patients with impending myocardial infarction. Although it may occasionally be delayed, these patients usually develop myocardial ischemia during the PTCA or within a few hours of its completion. The role of the cardiothoracic surgeon is especially important in the management of these patients.

Program Organization

During initiation of a new PTCA program, the incidence of complications requiring emergency myocardial revascularization is greater. This PTCA learning curve should be associated with a decreasing incidence of complications as the operator becomes more experienced in angioplasty. In this initial phase of development of a PTCA program, formal standby arrangements for emergency CABG are necessary. This usually means an operating room held in readiness with anesthesiologists, nurses, perfusionists, and surgeons on standby awaiting the outcome of the PTCA. This may be the continued method of management, especially if the level of open heart surgical activity in the institution is modest or the performance of PTCA infrequent.

During a routine pre-PTCA evaluation, any factor which might complicate CABG, especially an emergency procedure, should be discovered. The significance of these factors can then be discussed and their management resolved to the mutual satisfaction of the angiographer and the cardiothoracic surgeon. The patient should be an acceptable operative candidate for CABG from the standpoint of satisfactory distal vessels, significant proximal stenoses in a major vessel, significant symptoms, and a reasonable expectation of improving quality of life or longevity based upon the best current scientific evidence. Features such as prior CABG, poor left ventricular function, diffuse distal arterial disease, or unavailability of a suitable conduit should be elicited. A joint decision should be made concerning the advisability of PTCA and the potential for surgical treatment of complications. The patient should be informed that CABG, especially an emergency procedure, is more difficult and carries a potentially greater risk in those with prior CABG. Alternatively, depending upon the associated clinical conditions, it might be acceptable to perform PTCA as the sole treatment without operative intervention should a PTCA complication occur. This decision should be determined jointly by the angiographer and surgeon and communicated to the patient before PTCA is performed.

The key factors for the success of any PTCA program are communication, cooperation, and goodwill between the angiographer and the surgeon. Their joint efforts should be viewed as complementary and not competitive. As in any cooperative venture, familiarity with associates' opinions and technical capabilities will influence therapeutic decisions. As the invasive angiographer and surgeon become more familiar with each other's capabilities and have more experience in working together, this arrangement may become less rigid.

As experience with PTCA increases, if the level of open heart surgical activity in the institution is high the arrangements for emergency myocardial revascularization may become less formal. With some assurance that an operating room and associated personnel will be available as open heart surgical operations are completed during that day, it might be enough to send a list of the scheduled PTCA procedures to be performed on that day to the operating room and associated personnel the day before. The PTCA procedures should be listed on the operating room schedule as actual cases so that everyone is aware of the possibility that they may be operated upon should a complication occur. Notification of successful or unsuccessful completion of a procedure is given to the operating room and other personnel as the PTCA schedule progresses until the schedule is complete. The operating room alert can then be ended, assuming that there are no imminent problems. This more casual arrangement works well in institutions with a large open heart surgical volume and experienced invasive angiographers, but its success depends upon several factors. The primary one is communication. There must be communication among all parties regarding the progress in both the operating room and the angiography suite. Failure to communicate the progress of the schedules in both the operating room and the angiography suite effectively will generally result in dissatisfaction in one or several of the parties involved and may cause the arrangement to revert to the more rigid system used originally. It is best to discuss possible problems and resolve any potential conflicts prior to embarking upon a PTCA program. A protocol agreed to before institution of this program is exceptionally helpful. However, repeated discussions and resolution of potential problems on a continuing basis is an integral part of the success of this cooperative effort.

In the less formal arrangement, in which pre-PTCA surgical consultation may not be used routinely, it behooves the angiographer to be aware of any potential problems which might complicate CABG and notify the cardiothoracic surgeon of their presence. It also is necessary specifically to notify or engage the surgeon in patient management decisions if the anticipated PTCA procedure can be expected to be especially difficult or complex, or to have a high level of complication or failure. In a routine case for PTCA, it might be permissible for the angiographer to discuss the proposed PTCA, alone with the patient, especially as the angiographer and surgeon gain experience in working together. However, in more complex instances, it is imperative that the therapeutic options be discussed between the angiographer and the surgeon and then presented to the patient before the PTCA. Above all, the surgeon should not be presented with a fait accompli in a patient who is not a candidate for myocardial revascularization but who has had a PTCA complication requiring emergency CABG.

Preoperative Preparation

In a well-established program, routine extensive preparation for emergency CABG is unnecessary in patients about to undergo uncomplicated angioplasty. The need for operative intervention is infrequent in these patients. With a well-equipped operating room, experienced personnel, and a high level of open heart surgical activity, all that should be necessary is an open operating room and availability of the necessary personnel. When the personnel have been forewarned by posting of the PTCA schedule 24 h previously on the operating room schedule, if prompt notification of the need for an emergency CABG is made to that facility the necessary preparations can usually be made in the time that it takes to transport the patient to the operating room. This is predicated upon the fact that all personnel involved in standby preparation have been informed of the PTCA cases to be performed that day.

Extensive arterial and central venous cannulation for hemodynamic monitoring of every patient at the time of routine coronary angioplasty is not required. In an institution with a good level of experience, cardiopulmonary bypass can be undertaken in an unstable patient with the only monitoring line being the arterial pressure measured through the angiography catheter or sheath, which has been left in place. In these circumstances, additional lines may be placed after the operation has begun. If there is a strong likelihood based on clinical and angiographic factors that emergency CABG is more likely to be necessary or if experience in performing emergency CABG is slight, then more extensive cannulation of the patient prior to angioplasty is logical. This may include radial artery cannulation for systemic pressure monitoring and placement of at least a central venous sheath for insertion of a flow-directed pulmonary artery catheter should this become necessary. These are not routine procedures, however. Even in patients coming for emergency CABG, there is usually time for expeditious placement of the peripheral and central lines prior to performance of CABG. Insertion of a urinary catheter is not necessary prior to angioplasty, as it can also be placed during anesthetic induction after the decision for emergency operation has been made.

Patients scheduled for PTCA should have a blood type screen routinely as a precaution, in case of any problems with obtaining and cross-matching blood, should this become necessary. No blood is cross-matched until a patient is transferred to the operating room. Blood and blood products then will become available, if needed, before the conclusion of CABG.

Emergency CABG

Patients undergoing emergency CABG usually will be maintained with heparin until cardiopulmonary bypass is accomplished. Allowing the guidewire to remain across the troublesome coronary stenosis may sometimes reduce the possibility of total vessel occlusion during this interval. This is removed from the coronary artery after the institution of cardiopulmonary bypass and during the performance of the bypass graft. Whether the guidewire is left in place or not, the femoral arterial sheath through which the angioplasty catheters had been inserted is left in place until the patient has returned to the intensive care unit following CABG and is hemodynamically stable without bleeding and with normal coagulation. Administration of intracoronary streptokinase causes little difficulty if done appropriately. The lower dose administered into the coronary bed usually has little or no systemic effect. However, streptokinase administered systemically can result in significant impairment of the clotting mechanism, with excessive operative and postoperative hemorrhage. The major factor responsible for postoperative hemorrhage in patients undergoing emergency CABG for PTCA complications has been related to the platelet inhibitory drugs which are administered routinely in any patient undergoing PTCA. In this circumstance the bleeding can usually be managed by administration of platelets if necessary.

Intra-aortic balloon support is indicated in unstable patients following PTCA, whether it is due to coronary insufficiency or hemodynamic deterioration. Akins and Block advocate its prompt insertion routinely once myocardial ischemia unresponsive to intracoronary nitroglycerin is observed [1]. They suggest rapid transfer of the patient to the operating room for myocardial revascularization after intra-aortic balloon insertion as the keypoint in a program to reduce the incidence of permanent peri-PTCA myocardial injury. Furthermore, they decry prolonged attempts at reopening a closed artery in the cardiac catheterization laboratory as only delaying the revascularization procedure and thereby increasing the risk of permanent myocardial damage. Murphy et al. have demonstrated the use of intra-aortic balloon support to reduce the incidence of myocardial ischemia and myocardial damage associated with PTCA complications requiring CABG, even though at their institution these patients usually first undergo repeat angiography and remanipulation in the angiography suite if this appears feasible at that repeat angiography [2].

Intra-aortic balloon support is advised in instances of hemodynamic instability or for any unstable patient with severe myocardial ischemia uncontrolled by intracoronary nitroglycerin, systemic heparinization, or repeat angioplasty. It is not used routinely in all patients undergoing emergency CABG for PTCA complications. Once the intra-aortic balloon is inserted, the patient is rapidly transported to the operating room for emergency CABG. Under these circumstances, extracorporeal circulation can be instituted promptly using arterial monitoring through the intra-aortic balloon catheter or via the femoral arterial catheter or sheath which has been left in place. Insertion of a pulmonary artery flow-directed catheter or central venous sheath may be foregone until completion of the operation if necessary. Systemic heparinization may complicate central venous catheterization. In the presence of unrelieved myocardial ischemia, rapid revascularization is the primary therapy. Procrastination or any inordinate delay in achieving this goal only potentiates the probability of permanent myocardial damage. While several groups have reported successful reopening of an occluded coronary artery after PTCA in the angiography suite, it should be emphasized that selection of patients for such remanipulation requires exquisite judgement to avoid undue permanent myocardial damage [3–5].

Each clinical unit should follow the general procedures usually employed for routine CABG as the basic technique for managing these acutely ill patients. However, modifications will be required to adjust the procedure to the clinical condition of each patient presenting for an emergency revascularization procedure. The most urgent condition requiring modification of technique is hemodynamic instability. The routine hemodynamic monitoring procedures usually used may be abridged in the unstable patient. Intra-aortic balloon insertion or partial femoro-femoral cardiopulmonary bypass may be necessary in these patients. One or the other of these support techniques may be advisable when CABG is delayed or technical difficulties are encountered while achieving operative exposure, as might be expected, for example, in patients with prior CABG.

Adaptability by modification of the sequence of steps in performing CABG is also important. Early and prompt reestablishment of distal flow to the acutely obstructed vessel should have the highest priority. To achieve this, a distal anastomosis to this vessel should first be accomplished, with cardioplegia solution administered promptly through this conduit once the distal anastomosis is established. Only then should attention be directed to treating other stenotic vessels or constructing proximal anastomoses.

The etiology of the arterial occlusion generally does not affect the primary goal of rapid reinstitution of blood flow in the occluded coronary arterial bed. Whether occlusion is due to thrombosis, dissection, or both will usually not affect successful accomplishment of an effective more peripheral coronary bypass. In most instances the occlusion site at operation cannot be readily observed. It is unnecessary and generally meddlesome to attempt to find the occlusion site at operation, as this maneuver may worsen the lesion or result in a totally uncontrollable situation at that arterial site. Performance of more distal CABG is usually effective. In most instances, the arterial walls are intact and the distal lumen unoccluded. Occasionally, however, distal dissection of the arterial layers has been identified [6]. In these instances, it is important to repair this dissection meticulously at the site of graft insertion, to allow adequate distal perfusion.

Clinical Results

Collective published experience of emergency CABG for PTCA complications is shown in Tables 1 and 2. Emergency revascularization has been necessary in 4%–12% of the reported series (Table 1). The major clinical indication for immediate CABG has been prolonged unrelieved chest pain with or without ECG changes

Table 1. Emergency CABG for PTCA complications: Clinical and angiographic findings

	Patients	Chest pain[a]	ECG changes[b]	Hemo-dynamic instability[c]	Coronary artery	
					Occlusion	Dissection
	≠	%	%	%	%	%
Murphy et al. (1982) [7]	17	100	71	0	29	71
Dorros et al. (1983) [8]	102	17	4	2	29	31
Killen (1983) [9]	73	77	16	29	38	12
Murphy et al. (1984) [2]	32	100	–	41	38	62
Cowley et al. (1984) [10]	202	46	45	18	53	46
Akins and Block (1984) [1]	11	91	9	0	91	–
Roberts et al. (1984) [11]	14	100	100	0	45	40
Reul et al. (1984) [12]	70	81	74	29	43	46
McBride et al. (1984) [13]	33	67	48	0	52	33

[a] Persistent, prolonged or unrelenting chest pain
[b] ECG evidence of ischemia or myocardial infarction
[c] Hemodynamic instability as manifested by cardiac arrest, cardiogenic shock, or hypotension

Table 2. Emergency CABG for PTCA complications: Operative mortality and perioperative myocardial infarction

	Patients	PCTA series	Operative mortality	Perioperative myocardial infarction
	(*n*)	%	%	%
Murphy et al. (1982) [7]	17	4.8	0	47
Dorros et al. (1983) [8]	102	6.8	6.9	35
Killen (1983) [9]	73	–	8.2	47
Murphy et al. (1984) [2]	32	3.7	0	19
Cowley et al. (1984) [10]	202	6.6	6.4	45
Akins and Block (1984) [1]	11	8.8	0	9
Roberts et al. (1984) [11]	14	8.0	0	20
Reul et al. (1984) [12]	70	12.0	5.7	11
McBride et al. (1984) [13]	33	8.6	3.0	36

suggestive of persistent myocardial ischemia or myocardial infarction. Hemodynamic instability, as manifested by cardiac arrest, cardiogenic shock, or hypotension has been a less frequent, but also a significant indication for emergency operation (Table 1). The major angiographic observations in patients undergoing repeat angiography immediately before emergency CABG have been arterial occlusion, dissection or both. Emergency revascularization for these complications of PTCA has been accomplished with a generally low operative mortality, but greater than that observed for elective CABG (Table 2). The associated occurrence of permanent myocardial damage as indicated by evidence of transmural myocardial infarction has been greater than that reported for myocardial revascularization on a nonemergent basis (Table 2).

Operative Balloon Angioplasty

Following the development of PTCA, the use of balloon angioplasty during CABG has been evaluated [14–22]. In particular, its role in extending the benefits of bypass grafting has been investigated. It has been promoted as increasing the possibility of a higher degree of revascularization. It appears most useful in dilating lesions of the middle and distal parts of the left anterior descending coronary artery (LAD) and its branches. While its use has been evaluated in right coronary artery (RCA) lesions, its effectiveness in that location is questionable. The technique is effective in calcified or fibrotic vessels, in which endarterectomy is more difficult [23]. Whether the lesion ideally suited for management by this technique is discrete or diffuse remains unresolved. While there is a learning curve associated with its application, most investigators report an associated low incidence of significant operative arterial trauma, myocardial infarction, and death. Some have suggested that observed minor arterial trauma, such as has been observed with PTCA, may be inconsequential and not require repair. With increasing experience and improvements in catheter design and manufacture, significant arterial injury has decreased. While some workers have suggested the advisability of performing intraoperative coronary angiography following operative coronary artery balloon angioplasty [21], others have not felt this to be necessary, relying instead upon assessment of improvement by the ease of passing graduated intraluminal coronary artery probes [16–20]. Initial results evaluated early in the postoperative period have been encouraging, but caution has been advised against excessive optimism [22]. Almost one-third of the patients undergoing PTCA develop recurrent stenosis within 6 months, and it is highly likely that patients undergoing operative balloon angioplasty may have a similar incidence of recurrence [22]. For this reason, lesions amenable to either operative balloon angioplasty or sequential coronary artery bypass grafting should probably be managed with the latter [22].

For operative balloon angioplasty, the coronary arteriotomy is placed in an area selected on the basis of preoperative coronary angiography for insertion of a coronary artery bypass graft. The lesions to be dilated are determined preoperatively; they are identified externally and calibrated internally with graduated coronary artery probes. The angioplasty catheter is then passed through the lesion and inflated to the appropriate pressure. The balloon is actively deflated, moved one balloon length closer to the arteriotomy, and reinflated in a similar fashion. This process is repeated as many times as necessary to achieve maximum dilatation. Normal arteries should never be dilated, nor should the catheter be moved with the balloon inflated as an embolectomy catheter is. The changes created in the stenosis are measured by internal calibration. If possible, the artery is flushed to remove any debris. An appropriate bypass graft then is attached to the arteriotomy. Satisfactory dilatation may not be achieved in the case of proximal LAD and some RCA lesions. Further management of these lesions might include additional grafting or endarterectomy; in some cases further action might be unnecessary.

References

1. Akins CW, Block PC (1984) Surgical intervention for failed percutaneous transluminal coronary angioplasty. Am J Cardiol 53:108C
2. Murphy DA, Craver JM, Jones EL, Curling PE, Guyton RA, King SB, Gruentzig AR, Hatcher CR (1984) Surgical management of acute myocardial ischemia following percutaneous transluminal coronary angioplasty. J Thorac Cardiovasc Surg 87:332
3. Schofer J, Krebber H, Bleifeld W, Mathey DG (1982) Acute coronary artery occlusion during percutaneous transluminal coronary angioplasty: reopening by intracoronary streptokinase before emergency coronary artery surgery to prevent myocardial infarction. Circulation 66:1325
4. Hollman J, Gruentzig AR, Douglas JS, King SB, Ischinger T, Meier B (1983) Acute occlusion after percutaneous transluminal coronary angioplasty – a new approach. Circulation 68:725
5. Ischinger T, Zack P, Aker U (1984) Acute coronary occlusion during balloon angioplasty due to intracoronary thrombus and coronary spasm: a reversible complication. Am Heart J 107:1271
6. Murphy DA, Craver JM, King SB (1984) Distal coronary artery dissection following percutaneous transluminal coronary angioplasty. Ann Thorac Surg 37:473
7. Murphy DA, Craver JM, Jones EL, Gruentzig AR, King SB, Hatcher CR (1982) Surgical revascularization following unsuccessful percutaneous transluminal coronary angioplasty. J Thorac Cardiovasc Surg 84:342
8. Dorros G, Cowley MJ, Simpson J, Bentivoglio LG, Block PC, Bourassa M, Detre K, Gosselin AJ, Gruentzig AR, Kelsey SF, Kent KM, Mock MB, Mullin SM, Myler RK, Passamani ER, Stertzer SH, Williams DO (1983) Percutaneous transluminal coronary angioplasty: report of complications from the National Heart, Lung, and Blood Institute PTCA registry. Circulation 67:723
9. Killen DA (1983) The management of patients after streptokinase infusion or balloon dilatation or both. In: Syllabus postgraduate course on cardiac surgery. American College of Surgeons, pp 15–18
10. Cowley MJ, Dorros G, Kelsey SF, Van Raden MV, Detre KM (1984) Emergency coronary bypass surgery after coronary angioplasty: the National Heart, Lung, and Blood Institute's percutaneous transluminal coronary angioplasty registry experience. Am J Cardiol 53:22C
11. Roberts AJ, Faro RS, Knauf DG, Alexander JA, Feldman RL, Pepine C, Ellison D, LoPresti J, Staples EM, Rubin MR (to be published) Emergency coronary artery bypass graft surgery for evolving acute myocardial necrosis related to catheter-induced coronary artery disruption. Ann Thorac Surg
12. Reul GJ, Cooley DA, Ott DA, Duncan JM, Livesay JJ, Frazier OH (to be published) Coronary artery bypass for unsuccessful percutaneous transluminal coronary angioplasty. J Thorac Cardiovasc Surg

13. McBride LR, Aker U, Kaiser GC (to be published) Surgical management of PTCA complications
14. Wallsh E, Franzone AJ, Clauss RH, Bruno MS, Steichen F, Stertzer SH (1980) Transluminal coronary angioplasty during saphenous coronary bypass surgery. Ann Surg 191:234
15. Roberts AJ, Feldman RL, Conti CR, Selby JH, LaBrosse C, Knauf DG, Alexander JA, Watson WD, Pepine CJ (1982) Preliminary experience with intraoperative transluminal balloon-catheter dilatation and coronary artery bypass grafting for the treatment of symptomatic diffuse coronary artery disease. Ann Thorac Surg 34:504
16. Katz RJ, Leiboff RH, Aaron BL, Mills M, Wasserman AG, Ross AM (1982) Intraoperative retrograde balloon angioplasty of the left anterior descending coronary artery for reperfusion of jeopardized proximal branches. Circulation 66 [Suppl 1]:1–30
17. Mills NL, Doyle DP (1982) Does operative transluminal angioplasty extend the limits of coronary artery bypass surgery? A preliminary report. Circulation 66 [Suppl 1]:1–26
18. Wallsh E, Franzone AJ, Weinstein GC, Alcan K, Clavel A, Stertzer SH (1982) Use of operative transluminal coronary angioplasty as an adjunct to coronary artery bypass. J Thorac Cardiovasc Surg 84:843
19. Mills NL, Ochsner JL, Doyle DP, Kalchoff WP (1983) Technique and results of operative transluminal angioplasty in 81 consecutive patients. J Thorac Cardiovasc Surg 86:689
20. Roberts AJ, Faro RS, Feldman RL, Conti CR, Knauf DG, Alexander JA, Pepine CJ (1983) Comparison of early and long-term results with intraoperative transluminal balloon catheter dilatation and coronary artery bypass grafting. J Thorac Cardiovasc Surg 86:435
21. Ranier WG Discussion of 15
22. Jones EL, Kings SB (1983) Intraoperative angioplasty in the treatment of coronary artery disease. J Am Coll Cardiol 1:970
23. Mills NL Discussion of 15

Chapter 15. Complex Coronary Angioplasty: Multiple-Vessel/Multiple-Lesion Dilatation

GEOFFREY O. HARTZLER

The initial guidelines for the performance of percutaneous transluminal coronary angioplasty (PTCA) limited the technique to patients with ideal clinical status and anatomic features [1–3]. Consequently, patients with more than one obstructive coronary lesion were excluded, as were those with distal disease, advanced age, poor left ventricular function, previous bypass surgery and acute myocardial infarction. Certain anatomic factors were also felt to preclude or minimize the likelihood of successful PTCA, including eccentricity of lesions, presence of calcification within the lesion, or total obstruction. These selection criteria appeared to limit the potential application of PTCA to an estimated 5%–10% of patients undergoing coronary angiography [2–7].

However, increased and continued experience with the technique and, in particular, continued modification and refinement of angioplasty catheter systems have made it possible for many previously excluded patients to undergo dilatation safely and successfully [8–14]. For example, in our own institution approximately 50% of patients undergoing diagnostic coronary angiography are considered to be suitable candidates for a PTCA procedure, including patients with multiple-vessel disease. This gradual yet progressive evolution of the technique is again reflected in our own experience; of our first 100 patients undergoing PTCA, 92 had single lesions dilated, whereas over 70 of the last 100 patients had two or more stenoses dilated during the same procedure. Additionally, of the first 2000 patients undergoing PTCA, nearly 40% were considered to have one or more "high risk" clinical circumstances other than multiple-vessel disease.

Technical Considerations in the Performance of Complex PTCA

Experience

Without question, the single most important factor in the performance of successful single-lesion or multiple-lesion PTCA is the *experience* of the dilating cardiologist. Coronary angioplasty is a highly technical procedure best performed by the mature and skilled coronary angiographer who has gained PTCA experience slowly, cautiously, and under supervision. Early in this experience, it is inappropriate to select patient candidates who have complex clinical conditions including the presence of multiple-vessel disease. Rather, initial PTCA procedures should be limited to those patients with near-ideal coronary anatomy as the cardiologist gains familiarity and experience with a variety of guiding catheters, balloon catheters, and guidewires. Complications can and do occur with increased frequency in inexperienced hands, and are generally better tolerated by patients with single-vessel disease and no additional high-risk factors such as advanced age or poor left ventricular function. A distinct learning curve has been noted for all dilating cardiologists, demonstrating that with increasing experience the occurrence of complications decreases while the success rate rises [3, 15].

Imaging Requirements

Safely performed, successful multiple-lesion PTCA is clearly facilitated by prior study of a high-quality diagnostic coronary angiogram. It is inadequate to merely observe that a proximal, high-grade obstructive lesion is present. For successful PTCA, the lesions must be clearly delineated and characterized with definition of arterial origin, proximal and distal anatomy, eccentricity and the presence of adjacent branches. These factors, including features of lesion discreteness, diffuseness, or tubularity, influence the choice of guide catheter, balloon catheter and guidewires.

During PTCA, rapid acquisition of multiple fluoroscopic views is extremely important for the safe passage of guidewires. Biplane fluoroscopy is not essential.

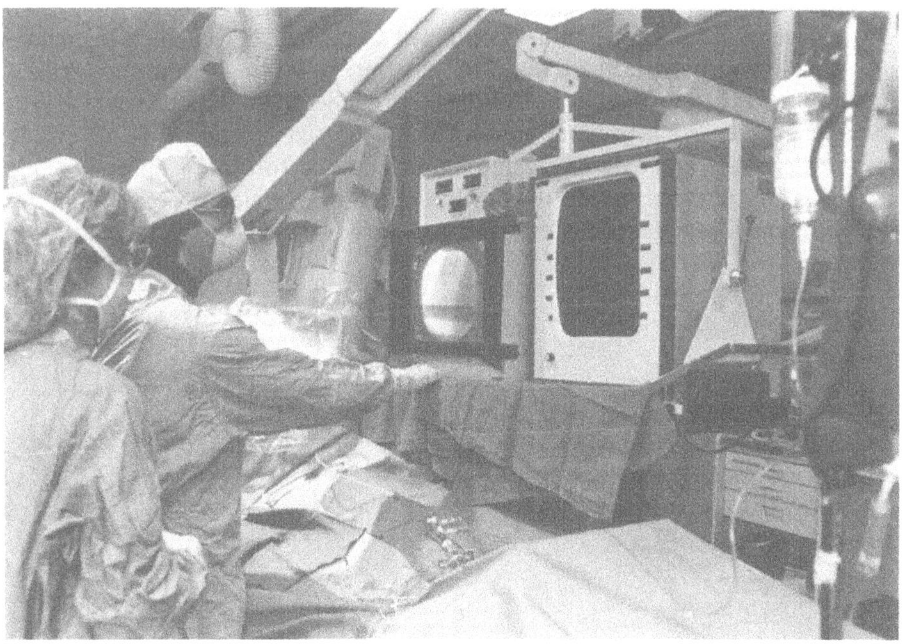

Fig. 1. Equipment in the author's angioplasty suite. General Electric LU-C X-ray system with MPX-125 generator and high-resolution video monitor having 1023 scan lines and 12 MHZ horizontal band width. An HPR-10 videotape system is utilized for recording and providing a frozen image when active fluoroscopy is not being performed. The television screen and adjacent physiologic display are mounted to allow close-proximity viewing and can be pulled to within several inches of the cardiologist's eyes

Rather, according to the present author's experience, it is clear that a monoplane X-ray system with the ability to rapidly obtain multiple standard and angled projections is adequate for the performance of complex PTCA (Fig. 1).

For successful dilatation, the vessel in which it is to be attempted must be visible. Consequently, it is extremely helpful to mount the television screen within the laboratory so that the dilating cardiologist can view the X-ray image from close proximity. High-resolution imaging by means of an X-ray system with an increased number of scan lines per screen is essential. This not only allows better resolution of small balloons and fine guidewires, but allows clearer definition of the lesion and adjacent arterial anatomy.

For multiple-lesion angioplasty, it has proven helpful to have an X-ray system capable of storing and displaying an immediately previous coronary injection. The "frozen" image can then be used as a continuous guide for balloon catheter and guidewire manipulation. In our laboratory, this static image is acquired with videotape and continuously displayed on the fluoroscopic screen, temporarily being replaced by the actual online image during active fluoroscopy. Consequently, additional "marker" catheters are not required or utilized during routine PTCA procedures.

Guide Catheter Selection

Our choice of guide catheters has continued to change as technological refinements have improved their qualities. At the time of writing, the author utilizes predominantly 8-F guides because of the their smaller outer diameter, which produces less potential peripheral and coronary arterial trauma while providing greater flexibility and ease of manipulation. These factors allow "propping" or folding of the catheter within the aortic root (Fig. 2), which is occasionally required to cannulate unusually oriented coronary ostia or to gain adequate sup-

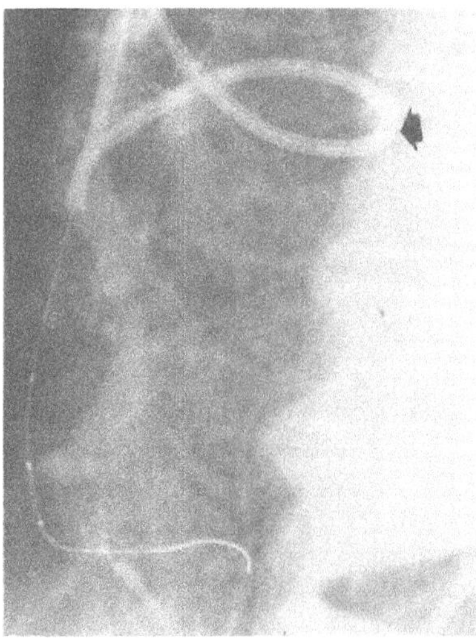

Fig. 2. Firm cannulation of the proximal right coronary artery with an 8-F Judkin's curve right coronary catheter. To facilitate passage of the balloon through a subtotal mid-right coronary stenosis, the guide catheter was propped against the opposite aortic wall (*arrow*). Note the very distal position of the guidewire

port for balloon passage through a tortuous or narrowed coronary segment. When required, deep insertion of the guide catheter is safer and more easily accomplished with smaller guides.

Standard Judkins curves have proved adequate for most dilatation procedures, including cannulation of vein grafts. However, owing to improved catheter designs and the introduction of guide catheters which approximate the more traditional Amplatz curves, and the creation of guides with less acutely angled yet flexible tips, such as the graft guide or multipurpose style, it is now possible to achieve adequate cannulation and support of unusually placed vein grafts, right and circumflex coronary arteries of anomalous origin, and coronary ostia in which the approach is complicated by marked ectasia or dilatation of the aortic root. Virtually all anatomic variations are approachable when these catheters are used via the transfemoral route, which is an inherently safer and technically easier approach than the brachial route.

The author rarely utilizes "out-of-plane" Judkins curves for selective cannulation of the LAD. Rather, the standard Judkins left coronary catheters can be directed toward the LAD by counterclockwise rotation and advancement of the guide. Conversely, the circumflex artery can be selected by clockwise rotation of the guide catheter, frequently combined with slight withdrawal. Other approaches for guide catheter cannulation exist. Following selection of the proximal vessel by use of a directionally changeable guidewire, the guide catheter can be more deeply advanced over the wire or balloon catheter for deep engagement.

Special circumstances may require a trial of several different guide catheters, particularly for anomalously originating right coronary arteries and for stable engagement or approximation of right coronary ostial lesions. Frequently, a left Amplatz guide is most effective for stable engagement or direction of a guidewire and balloon catheter into the proximal right coronary artery. Cannulation of a left internal mammary artery (LIMA) bypass graft for dilatation of the graft or native vessel through the graft can be extremely difficult (Fig. 31). In our experience, a most effective approach is first to cannulate the LIMA with a standard 7- or 8-F LIMA angiographic catheter, and then to place a 0.035 exchange wire in the internal mammary artery. A standard 8-F Judkins style right coronary guiding catheter may then be passed over the exchange wire for LIMA engagement.

This can be facilitated by first heating the catheter and bending the guide catheter tip to a more acute angle. Right internal mammary arteries have been most easily cannulated with a standard Judkins right coronary curve guide with or without a guidewire as described.

Guidewires

The guidewire approach to coronary angioplasty has revolutionized the procedure. Directionally changeable or "steerable" guidewires with flexible or floppy tips not only allow access to virtually all segments of the coronary circulation but have increased the safety of the procedure. In our experience, dissection or disruption of the plaque and vessel wall occur far less commonly than with the original

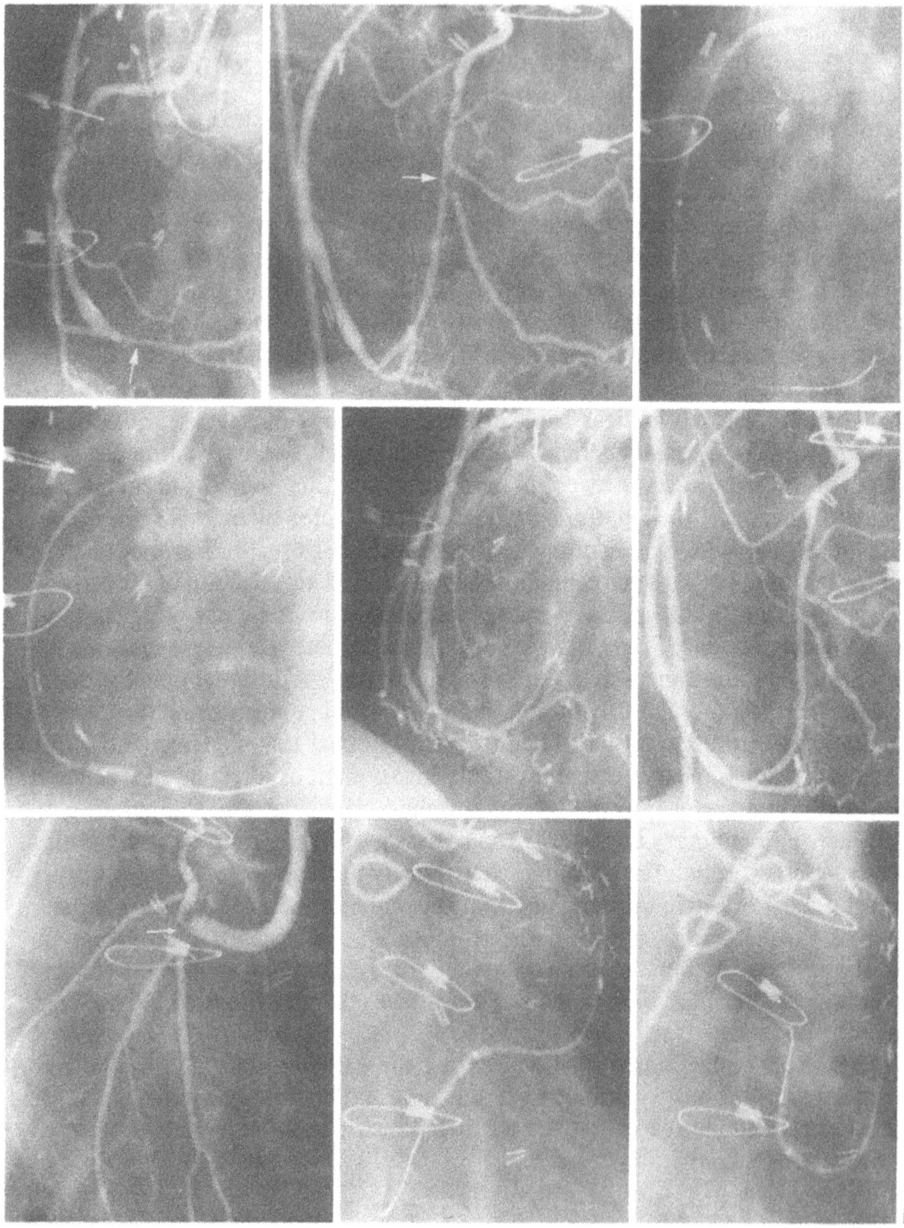

a, b c d, e f g, h i

Fig. 3 a–t. Multiple-lesion angioplasty in a 55-year-old man with functional class III angina 4 months after bypass surgery. The cineangiographic frames are displayed in sequence of the actual PTCA procedure. All guide catheters are 8 F in diameter, from United States Catheter and Instrument, Billerica, Mass. All balloon catheters and guidewires are products of Advanced Cardiovascular Systems, Mountain View, Calif. **a** Right coronary injection in LAO projection demonstrates stenosis distal to vein graft insertion site. Backfilling of the vein graft shows diffuse proximal narrowing. **b** Right coronary injection in RAO projection demonstrates an additional (Legend cont. p. 256)

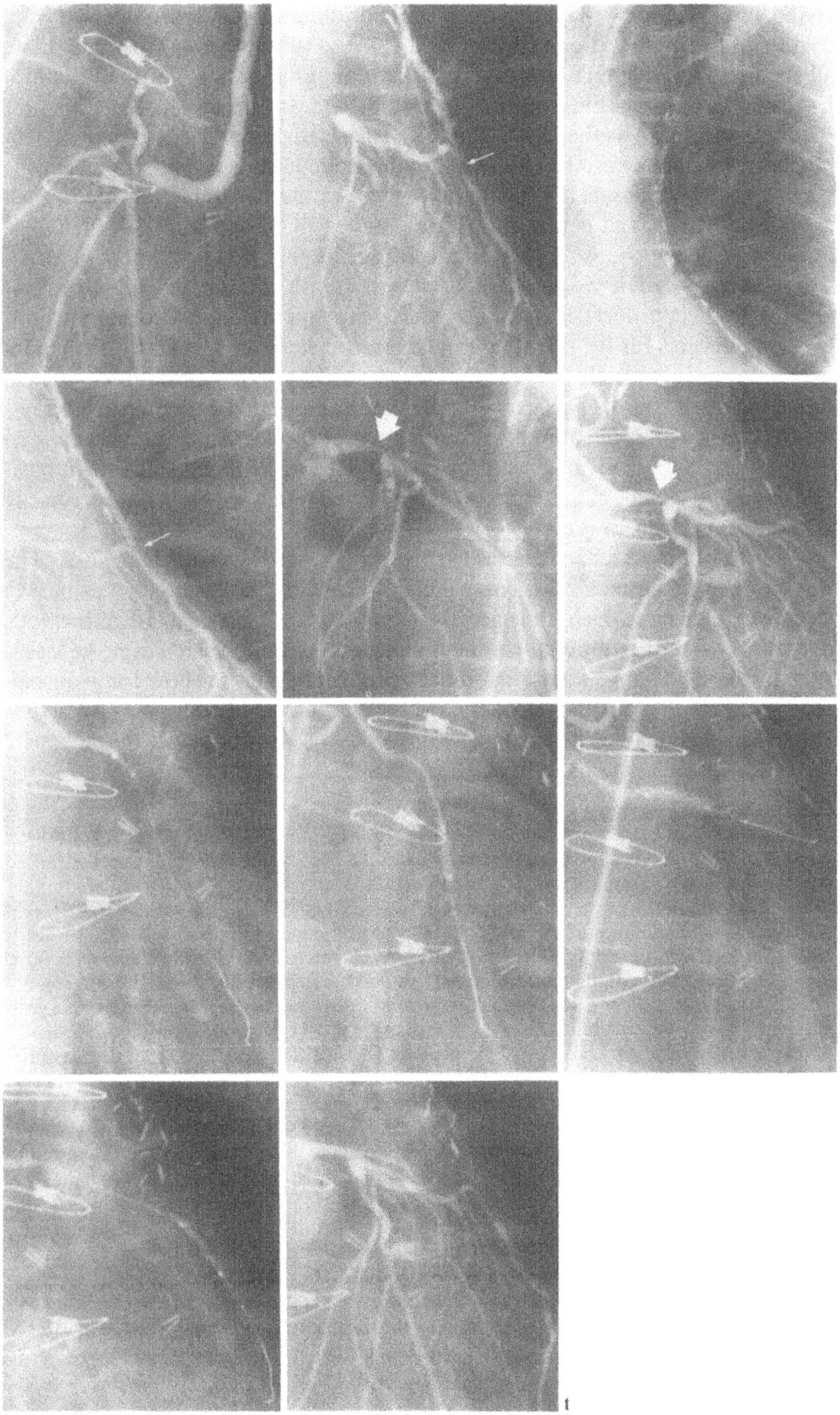
j, k
l
m, n
o
p, q
r
s
t

"fixed wire" balloon catheters. Still, a range of different guidewires with varying degrees of flexibility, torque control, and stiffness is required to cross and dilate all stenoses. For example, a subacute or chronic total occlusion usually cannot be readily crossed with a floppy tipped guidewire. In this case, we use a stiffer steerable wire, such as the USCI (United States Catheter and Instrument) 0.016-in. platinum guidewire. Although ideal in these circumstances, the stiffness of the wire makes its use unsafe for negotiation of many other anatomic variations, such as series of curves and bends, which are more easily passed with a flexible platinum wire such as the ACS (Advanced Cardiovascular Systems) Sof-T or High-Torque Floppy guidewires. These latter wires, with extremely flexible tips but varying in their properties of torque and shaft support, have become our preferred guidewires for the initial approach to most stenoses. Generally, the guidewire is passed completely through the stenosis and positioned several centimeters distally (Figs. 2 and 3). This lends support to the guide and balloon catheters, allowing consistent and maintained cannulation of the coronary ostium and relatively rapid balloon advancement for prompt PTCA. With a distal wire in position, should the guide catheter become disengaged total support is not necessarily lost and reengagement is easier.

We seldom use exchange wires for the purpose of recrossing a stenosis. The need for this has been almost completely obviated by the extremely flexible yet steerable guidewire which, in general, can be redirected across a site of previous dilatation without additional trauma or plaque disruption. However, we occasionally place exchange wires after initial balloon inflations to allow complete balloon withdrawal from the coronary artery and guide catheter, and give a subsequent, relatively unobstructed injection of contrast medium over the guidewire

---

Fig. 3 a–t (continuied)
mid-vessel stenosis. **c** A 2.5-mm balloon is inflated in the mid-right coronary artery. Note distal position of an 0.18-in. High-Torque Floppy guidewire. **d** The 2.5-mm balloon has been advanced into the distal right coronary artery. **e** Wide patency of the distal right coronary artery after PTCA. **f** Wide patency of the mid-right coronary artery after PTCA. **g** Injection into the vein graft to the mid-circumflex artery in an RAO caudal projection. There is diffuse stenosis of the circumflex artery at the vein graft insertion site. **h** A 2.5-mm balloon is inflated across the junction of the vein graft with the mid-circumflex coronary artery oriented into the distal vessel. **i** The 2.5-mm balloon has now been directed superiorly across the proximal aspect of the vein graft anastomosis with the circumflex artery. **j** Immediate post-PTCA result, showing wide patency of the circumflex artery. **k** Left internal mammary artery injection in an RAO view demonstrates subtotal occlusion at its distal anastomosis with the left anterior descending coronary artery. **l** A 4-F guide has been passed over an exchange wire into the left internal mammary artery. A 2.5-mm low profile steerable balloon catheter is inflated in the distal anastomotic lesion. **m** Immediate post-PTCA result, showing wide patency of the distal internal mammary artery anastomosis with LAD; **n** LAO injection into a native left coronary artery demonstrates high-grade distal left main coronary stenosis. **o** Left coronary injection in RAO view demonstrates high-grade distal left main coronary stenosis. **p** A 2.5-mm balloon is first inflated in the left main coronary stenosis. Note distal circumflex position of the high-torque floppy guidewire. **q** The 2.5-mm balloon has been advanced distally to redilate the circumflex artery at the site of vein graft insertion. **r** 3-mm balloon is subsequently used to redilate the left main coronary artery. **s** The 3-mm balloon has been advanced into the LAD to redilate the site of internal mammary artery anastomosis and LAD stenosis. **t** Final left coronary injection showing markedly improved patency of the left main coronary artery. The circumflex artery is widely patent, as is the left anterior descending coronary artery with competing flow present at the site of internal mammary artery anastomosis

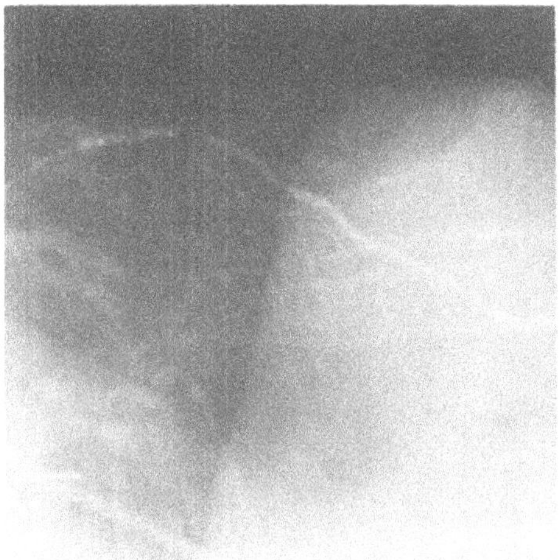

Fig. 4. An end-hole injection of contrast through an Advanced Cardiovascular Systems' 2.5-mm balloon during balloon inflation in a proximal lesion with guidewire withdrawn. This technique allows enhanced visualization of the distal circulation and is particularly useful in situations where distal anatomy has not been clearly delineated or is difficult to image

for a more complete angiographic assessment of the dilatation result while maintaining access to the artery.

In the author's opinion, a most important property of any guidewire is that the wire itself move freely through the balloon catheter. Unrestricted steering and passage of the wire through the stenosis and coronary artery as an independent motion is preferable to passage of a guidewire by movement of the balloon and wire en bloc. A freely moving guidewire transmits sensations of torque, resistance, and obstruction to the hands of the dilating cardiologist. This quality of unrestricted motion facilitates steering and balloon passage while reducing the potential for trauma to the arterial wall.

No presently available guidewire system allows rapid, accurate measurement of distal arterial pressures or injection of adequate distal contrast medium. Consequently, when distal pressure or dye injections are required, we prefer to remove the guidewire completely and record or inject directly through the unobstructed central lumen of the balloon catheter (Fig. 4). This technical and philosophical evolution of our approach further simplifies complex angioplasty by obviating the need for routine use of two injection syringes and two multiple stopcock manifolds.

Balloon Catheters

For dilatation of distal lesions and those located beyond angles and bends within the coronary tree, a highly flexible balloon catheter which moves freely over a guidewire is required. Consequently, we prefer and routinely utilize polyethylene catheters such as those manufactured by Advanced Cardiovascular Systems, Inc. (Mountain View, Calif.). When introduced through a nonbinding and minimally restrictive Y connector attached to the guiding catheter (Fig. 5), polyethylene balloon catheters move easily and readily transmit sensations of obstruction or resistance. As with a freely moving guidewire, the tactile awareness of movement and

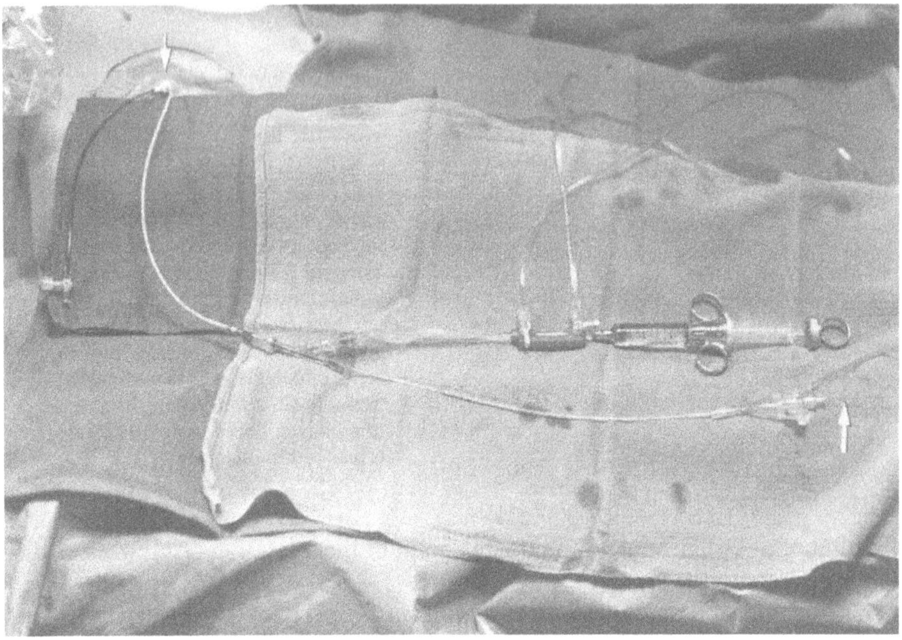

Fig. 5. The "basic" catheter-manifold setup for routine angioplasty. At the top left (*arrow*) an 8-F side-arm sheath has been inserted into the right femoral artery. The 8-F guide catheter is attached to a Y connector through which the balloon catheter has been passed. The side-arm of the Y connector is attached to a simple two-stopcock manifold, which allows pressure flushing and contrast injections through the Y connector around the angioplasty catheter. The manifold is attached to a standard 10-cm^2 glass control syringe. The guidewire (*arrow extreme right*) is allowed to move freely through the central lumen of the balloon catheter without attempts to infuse or inject around the wire, which is controlled by external rotation and advancement

restriction within the coronary artery adds an extremely important dimension to complex coronary angioplasty.

The manufacturing industry has made countless modifications and improvements in balloon catheter systems. Consequently, the delicate and expensive instruments used for PTCA today are clearly superior to the original balloon catheters. A multiplicity of sizes exist, both for the deflated and inflated states. Extremely low profile, highly flexible, and freely moving balloons tend to seek their way more readily through tortuous coronary arteries, around angles within the coronary tree, and through tight stenoses.

It is extremely important to utilize a balloon which is properly matched to the native coronary dimension, avoiding overexpansion and minimizing disruption of the plaque and vessel wall. In our experience, formal quantitative angiographic measurements of the coronary arterial caliber do not enhance the selection of an appropriately sized balloon. Subjective assessment by an experienced dilating cardiologist at the time of initial and repeat angiography, including comparison of coronary dimension with that of the standard guiding catheter, has proven optimal. Fluoroscopic visualization of the balloon during initial low-pressure (3–

4 atm) inflation allows an immediate judgment regarding the appropriateness of balloon size relative to the lesion and artery being dilated. We do not hesitate to change the balloon catheter immediately should it appear to be too large. This minimizes one of the most common complications of PTCA – overexpansion of the coronary artery with localized or dissecting disruption and ultimate closure.

Strategy for Complex Coronary Angioplasty

In selection of patients for multiple-lesion angioplasty, the diagnostic coronary angiogram is carefully reviewed and each stenosis is considered individually. Questions asked include whether or not the stenosis is accessible to a guidewire and balloon; what the native coronary arterial size is; and what size balloons will be required. It is also important to ask whether the particular anatomy requires an unusually low profile balloon or perhaps an investigational device; whether the stenosis involves adjacent branches and if so, what their relative importance is; whether a two-balloon or two-guidewire technique should be used to preserve patency and access to a threatened side branch; how large the distal arterial bed is and whether the myocardium subserved by the artery is viable; and whether there are particular clinical or anatomic features that require modification of the routine approach, such as placement of an intra-aortic balloon pump prior to PTCA.

In general, the clinically most significant stenosis is crossed and dilated first. At times, it may not be obvious which this is. If multiple stenoses are present within the same vessel the guidewire is first directed through all lesions, followed by sequential dilatation commencing from proximal to distal. In the process, it may be necessary to exchange the balloon catheter for a narrower one as dilatation progresses into smaller arterial segments. The adequacy of dilatation is judged by fluoroscopic monitoring of full balloon expansion; contrast injections performed through the guide catheter over the balloon catheter and guidewire; contrast injections performed over an exchange wire with the balloon catheter removed; and distal pressure measurements in some instances. However, the very best assessment of adequate dilatation comes from repeat coronary angiography, the guide catheter being used as the angiographic catheter with balloon and all guidewires completely removed. In the majority of instances, this last assessment is our definitive assessment, which may be the basis for a decision to recross and redilate a stenosis which appears to be inadequately dilated, i.e., more than 40% obstructed in multiple views.

In exceptional circumstances, stenoses and arteries of lesser functional magnitude merit initial dilatation. For example, this approach may be indicated when collateral circulation is present, from the artery of lesser magnitude or arteries supplying a previously infarcted zone to the more important or major vessel containing a high-grade stenosis. A high-grade proximal LAD lesion may be dilated *after* PTCA of a totally occluded mid-right coronary artery, even if the distal right coronary circulation is small or if the inferior wall is akinetic. This approach should be considered if upon either left or right coronary injection collateral circulation is evident between these two arteries. Following successful dilatation of the lesser artery, pressure and flow within the collateral circulation may be enhanced, providing a degree of "protection" should there be a complication or acute occlusion of the more dominant artery. Obviously, there are many clinical and anatomic variations that require individual consideration.

Poor Left Ventricular Function

In the presence of poor left ventricular function, which can be secondary to prior myocardial infarction, ischemic or nonischemic cardiomyopathy or chronic valvular disease, the elective placement of an intra-aortic balloon pump can support the left ventricle and coronary flow. In these circumstances, even brief occlusion of a moderate-sized coronary artery can result in prompt ischemic regional wall dysfunction, a reduction in cardiac output, and a decline in systemic blood pressure. These transient sequelae of PTCA can prevent an otherwise successful outcome. Consequently, a left ventricular angiogram or noninvasive assessment of global and regional left ventricular function performed before hand provides invaluable information pertinent to the PTCA procedure.

Left Main Coronary Dilatation

In general, significant left main coronary arterial obstruction remains a relative contraindication for PTCA. Isolated left main coronary disease is uncommon. When associated with additional distal obstructive lesions, left main coronary disease contributes to a technically and hemodynamically complex procedure. Nonetheless, there are many clinical circumstances in which PTCA may be the best therapeutic approach for a patient with left main obstruction. These include selected patients at high risk of complication during elective surgery, such as the very elderly, those with extremely poor left ventricular function, and those with diffuse distal disease that might otherwise be judged inoperable. Obviously, if prior bypass surgery has been performed with patent grafts to the circumflex or left anterior descending coronary artery, left main PTCA carries less risk, as the total left coronary circulation will not be compromised during balloon inflation. Also, if collateral supply to the anterior or lateral wall is present from an uncompromised right coronary circulation, the risks of left main dilatation may be reduced.

In general, we prefer to place an intra-aortic balloon pump prior to left main coronary dilatation. This increases the patient's hemodynamic stability and generally allows longer balloon inflation times. Coronary flow is augmented immediately after balloon deflation, a period during which systemic hypotension may be present as a result of the prolonged ischemic period induced by balloon inflation within the left main coronary artery.

In general, we use shorter balloon inflation times (15–20 s) during left main PTCA and frequently remove the balloon and guide catheter from the left main ostium following each dilatation, while maintaining access to the artery with a distally placed guidewire.

Despite the relative technical ease of passing a wire and balloon across a left main coronary stenosis, we have been struck by the frequent inadequacy of left main dilatation despite full balloon expansion. Stenoses in this location frequently do not dilate as completely as do those within true epicardial coronary segments.

Advanced Age

Advanced age is associated with increased procedure-related morbidity and mortality, just as risks of coronary artery bypass surgery are increased in this subgroup. With acceptance of these facts and a full discussion of the goals and risks of PTCA with the elderly patient and the family, both single- and multiple-lesion angioplasty can be performed with reasonable expectation of benefit. In all likelihood, many factors contribute to this generally increased risk which we have experienced in the aged population (see "Results"). Still, PTCA is inherently more attractive than coronary bypass surgery for the elderly patient, who has a greater prevalence of medical disorders and in whom the capacity for recovery is not so great as in the younger population.

Results: Multiple-Lesion/Multiple-Vessel Coronary Angioplasty

Dilatation of two or more coronary stenoses during the same PTCA procedure remains controversial. However, this "aggressive" approach to the treatment of coronary disease is now far more acceptable than in the early 1980s, when the "classical" indications for PTCA limited the procedure to patients with single coronary stenoses. New catheter technologies and increasing experience with PTCA have allowed this corresponding evolution, and it is supported by experience within our own institution and reports from others [12, 13, 16, 17]. Clearly, with experience and with proper patient selection, multiple-lesion PTCA can be performed with a primary success rate and a low incidence of complications approaching those reported for single-lesion coronary angioplasty.

Of the first 2000 consecutive PTCA procedures performed by a group of four dilating cardiologists at the Mid-America Heart Institute of St. Luke's Hospital in Kansas City, Mo, USA, multiple high-risk subsets were included. There were 274 patients 70 years of age or older; 197 patients with poor left ventricular function defined as ejection fraction of less than 40%; 204 patients with prior coronary bypass surgery; 22 patients undergoing left main coronary dilatation; and 143 patients with acute myocardial infarction as the indication for PTCA. In addition, there were 835 patients who underwent dilatation of two to ten coronary stenoses during the initial PTCA procedure (Table 1).

The patients undergoing multiple-lesion PTCA were 691 men and 144 women, with an age range of 22–84 years. This included 479 patients having two lesions attempted, 212 patients having three lesions attempted, 76 patients having four lesions attempted and 68 patients having five or more stenoses dilated during the initial PTCA procedure.

Table 1. Multiple-lesion PTCA in 835 patients

		Number
	Males	691
	Females	144
		835
Ages 22–84 years		
Lesions attempted		
	Two	479
	Three	212
	Four	76
	Five–ten	68
Lesions successfully dilated		2105 (93%)
Complications		
	Urgent surgery	13 (1.6%)
	Transmural infarction	12 (1.4%)
	Death	8 (1.0%)

Of all stenoses attempted, 93% were successfully dilated to 40% residual obstruction or less according to assessment in two or more angiographic views.

Procedural complications included the need for urgent coronary bypass surgery due to vessel occlusion or disruption in 13 patients (1.6%), transmural myocardial infarction in 12 patients (1.4%), and 8 deaths, giving a 1% overall mortality. These data compare favorably with the results of PTCA in the total series of 2000 patients in which 90% of stenoses attempted were successfully dilated and in which there was a 2.3% requirement for urgent bypass surgery and a 1.4% incidence of transmural myocardial infarction and 17 deaths giving a procedure-related mortality of 0.9%.

Multiple-Lesion PTCA in Complex Subgroups

With increasing experience, we have attempted multiple-lesion PTCA in a variety of patients with additional high-risk factors. Many patients had clinical features associated with increased surgical morbidity and mortality. Several multiple-lesion PTCAs were performed in patients considered to be poor surgical candidates or who had been judged "inoperable" at our institution and others. However, following review of their clinical circumstance and previous coronary angiography, it was felt that a judicious attempt at multiple-lesion PTCA was warranted and justifiable as a definitive or at least palliative procedure.

Comparison of Results of Multiple-Lesion Versus Single-Lesion PTCA in High-Risk Subsets (Table 2)

Prior Coronary Bypass Surgery

Multiple-lesion PTCA was attempted in 123 patients who had prior coronary bypass surgery. The primary success rate was 91% with no requirement for urgent

Table 2. Multiple-lesion PTCA in "high-risk" subgroups Complications

	Multiple lesions	Single lesions
Prior CABG	123	81
Infarction	0	0
CABG	0	0
Death	1 (0.8%)	0
Poor LV function	61	136
Infarction	0	3 (2.2%)
CABG	2 (3.3%)	3 (2.2%)
Death	2 (3.3%)	3 (2.2%)
Acute MI	31	112
Infarction	–	–
CABG	3 (9.6%)	1 (0.8%)
Death	2 (6.5%)	4 (3.5%)
Advanced age	124	150
Infarction	3 (2.4%)	2 (1.3%)
CABG	0	3 (2.0%)
Death	6 (4.8%)	4 (2.6%)

bypass surgery, no transmural myocardial infarctions, and with one death, giving a procedure-related mortality of 0.8%. There were no significant differences between primary success rate or incidence of complications in this group and after single-lesion PTCA in 81 patients with prior coronary bypass surgery.

Poor Left Ventricular Function

Multiple-lesion PTCA was attempted in 61 patients with poor left ventricular function as previously defined. Although 2 patients (3.3%) required urgent bypass surgery and there were 2 procedure-related deaths (3.3%), these data did not differ significantly from the results of single-lesion angioplasty in 136 patients with poor left ventricular function. In this latter group, there were 3 patients requiring urgent bypass surgery (2.2%) and 3 deaths (2.2%).

Left Main Coronary Dilatation

Multiple-lesion PTCA was attempted in 11 patients with left main coronary disease, and the results were compared with those of single-lesion (left main) dilatation in 11 patients. There were two deaths in the multiple-lesion subgroup. However, one death occurred in a patient in cardiogenic shock who underwent attempted recanalization of a totally occluded left main coronary artery late in the course of an anteroseptal/lateral myocardial infarction. The small size of the left main coronary subgroups prevents statistical analysis and comparison.

Acute Myocardial Infarction

Multiple-lesion PTCA was performed in 31 patients experiencing acute myocardial infarction, and the results were compared with those of single-lesion PTCA in 112 patients with acute infarction. Although primary success rates were similar, the morbidity and mortality in the multiple-lesion subgroup were increased relative to those in patients with acute infarction undergoing single-lesion PTCA. Three multiple-lesion patients (9.6%) required urgent bypass surgery, as against one (0.8%) single-lesion patient. In each instance, the urgent surgical procedure was required because of a complication resulting from attempted dilatation of a noninfarcted artery. Added myocardial dysfunction was poorly tolerated in this complicated group of patients, who underwent multiple-lesion PTCA relatively early in our angioplasty experience. The mortality was also increased, with two deaths (6.5%), but was not of greater statistical significance than the 3.5% mortality (4 deaths) in the population undergoing single-lesion dilatation.

This experience has led to changes in our practice policies: in general, we dilate only the infarcted artery during the acute incident. Assuming that the patient stabilizes and remains free of further ischemic events, additional stenoses are dilated 7–10 days later, following medical management and recovery of regional wall function. At this time, during a second procedure, left ventricular function and the acutely dilated coronary segment are reassessed. Additional stenoses are electively dilated at that time, following a review of the previous diagnostic coronary angiogram when procedural complications would be better tolerated.

There are many potential problems in comparison of the multiple-lesion and single-lesion PTCA subgroups in the acute infarct setting. It could be argued that the multiple-lesion population was a "sicker" subgroup requiring more aggressive dilatation, and that this subgroup would have experienced a higher morbidity related to medical management or urgent bypass surgery. Still, for the reasons discussed above, we feel that the preferred management of the acute infarct patient involves single-lesion dilatation followed by medical management and subsequent reassessment.

Advanced Age

Multiple-lesion PTCA was attempted in 124 patients 70 years of age or older and the results were compared with those of single-lesion PTCA in 150 patients of similar age. Procedure-related mortality was significantly elevated in both subgroups, at 3.2% for multiple-lesion PTCA and 4% for single-lesion PTCA. The multiple-lesion group was further analyzed by excluding additional risk factors of acute myocardial infarction, poor left ventricular function, prior bypass surgery, and left main coronary disease. For this subgroup of 100 patients with advanced age and multiple-lesion PTCA as the only risk factors, the mortality remained significantly elevated at 4%, compared with a 0.2% mortality for 504 patients without additional risk factors but less than 70 years of age. Consequently, in this experience, advanced age clearly increased risk for both single- and multiple-lesion PTCA. However, advanced age also identifies patients at increased risk of complication and death resulting from coronary bypass surgery.

Discussion

Multiple-lesion coronary angioplasty is emerging as a viable and realistic alternative to multiple-vessel coronary bypass surgery in selected patients. With experience, single- and multiple-lesion PTCA in several subgroups previously considered to be at high-risk can be performed successfully and safely. Relatively contraindicated in the late 1970s and early 1980s, these forms of complex PTCA now deserve special consideration by individuals and institutions with extensive angioplasty experience.

Although a few studies are in progress, to date there has been no direct comparison of the results of multiple-lesion PTCA and the long-term results of multiple-vessel bypass surgery. Such investigations will be difficult to perform and perhaps more difficult to interpret. Clearly, the incidence of restenosis reported by major centers exceeds the incidence of vein graft occlusion. Consequently, on assessment at 6 months or 1 year after the procedure, it is likely that PTCA will appear to be "less complete" as a single revascularization procedure. Still, there are many attributes of single- and multiple-lesion PTCA that cannot be overlooked or minimized in such a comparison and will weigh in favor of nonsurgical revascularization.

PTCA is less invasive and thereby associated with a lesser morbidity and mortality. PTCA requires a shorter hospitalization and less intense use of less expensive hospital facilities, and as a consequence is less costly for the patient and health care system than is coronary bypass surgery [18, 19]. The period of disability following PTCA is shorter than that required for recuperation from bypass surgery. Consequently, patients can be returned to a productive life and to employment more rapidly than those undergoing surgery. Angioplasty can be repeated with relative ease, low morbidity and mortality, and with lesser expense than a repeat bypass operation.

Nonetheless, the clinician must recognize that single- or multiple-lesion PTCA represents only one additional, potential mode of therapy for patients with the progressive disease of coronary atherosclerosis. Because of widespread lack of technical skills and experience and because of varying clinical and anatomic circumstances, many patients are not suitable for coronary angioplasty, just as they may not be suitable for coronary bypass surgery. Such judgments need individualization and collaboration between clinician, invasive cardiologist, and surgeon to plan the optimal course for management of patients with obstructive coronary disease. It would be far healthier for cardiovascular physicians to view angioplasty and bypass surgery not as competitive procedures but as complementary therapies, both of which may play a role in the management of a particular patient during the evolution of his disease process. The ultimate goal should remain that of providing the most effective, least hazardous, least expensive and least emotionally and physically disabling course of diagnostic and therapeutic procedures to the individual patient.

Acknowledgement. The author wishes to thank his professional colleagues and the Catheterization Laboratory staff of St. Luke's Hospital, Kansas City, Mo, for their support and participation in the care of patients undergoing coronary angioplasty.

References

1. Myler RK, Gruentzig AR, Stertzer SH (1981) Technique and clinical indications for percutaneous transluminal coronary angioplasty. In: Mason DT, Collins JJ Jr (eds) Myocardial revascularization. Yorke Medical, New York, pp 431–444
2. Hamby RI, Katz S (1980) Percutaneous transluminal coronary angioplasty: its potential impact on surgery for coronary artery disease. Am J Cardiol 45:1161–1166
3. Levy RI, Mock MB, Willman VL et al. (1981) Percutaneous transluminal coronary angioplasty: a status report. N Engl J Med 305:399
4. Mock MB, Levy RI (1980) Percutaneous transluminal coronary angioplasty. J Cardiovasc Med pp 31–34
5. King SB (1983) Indications for coronary arteriography and coronary angioplasty. Cardiovasc Rev Reports 4:625–632
6. Berger SM, Gorfinkel HJ (1981) Candidates for transluminal coronary angioplasty. Am J Cardiol 48:810
7. Gosselin AJ, Fisher L, Judkins M (1980) Percutaneous transluminal coronary angioplasty – an estimate of the number of possible candidates from the CASS Registry. In: Proceedings of the workshop on percutaneous transluminal coronary angioplasty, June 15–16, 1979. US DHEW publ no 80–2030, pp 89–100
8. McCallister BD, Hartzler GO, Rutherford BD, McConahay DR (1981) Palliative percutaneous transluminal coronary angioplasty for unstable angina in patients over 70 years of age. Circ 64[Suppl 1V]:225 (abstract)
9. Hartzler GO, Rutherford BD, McConahay DR (1983) Percutaneous transluminal coronary angioplasty with and without thrombolytic therapy for treatment of acute myocardial infarction. Am Heart J 106:965–973
10. Hartzler GO, Rutherford BD, McConahay DR (1984) Percutaneous transluminal coronary angioplasty: application for acute myocardial infarction. Am J Cardiol 53:177C–121C
11. Douglas JS, Gruentzig AR, King SB (1983) Percutaneous transluminal coronary angioplasty in patients with prior coronary bypass surgery. J Am Coll Cardiol 2:745–754
12. Dorros G, Stertzer SH, Cowley M, Kent K, Williams D (1982) Complex transluminal coronary angioplasty: Multivessel disease and multiple dilatations. Circulation [Suppl 11]:329 (abstract)
13. Hartzler GO (1983) Percutaneous transluminal coronary angioplasty in multivessel disease. Cathet Cardiovasc Diagn 9:537–541
14. Giorgi LV, Hartzler GO, Rutherford BD, McConahay DR (1983) Angina following total coronary occlusion – definitive treatment with percutaneous coronary angioplasty. J Am Coll Cardiol 1:656 (abstract)
15. Jones EL, Craver JM, Gruentzig AR (1982) Percutaneous transluminal coronary angioplasty: role of the surgeon. Ann Thorac Surg 34:492–503
16. Hartzler GO, Rutherford BD, McConahay DR, McCallister SH (1982) Simultaneous multiple lesion coronary angioplasty. A preferred therapy for patients with multiple vessel disease. Circulation 66 [Suppl 11]:11–5 (abstract)
17. Hartzler GO, Rutherford BD, McConahay DR (1984) Multiple lesion coronary angioplasty in "High-Risk" patient sub-groups. J Am Coll Cardiol 3:469 (abstract)
18. Jang G, Block PC, Cowley MJ (1982) Comparative cost analysis of coronary angioplasty and coronary bypass surgery: results from a national cooperative study. Circulation [Suppl] 66:2–124
19. Jang G, Gruentzig AR, Block PC (1982) Work profile of patients following coronary angioplasty or coronary bypass surgery: results from a national cooperative study. Circulation [Suppl] 66:11–123

Chapter 16. Coronary and/or Saphenous Vein Graft Angioplasty in Patients with Prior Coronary Artery Bypass Graft Surgery

GERALD DORROS

Introduction

Percutaneous transluminal coronary angioplasty (PTCA) is a safe and effective treatment for selected patients with obstructive coronary disease, usually without prior bypass surgery, who have isolated proximal coronary stenoses [1]. Coronary artery bypass graft surgery (CABG) has also proven to be an effective treatment of obstructive coronary artery disease which has enabled the vast majority of patients to obtain 5–10 years of useful life with the anginal syndrome relieved or improved in over 80% of these bypass patients [2]. However, direct myocardial revascularization surgery (CABG) is not a cure for coronary atherosclerosis. Atherosclerosis continues to progress as long as the patients continue to survive.

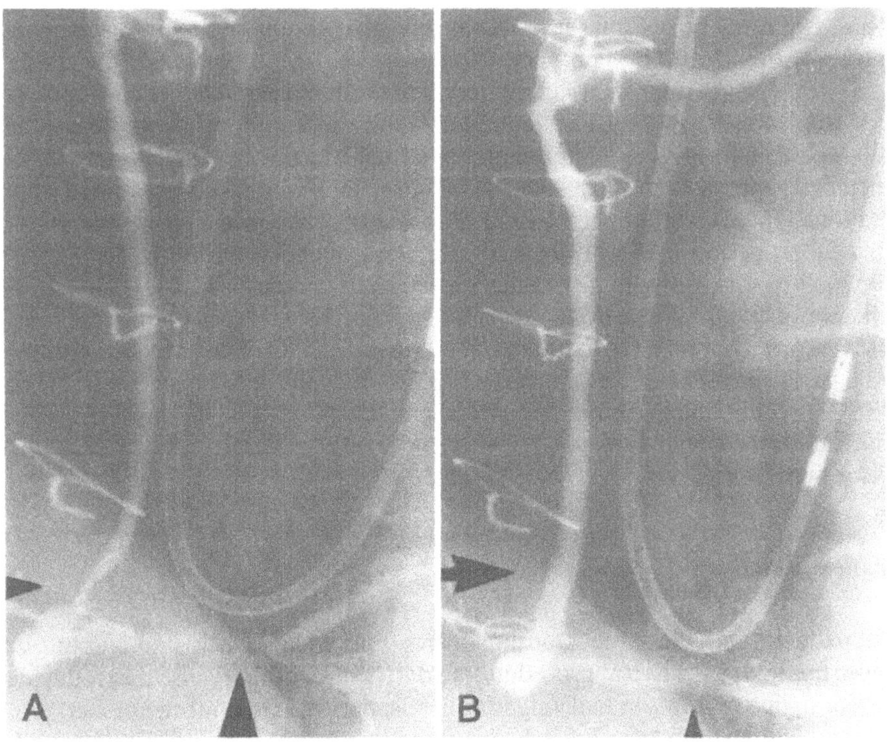

Fig. 1 A, B. Dilatation of shaft and distal anastomotic vein graft stenoses before (**A**) and after (**B**) angioplasty

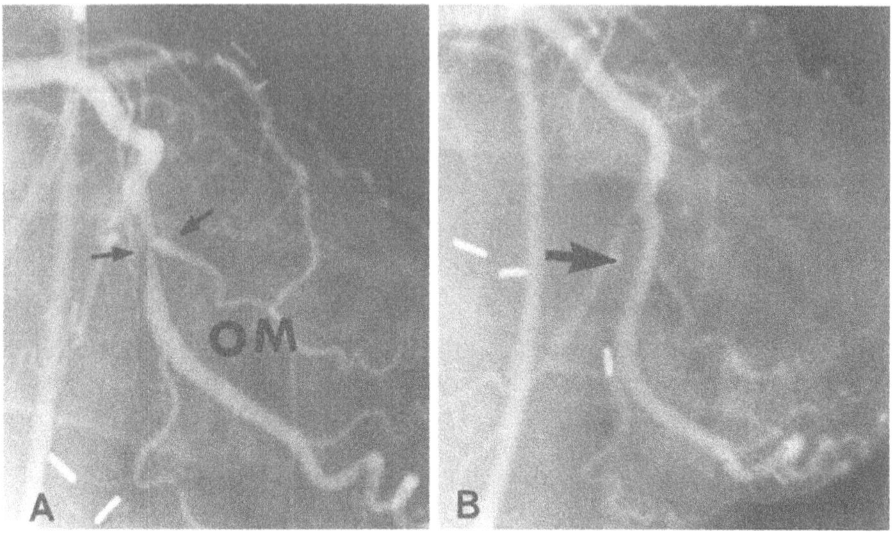

Fig. 2 A, B. Dilatation of a nonbypassed native arterial stenosis (the circumflex obtuse marginal, *OM*) in a 73-year-old woman with prior bypass surgery before (**A**) and after (**B**) angioplasty

Thus, symptoms of ischemic heart disease reappear as atherosclerotic disease progresses within the native coronary artery (whether or not previously bypassed), and/or saphenous vein graft failure occurs with the development of a stenosis or occlusion. Repeat myocardial revascularization procedures can be performed in these patients, but with symptomatic relief achieved in only 60%–70% [3] of them, as opposed to the 80%–90% in whom relief is obtained after primary operations [4]. In addition, the complications associated with repeat operations (mortality, perioperative myocardial infarction, reoperation for bleeding, etc.) are significantly more frequent than with primary operations [5–11]. Therefore, alternative forms of therapy have been sought with the aim of avoiding repeat bypass surgery. Angioplasty has been utilized in patients with prior bypass grafting who had stenosis(es) of the vein graft (Fig. 1) and/or the native artery (Fig. 2) [12, 13]. This communication will discuss patient selection, technical considerations, the results, the advantages, and the disadvantages of angioplasty in patients with prior bypass surgery.

Patient Selection

All patients who underwent transluminal coronary angioplasty had had one or more prior bypass surgical procedures, had ischemic coronary disease producing severe angina pectoris, or had a significant coronary or vein graft stenosis(es) producing significant myocardial ischemia that was confirmed by noninvasive studies (i.e., exercise stress testing and/or myocardial scintigraphy). The patient's coronary anatomy, including the site of the coronary lesion(s), was the determinant of whether or not transluminal angioplasty would be attempted; in addition, the site of the lesion(s) influenced the choice of approach for the guide catheter (brachial or femoral artery).

Each patient agreed to an attempted angioplasty with the proviso that, if necessary, immediate myocardial revascularization or intra-aortic balloon counterpulsation, or both, could be performed. Certain patients, very high risk surgical patients (i.e., patients with an anticipated high surgical mortality and morbidity which could range between 5% and 50%, because of prior surgical procedures and/or concomitant or concurrent medical problems), were informed that emergency revascularization would be performed only in the event of a catastrophe or not at all. In certain patient situations, a coronary occlusion which produced a myocardial infarction would be managed medically and would not be an indication for emergency bypass graft surgery.

Some patients were referred by cardiovascular surgeons or cardiologists for angioplasty of rather complex situations in which a poor immediate surgical result had occurred which led to deterioration of the patient's clinical condition. In some cases multiple lesions were present in bypasses and/or native vessels which would have been amenable to surgery, but the patients were considered more suitable for angioplasty because of a previous complicated and prolonged postoperative course (respiratory failure, renal failure, stroke, or multiple postoperative procedures); because mammary artery grafts were present whose function might be lost at repeat surgery; because of the absence of any obvious remaining sources of vein graft; or because of concomitant medical problems (chronic obstructive lung disease, thrombocytopenia, severe renal disease with chronic renal failure, severe diabetes mellitus with marked end-organ damage, or prior cerebrovascular accidents). Patients who had had prior coronary endarterectomy (Fig. 3) or more than two prior bypass procedures were not considered good candidates for repeat surgery; angioplasty was the chosen technique when the stenosis considered critical could be approached by the dilatation catheter.

Each patient received maintenance treatment with an antiplatelet regimen of aspirin (10 grains) and dipyridamole (150 mg) for 1 or 2 days before, and indefinitely after, the procedure. A calcium antagonist (nifedipine 40 mg daily or diltiazem 120 mg daily) was empirically continued for 1 week after angioplasty unless clinically required for longer.

Each patient was seen by a cardiac surgeon, who reviewed the medical history and cinearteriograms prior to the procedure. The cardiovascular surgical team was available during all procedures. The operating theater was not reserved.

Coronary angioplasty was considered successful when all the lesions attempted were dilated, or when the area of stenosis considered critical was successfully dilated and there was evidence of significant clinical improvement.

Followup was accomplished noninvasively by exercise treadmill testing (Bruce protocol), within 1 week and then at 3-month intervals for 1 year. Angiographic followup was timed differently for vein graft and native artery dilatation. When vein graft stenoses were dilated angiography was performed at 5–6 months and at 12–18 months after the procedure unless clinically indicated before. When a native artery was dilated angiograms were performed about 12 months after the angioplasty unless clinically indicated before. This strategy for angiographic fol-

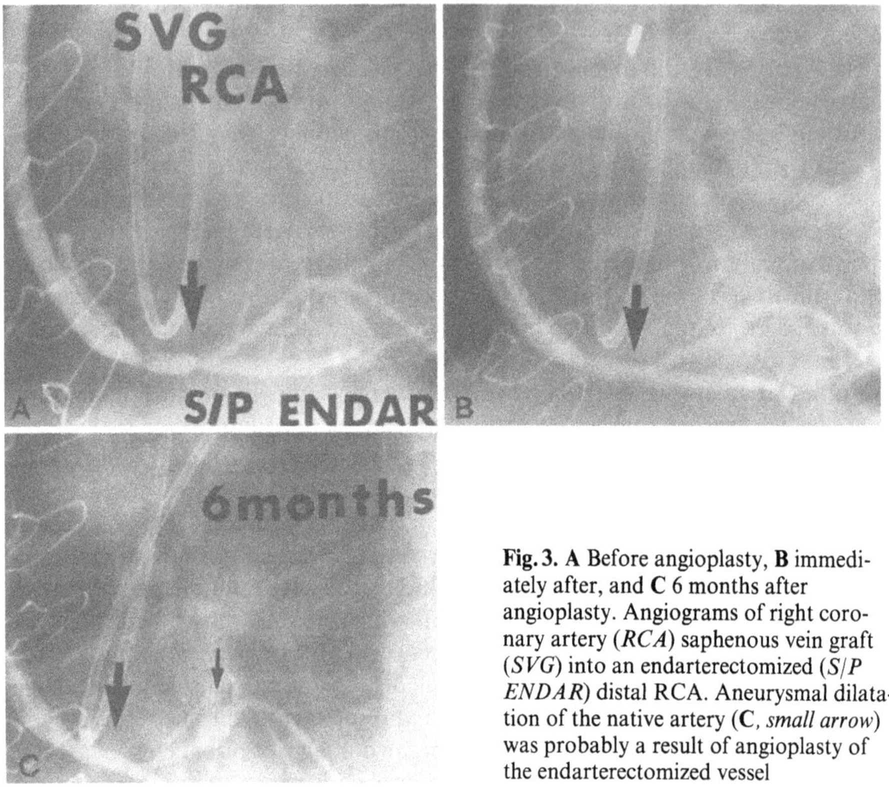

Fig. 3. A Before angioplasty, **B** immediately after, and **C** 6 months after angioplasty. Angiograms of right coronary artery (*RCA*) saphenous vein graft (*SVG*) into an endarterectomized (*S/P ENDAR*) distal RCA. Aneurysmal dilatation of the native artery (**C**, *small arrow*) was probably a result of angioplasty of the endarterectomized vessel

lowup was determined by our past experience [10] of an increased incidence of restenosis.

Technical Considerations

The choice of guide catheters is determined by multiple factors: (a) the coronary lesion which was the stenosis considered critical and the number and types of additional lesions to be dilated; (b) the extent of iliofemoral peripheral vascular disease; (c) the number of previous brachial cutdowns; (d) whether the brachiocephalic system is tortuous; (e) whether the abdominal/thoracic aorta is tortuous and/or dilated; (f) whether the right innominate artery arises distally on the transverse aorta; and (g) whether there has been previous peripherovascular bypass surgery. A right coronary artery lesion is preferentially approached via the brachial artery, while the left anterior descending and the intermediate branch can be approached by either the brachial or the femoral technique (difficulties encountered during the diagnostic procedure must always be taken into account), while for a circumflex lesion the femoral technique is initially used. A saphenous

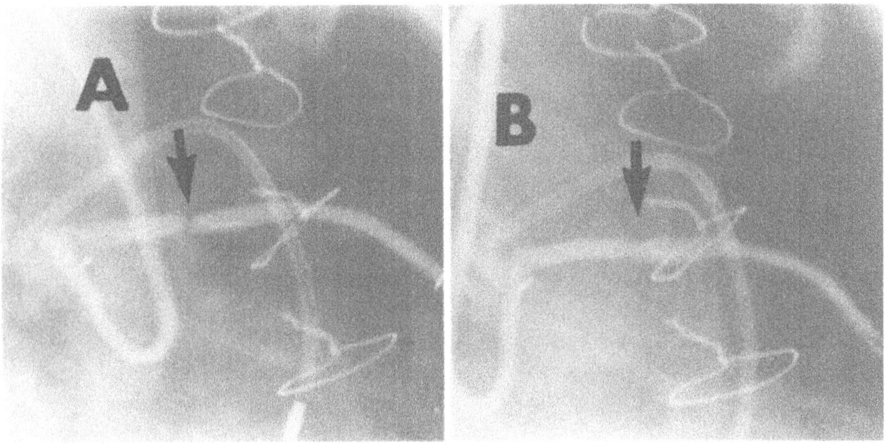

Fig. 4. A Pre- and **B** postangioplasty angiograms of proximal saphenous vein graft stenosis

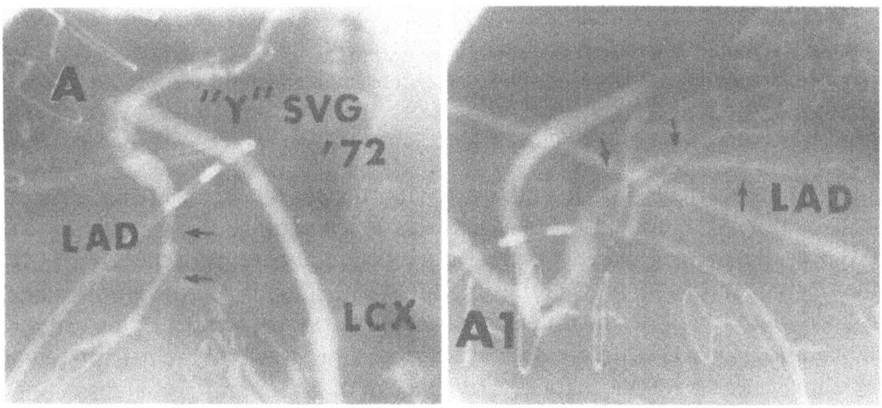

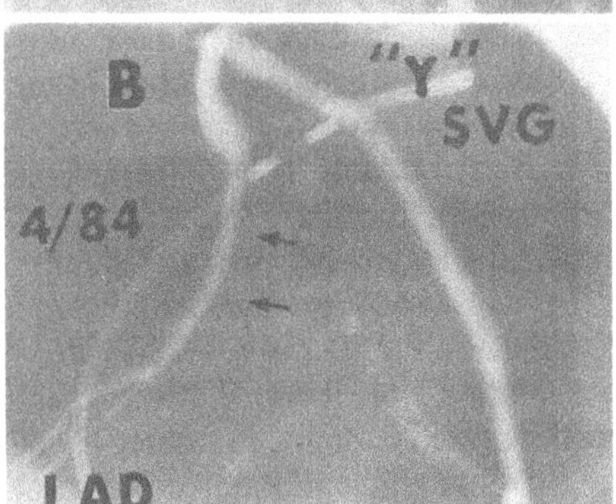

Fig. 5 A, B. Successful dilatation was achieved in a 14-year-old Y saphenous vein graft (*SVG*) in a 68-year-old man with class III angina who had undergone two prior bypass operations. The left anterior oblique projection shows (**A**) the SVG limb going to the left anterior descending artery (*LAD*) with a shaft stenosis and with severe cranial angulation (30°) in the anteroposterior projection (**A1**) the distal anastomotic stenosis is seen; the postangioplasty angiograms (**B**) show a successful result. The patient became clinically symptomfree

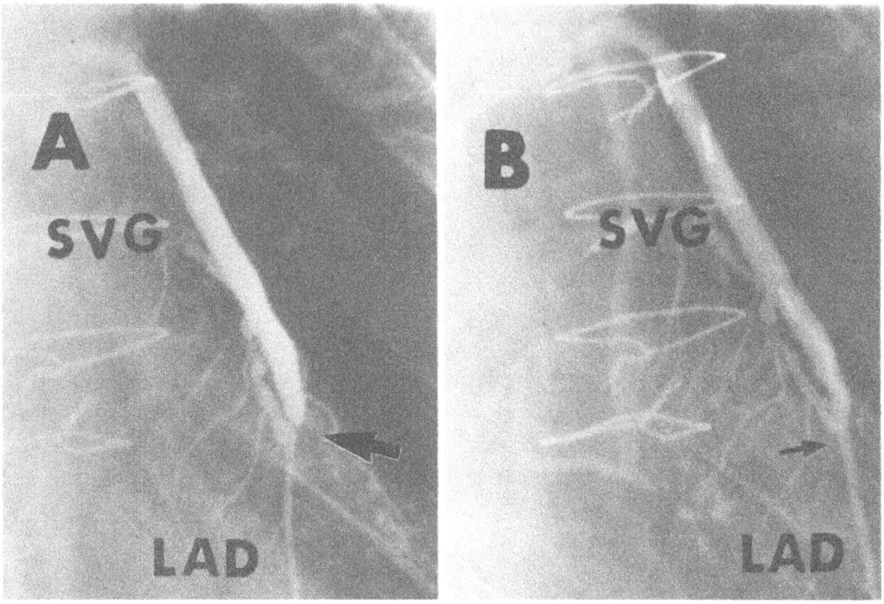

Fig. 6 A, B. Dilatation of a (distal) saphenous vein graft (*SVG*) stenosis at the anastomotic site with the left anterior descending artery (*LAD*). **A** Before and **B** after angioplasty

vein graft stenosis may perferentially be approached via the brachial artery, usually with a 9-F modified Amplatz catheter which permits easy cannulation of the vein graft ostium, good guide catheter stability, and passage of the larger (3.7-mm, 4.2-mm, and 5.0-mm) steerable dilatation catheters. When the graft ostium has been placed high on the anterior ascending aorta, or posteriorly on the ascending aorta for a graft to cross the transverse sinus, the left brachial approach may allow easier ostial intubation. The creation of a vein graft ostial dissection with these Amplatz shaped guiding catheters is less likely than when these same stiff-tipped catheters are used in the native artery. The aortic anastomotic site has healed with a firm fibrotic scar.

In proximal (aortic) anastomotic (Fig. 4) and shaft stenosis (Fig. 5) (regardless of the age of the graft) a larger balloon catheter is initially utilized, often a 4.2-mm dilatation catheter, unless the vein graft appears very small, when a 3.0-mm catheter is used. Normally, the catheter will traverse these stenoses readily, and once in place will be inflated to between 5 and 8 atm for 60–180 s. Higher inflations are usually not necessary with larger dilatation catheters [11]. Multiple inflations may be necessary to produce a significant reduction ($\leq$20 mmHg residual gradient) or abolition of the mean trans-stenotic gradient. After withdrawal of the dilatation catheter angiography is performed with the guide catheter.

A distal anastomosis stenosis (Fig. 6) and a lesion in the native artery beyond the distal anastomosis are approached differently. When the vein graft is anastomosed into a large coronary artery and the lesion is not too severe a 3.7-mm steerable catheter is usually chosen, or when the stenosis is very severe, a 3.0-mm low-

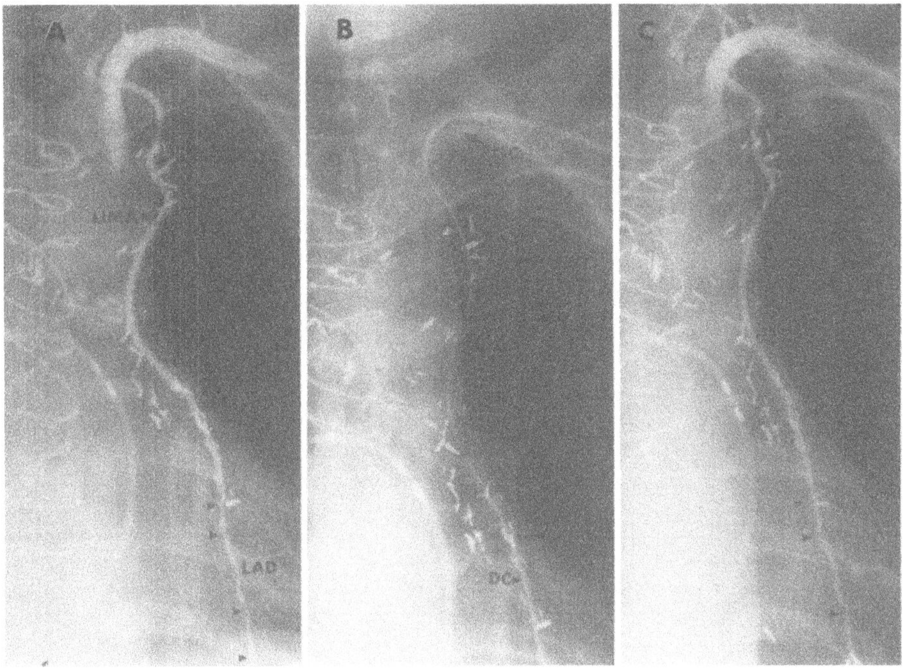

Fig. 7 A–C. The dilatation of multiple stenoses in the left anterior descending artery (*LAD*) with the dilatation catheter (*DC*) traversing the left internal mammary artery (*LIMA*) using the left brachial artery approach. **A** before dilatation; **B** guide catheter (*GC*) in place and dilatation catheter (*DC*) positioned across the left anterior descending artery stenosis; **C** postangioplasty results

profile catheter is used. If the stenosis does not permit passage of any steerable catheter, including the 2.5-mm or 2.0-mm balloon, the finely tapered nonsteerable USCI DG-20-20 catheter usually crosses the lesion without hindrance. But this catheter, with its dagger-like tip, will require the lesion to be recrossed with a larger catheter in the same session or a future session. Lesions in the native artery distal to an open distal anastomosis are approached with a steerable 3.0-mm balloon catheter. Occasionally, a guide catheter has been threaded down the graft to supply sufficient support for the lesion to be crossed. In a similar manner, lesions in the native artery distal to the mammary artery insertion may be approached and dilated via the mammary artery (Fig. 7).

Results

The results of angioplasty performed in patients with prior bypass surgery must be viewed with reference to the patient's age and clinical status, the failure of medical management, the results of alternative therapies (repeat bypass surgery), and concomitant medical problems.

Table 1. Patient characteristics

		No.		%
Total no. of procedures		140		
1. Patients		114		
Male		92		(81)
Female		22		(19)
Age (years)		59		
2. Extent of coronary disease				
Multivessel		131		(94)
Single vessel		9		(5)
3. Prior myocardial infarction		84/140		(60)
4. Diabetes		20/140		(14)
5. Hypertension		54/140		(39)
6. Anginal class 0		19/140		(13)
I		12/140		(9)
II		39/140		(28)
III		38/140		(27)
IV		32/140		(23)
7. Prior revascularization procedure (140 cases)				
No. of procedure	1	2	3	4
No. of pts	117	17	4	2

During the 65 months from 12/78 to 4/84, in all 114 patients underwent 140 separate procedures, during which 215 angioplasties were attempted. The baseline characteristics are shown in Table 1. The interval between bypass surgery and the angioplasty procedure varied between about 2 weeks and 180 months (mean of 39 months). In 34 cases (33 patients) the surgical risk was considered very high because of the number of prior surgical operations, diminished left ventricular ejection fraction (≦40%), or accompanying medical problems.

The results of PTCA are shown in Table 2 with 180/215 (84%) stenoses successfully dilated. A successful clinical improvement at hospital discharge, excluding emergency bypass patients and including those with/without complications, was recorded in 112/140 (80%) of cases. No complications were encountered in 121/140 cases (86%). When complications occurred they often appeared in clusters [14], i.e., more than one occurred in the same patient, and tended to be serious problems.

There were 5 deaths (5/114 pts, 4.4%), 3 in patients with a prohibitively high surgical risk (>50%, or reoperation impossible). Patient 1 (a 53-year-old man) had been hypotensive for 1 month and required intra-aortic balloon pump support (20 days); he had renal and hepatic failure and adult respiratory distress syndrome. He underwent successful angioplasty of the left main coronary stenosis, which permitted removal of the intra-aortic balloon pump, and discontinuation of the i.v. cardiovascular supporting medication; hemodynamic stabilization was achieved within 12 h of the angioplasty. The patient died of asystole during endotracheal suctioning 5 days after angioplasty. Patient 2 (a 50-year-old man) had class III angina; he had undergone three unsuccessful attempts at bypass surgery and underwent apparently successful dilatation of multiple circumflex stenosis

Table 2. Angioplasty data

	No.	%
1. Results		
a) Angioplasty attempts	215	
Successes/total lesions	180/215	(84%)
Successes/total patients	112/140	(80%)
b) Complications		
Myocardial infarction	5	(3.6% per case) (2.3% per lesion)
Emergency bypass surgery	3	(2.1% per case) (1.2% per lesion)
Death	5	(4.4% per patient)
Neurological complications	0	
c) Angiographic changes		
Mean diameter stenosis		
Before	84% ± 14%	
After	8% ± 20%	
d) Mean trans-stenotic gradient change		
Before	33.2 mmHg	
After	6.3 mmHg	
e) Percentage of cases with number of dilatations		
1 Lesion	(63%)	
2 Lesions	(27%)	
3 Lesions	(8%)	
4 Lesions	(2%)	

without incident. Upon leaving the catheterization laboratory the patient had a cardiac arrest and could not be resuscitated. The presumptive cause of death was coronary spasm producing coronary occlusion following the initially successful dilatation which was documented angiographically. Patient 3 (a 62-year-old man) had class III angina and had undergone two previous surgical operations complicated by difficult postoperative courses. He had an occluded left anterior descending artery with a functioning saphenous vein graft. The left main artery was severely stenosed but supplied a large marginal artery which had not previously been bypassed. During the actual dilatation of the left main stenosis, electromechanical dissociation occurred. External cardiopulmonary resuscitation provided good support. The patient was taken to the operating room alert but without any effective intrinsic cardiac output. He did not survive a difficult third bypass operation. Thus, 3 deaths occurred in this group of 33 patients who underwent 34 procedures, all of whom were considered very high risk surgical cases. This means an angioplasty-associated mortality of 8.8% (3/34) per intervention, or 9.1% (3/33) per patient. If these difficult cases are excluded from the series the mortality associated with angioplasty is 1.9% (2/106) per intervention, or 2.5% (2/81) per patient. Thus, the operative risk for angioplasty in most patients with prior bypass surgery ranges between 2.0% and 3.0%.

Table 3 analyzes the success rate with the angioplasty procedure by the site of the lesion(s) attempted. Dilatation of 39 saphenous vein graft stenoses alone was attempted in 33 cases, with success achieved in 33 (85%) of the grafts and

Table 3. Distribution of procedures performed by site of stenosis

	Success/Total lesions	Success/Total cases
All angioplasty procedures	180/215 (84%)	112/140 (80%)
a) Vein graft alone	33/ 39 (85%)	28/ 33 (85%)
b) Vein graft and native artery	67/ 78 (86%)	33/ 37 (89%)
c) Native artery alone	80/ 98 (82%)	51/ 70 (73%)

Table 4. Analysis of lesions attempted by site of stenosis

	Success/Total lesions	Restenosis[a]
Individual lesion analysis		
a) Saphenous vein graft	74/ 82 (90%)	15/ 74 (20%)
(I) Proximal (aortic) anastomosis	27/ 30 (90%)	–
(II) Body (shaft)	16/ 16 (100%)	–
(III) Distal anastomosis	31/ 36 (86%)	–
b) Native stenosis	106/133 (80%)	26/106 (25%)
(I) Left anterior descending	37/ 47 (79%)	–
(II) Left circumflex	23/ 32 (72%)	–
(III) Right coronary	37/ 44 (84%)	–
(IV) Left main coronary	9/ 10 (90%)	–

[a] Clinically evident restenosis

clinical success achieved in 28 (85%) of cases. Saphenous vein graft stenosis(es) was dilated in conjunction with native coronary artery stenosis(es) in 37 cases. The native artery had been bypassed previously in some cases. Successful dilatation was achieved in 67 of 78 lesions (86%). Clinical success was achieved in 33 cases (89%).

In 70 patients angioplasty of native coronary artery stenosis(es) was attempted, and 80 of the 98 stenoses (82%) were successfully dilated. Clinical success was achieved in 51 (73%) of the cases.

An analysis of the lesions attempted according to the site of stenosis is shown in Table 4. Of the 82 saphenous vein graft stenoses, 74 (90%) were successfully dilated, with clinical restenosis occurring in 15 (20%). The position of a stenosis in a vein graft did not affect the result of dilatation.

Of 133 native artery stenoses, 106 (80%) were successfully dilated, with clinically evident restenosis occurring in 26 (25%). The specific arterial site, the success rate at each site, and the restenosis rates are shown.

There is no statistical difference in the success rates achieved between the saphenous vein grafts and the native arteries. There is no statistical difference in the restenosis rates between a saphenous vein graft and a native artery.

Followup data (Table 5) of all the angioplasty patients (114) show: 85 patients (75%) remain clinically well as a result of the initial angioplasty procedure or a repeat procedure. An improved anginal status compared with that before angioplasty was present in 51 patients (60%). Twenty-one patients (18%) under-

Table 5. Followup of all angioplasty patients (114)[a] (mean followup 18 months)

	Medical treatment ($n=73$)	2nd/3rd TCA ($n=15$)	Elective CABG ($n=21$)
Angina[b]			
Same	8	1	2
Worse	1	0	1
Improved	48	14	18
No record	13	0	0
Late MI	2	0	0
Death	3	0	0

[a] Five patients died before hospital discharge
[b] Anginal status compared with that prior to angioplasty

went elective coronary artery bypass surgery during the followup period because of failure of the initial angioplasty procedure, lesion recurrence, and/or progression of disease. Within the medical treatment group there were 2 late infarctions and 3 late deaths. Repeat angioplasty was performed in 15 patients with 17 stenoses [restenosis rate of 15% (17/114)], 15 being treated for the second time and 2 for the third time. The mean interval between the initial angioplasty and the second procedure was 4.5 months, with 14/15 patients (93%) having a successful dilatation. However, 4 of the 15 patients (27%) subsequently underwent elective bypass surgery after a restenosis angioplasty. Thus, 81 patients (71%) continued to be successfully managed with or without medication and/or a subsequent angioplasty procedure.

Discussion

The introduction of coronary bypass surgery to alleviate the symptoms of patients with ischemic coronary disease has enabled the vast majority of these patients to have 5–10 years of useful and productive life, the anginal syndrome being dramatically relieved or improved in 80%–90% of them. These people continue to survive and function, while at the same time their illness, atherosclerosis, continues to progress. The progression of coronary atherosclerosis will cause angina to recur or worsen in about 5% of patients per year. Therefore, as we enter the second decade of bypass surgery, many prior coronary artery bypass patients are beginning to have worsening or the recurrence of symptoms of ischemic heart disease. The cause of the problem may be related to atherosclerotic disease within the native coronary artery (whether or not it has previously been bypassed) and/or saphenous vein graft failure secondary to atherosclerosis or intimal hyperplasia.

Symptoms can recur within 6–12 months following bypass surgery for various reasons. Early operative "failure," (i.e., significant symptomatic recurrence within 6–12 months of surgery) is often related to vein graft failure: incorrect surgical manipulation of a vein graft, inadequate operating technique or surgical ex-

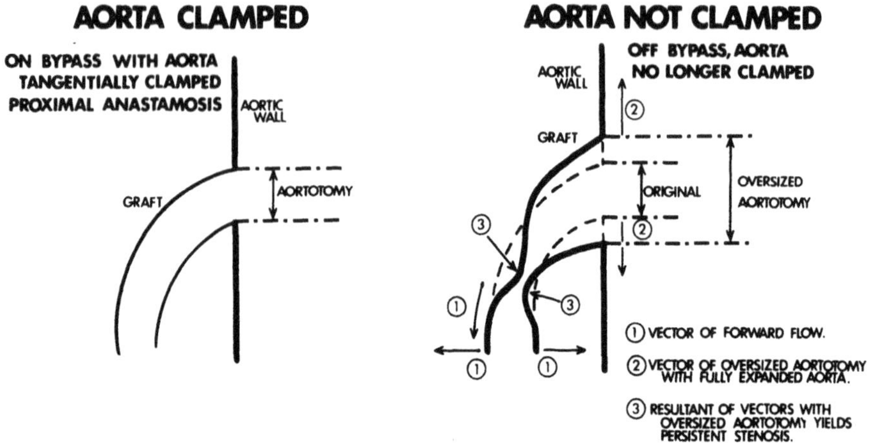

Fig. 8. Schematic showing how too large an aortotomy could create proximal vein graft constriction

Table 6. Significant complications related to repeat myocardial revascularization

	Reoperation/ all CABG pts	Perioperative infarction	Deaths	
			#	%
Reul et al. (1979)	168/13 049	2%	8	4.8
Loop et al. (1968)	219/ 2 613	9%	8	3.7
Johnson (personal communication, 1983)	636/ 6 258	–	51	8.0
(a) Good ventricle (E. F.[a] >35%)	514		30	5.8
(b) Bad ventricle (E. F. <35%)	111		19	17.1
(c) Unknown (unknown E. F.)	11		2	18.2

[a] Left ventricular ejection fraction

perience, unsuitable size of anastomosis [i.e., too large an aortotomy (Fig. 8) or too small a coronary arteriotomy], a short vein graft which pulls or dents the coronary artery, use of an unsuitable conduit, and poor arterial runoff or vein graft flow rate can all prejudice the result of angioplasty. These early postoperative problems are in contradistinction to those occurring years after the procedure, which are usually related to atherosclerosis or hyperplasia within the vein graft, progression of disease in grafted and/or ungrafted vessels, or inadequate or incomplete revascularization. Dr. W. Dudley Johnson, the innovator of bypass surgery, has repeatedly stated that failure to bypass less than "critical" vessels or those in which bypass is technically difficult because of beaded lesions or diffuse atheroslerotic disease results in inadequate or incomplete revascularization and will eventually lead to repeat surgery, which can usually be avoided by complete revascularization at the first operation.

Repeat coronary artery bypass surgery even at a second operation is associated with higher morbidity and mortality rates (Table 6) than are associated with primary operations. The number of published reports of the results of repeat bypass surgery are few [3, 5–11], only two reports dealing with more than 100 cases [3, 5]; Reul [5] excluded all repeat surgery (another 160 cases) from the report when his group had not done the primary operation. the largest series of repeat operations is described in a personal communication from W. Dudley Johnson (1983), which not only lists 636 repeat operations but also subdivides the cases in relation to ventricular function. The perioperative myocardial infarction rate varied among the different surgical reports from 2% to 11.5%, the mortality rate varied from 1.2% to 17.1%, and the incidence of reoperation for bleeding and other complications was not insignificant. This can be compared with the 0.5% –2% mortality for patients with normal or mildly impaired ventricular function and a perioperative infarction rate (presence of new electrocardiographic Q waves) of less than 5% during the primary surgical experience. What is of importance is that even though repeat direct myocardial revascularization can be accomplished with a low but not insignificant mortality and morbidity, the achievement of symptomatic relief, i.e., operative success as determined by the patient's clinical response, is only 60%–70%, as against the 80%–90% success rate after primary operations.

Clearly, the results of angioplasty in the patient with prior bypass surgery are gratifying, especially compared with the results of repeat bypass surgery, with regard to success rates, recurrence rates, complication rates, and long-term clinical improvement.

Angioplasty of vein grafts more than 6 months old that had developed diffuse or even localized disease was formerly criticized by some surgical colleagues, whose descriptions of the graft appearance at operation, with its intimal hyperplasia, fibrin and clot deposition, and atherosclerotic grumous material, gave credence to their pronouncement that in these grafts angioplasty should not be attempted [13]. However, these strong reservations against angioplasty in these particular cases were reversed by the same colleagues after they had referred patients for angioplasty with these same severe lesions except that the surgical risk was considered prohibitive and the angioplasty results were satisfactory and did not bear out their prior objections.

The results of these procedures were most interesting, since all the shaft lesions were successfully dilated. But, as had been predicted, distal embolization (Fig. 9) occurred in three patients and all had chest pain, modest (two-fold) CPK enzyme elevations, and transient ST segment changes without the development of any new Q waves. These three patients became clinically asymptomatic. Followup angiography in two patients showed no evidence of any residual embolization *or* loss of any arterial branches. One patient had progression of disease and subsequently underwent elective bypass surgery.

Myocardial infarction is not a desirable outcome of any procedure. However, this complication may have to be accepted by the operator and treated in a vigorous and cffective manner without subjecting the patient to emergency bypass surgery with its attendant high mortality [15]. Therefore, if an arterial occlusion occurs or a vein graft dilatation produces distal debris embolization, in most cases standard medication, arrhythmia monitoring, and perhaps percutaneous intraaortic balloon pump counterpulsation would be preferable to emergency bypass surgery for management of the patient.

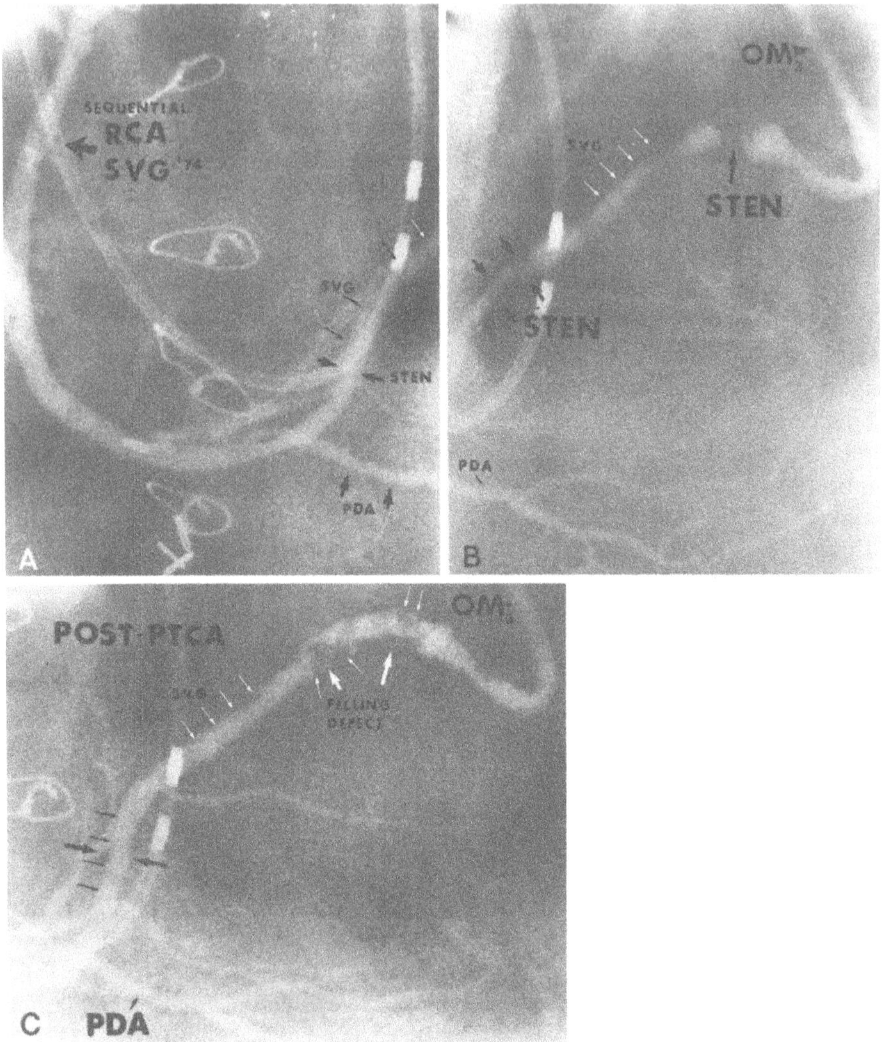

Fig. 9 A–C. Dilatation of a 10-year-old saphenous vein graft stenosis in a 76-year-old man with class III angina. Results were distal embolization, a small subendocardial infarction, and the patient becoming asymptomatic. **A** The sequential right coronary artery (*RCA*) saphenous vein graft (*SVG*) with a side-to-side anastomosis to the posterior descending artery (*PDA*), affected by multiple stenoses (*STEN*) between the *PDA* and the third obtuse marginal (OM_3) anastomoses (**B**). The postangioplasty angiogram (**C**) shows successful result following dilatation of the stenoses and the presence of an intraluminal filling defect recorded by cinearteriography as it migrated distally down the vein graft

This approach requires an assessment of the desired goals and of the risks of alternative management methods for the patient, and the psychological readiness of the interventional angiographer to accept these problems without sending an unstable patient to the surgeon. The technical skill, dexterity, and expertise of the interventional angiographer must be refined before he treats such patients, just as the surgeon's operative technique and experience must mature before the difficult cases are attempted. The interventional angiographer must be technically adept at dealing with cardiovascular complications, and at percutaneous insertion of the intra-aortic balloon counterpulsation device. The interventional angiographer must accept that he can create a major complication that can lead to the patient's demise, without any further interventions being offered. The internist and cardiologist have not been trained to accept that they might do something that will directly precipitate the immediate death of a patient. The interventional angiographer cannot utilize the cardiovascular surgeon to psychologically relieve him of the responsibility of precipitating that patient's death. Obviously, the performance of any therapeutic intervention, including angioplasty, will produce situations over which the interventionist has no control. He/she must accept this. This factor alone will be a significant reason for many patients not to undergo angioplasty in such critical, high-risk situations. However, these patients can and should be referred to individuals who deal with such high-risk cases on a daily basis.

The problem of restenosis has yet to be solved. The vast majority of lesions, when carefully selected, can not only be approached, but can also be successfully dilated. Thus, the restenosis rate becomes an extremely important consideration. What causes the restenosis to occur has not been defined. The differences between the rates of restenosis in vein grafts and native arteries may be related in part to the anatomic distinctions between a low-pressure conduit, the vein, placed into a high-pressure system, the vein graft and the high-pressure native coronary artery. The surgical technique itself is important. If the size of the proximal aortic anastomosis (Fig. 8) is inappropriate this may produce early stenoses which will rapidly recur following dilatation. If the aortotomy is significantly larger than the vein graft lumen, and when the aorta is fully expanded after being unclamped and the patient has been taken off bypass, it will result in proximal vein graft constriction. If this is the problem, recurrence after angioplasty is probable. However, if the proximal stenosis is secondary to inappropriate vein graft manipulation this lesion may be more amenable to angioplasty. The differentation of these problems appears insoluble at present.

The modification of angioplasty techniques and equipment may overcome or attenuate the problems of restenosis. The use of larger dilatation catheters (4.2-mm and 5.0-mm balloons), longer inflation times (60–180 s), prolonged and moderately higher pressures during these longer inflation times (5–12 atm), and antiplatelet medication regimens (acetylsalcytic acid in conjunction with dipyridamole, and/or sulfinpyrazone) may help lower the restenosis rate. In addition, the referring physician, as well as the patient, must be made to realize that the restenosis rate is significant. During the initial patient interview the patient must be made aware that a second dilatation may well be necessary and should not be unexpected. We must learn whether or not the second dilatation, or perhaps even a third dilatation, may be necessary for angioplasty to be effective in vein graft stenosis. This has been shown to be effective in the restenosed native coronary artery lesion.

The rate of restenosis within the native coronary arteries is similar to that previously reported. The results of repeat angioplasty in this group are satisfying and acceptable. Thus, repeat angioplasty of a native coronary artery should be undertaken whenever clinically possible.

Rapid or "significant" progression of "malignant" atherosclerosis occurs in a subset of patients for which angioplasty may not provide a solution. At present, surgery, and in particular newer surgical techniques, such as extensive coronary endarterectomy, may be the best therapeutic approach in these patients.

Summary

Direct myocardial revascularization not only provides symptomatic relief but also prolongs life in the majority of patients. Repeat direct myocardial revascularization provides symptomatic relief in a smaller number of patients and is associated with higher morbidity and mortality than primary operations. Angioplasty is an interventional, therapeutic catheter technique that can be used in a large number of prior bypass patients who have sufficiently severe symptoms to require another revascularization procedure. The initial results of successful lesion dilatation coupled with clinical improvement, the associated mortality and morbidity statistics, and the long-term symptomatic relief are comparable to those published for repeat coronary bypass graft surgery. In addition, technological advances in angioplasty equipment and more experienced interventionists will enable more lesions to be successfully reached, traversed, and dilated with a concomitant lower morbidity. I estimate that 30%–40% of patients now requiring repeat operation can undergo a coronary angioplasty procedure with comparable clinical results to those achieved with repeat bypass surgery and with comparable or better morbidity and mortality statistics, bearing in mind that more than two-thirds of the angioplasty patients will be clinically improved in the long term.

Finally, a word of admonition. Coronary angioplasty is a deceptive procedure because of its apparent simplicity and elegance. Yet, angioplasty eloquently appeals to human ingenuity, which can identify and solve a problem and then continually refine the solution.

Angioplasty is a dramatic illustration of the changes that can occur in therapeutic medicine when technology is combined with ingenuity and daring. However, angioplasty's alluring simplicity when demonstrated by a skilled and dedicated interventionist can deceive the novice into believing he or she can do it as easily. Ultimately, this false confidence can result in catastrophe. Angioplasty can be like Heinrich Heine's Lorelei, the beautiful siren who lured the sailors to their deaths on the rocks of the River Rhine just above Koblenz, at St. Goar. It is a technical skill which can be learned, but should not be learned totally at the patient's expense. The cardiovascular surgeon does not want a dilettante colleague who comes into the operating room to do an occasional procedure. Repeat bypass surgical procedures are different and more difficult than primary procedures and should not be done by a surgeon once, twice, or three times a year. Similarly, cardiologists should realize that cardiology has become so diffuse and segmented that no cardiologist cannot provide all services to the patient. The performance of diagnostic angiography does not give the angiographer interventionist's privileges. Interventional angiographers do not desire to see the occasional "angioplasterer." Angioplasty is itself a technical discipline which must be exercised continuously to provide the patient with the best likelihood of success and the least likelihood of complication.

References

1. Kent KM, Bentivoglio LG, Block PC, Cowley MJ, Dorros G, Gosselin AJ, Gruentzig A, Myler RK, Simpson J, Stertzer SH, Williams DO, Fisher L, Gillespie MJ, Detre K, Kelsey S, Mullin SM, Mock MB (1982) Percutaneous transluminal coronary angioplasty. Report from the Registry of the National Heart, Lung and Blood Institute. Am J Cardiol 49:2011–2020
2. Loop FD, Sheldon WC, Lytle BW, Cosgrove DM, Proudfit WL (1981) The efficacy of coronary artery surgery. Am Heart J 101:86
3. Loop FD, Thurer RL, Lytle BW, Cosgrove DM (1968) Reoperation for myocardial revascularization. World J Surg 2:719–729
4. Anderson RP, Rahimtoola SH, Bonchek LI, Starr A (1974) The prognosis of patients with coronary artery disease after coronary bypass operations. Circulation 50:274
5. Reul GJ, Cooley DA, Ott DA, Coelho A, Chapa L, Eterovic I (1979) Reoperation for recurrent coronary artery disease. Arch Surg 114:1269–1275
6. Krause AH, Page VS, Bigelow JC, Okies JE, Dunlop SF (1978) Reoperation in symptomatic patients after direct coronary artery revascularization. J Thorac Cardiovasc Surg 75:499–504
7. Keon WJ, Bedard P, Akyurekli Y, Brais M (1977) Experience with reoperation following coronary bypass grafting. Can J Surg 20:142–146
8. Allen RH, Stinson EB, Oyer PE, Shumway NE (1978) Predictive variables in reoperation for coronary disease. J Thorac Cardiovasc Surg 75:186–192
9. Culliford AT, Girdwood RW, Isam OW, Krauss KR, Spencer FC (1979) Angina following myocardial revascularization. J Thorac Cardiovasc Surg 77:889–895
10. Vouhe P, Grondin CM (1979) Reoperation for coronary graft failure. Clinical and angiographic results in 43 patients. Ann Thorac Surg 27:328–334
11. Norwood WI, Cohn LH, Collins JJ (1977) Results of reoperation for recurrent angina pectoris. Ann Thorac Surg 23:9–13
12. Douglas JS, Gruentzig AR, King SB, Hollman J, Ischinger T, Meier B, Craver JM, Jones EL, Waller JL, Bone DK, Guyton R (1983) Percutaneous transluminal coronary angioplasty in patients with prior coronary bypass surgery. J Am Coll Cardiol 2:745
13. Dorros G, Johnson WD, Tector AJ, Schmahl TM, Kalush SL, Janke L (1984) Percutaneous transluminal coronary angioplasty in patients with prior coronary artery bypass grafting. J Thorac Cardiovasc Surg 87:17
14. Dorros G, Cowley MJ, Simpson J, Bentivoglio LG, Block PC, Bourassa M, Detre K, Gosselin AJ, Gruentzig AR, Kelsey SF, Kent KM, Mock MB, Mullin SM, Myler RK, Passamani ER, Stertzer SH, Williams DO (1983) Percutaneous transluminal coronary angioplasty: report of complications from the National Heart, Lung and Blood Institute PTCA Registry. Circulation 67:723
15. Cowley MJ, Dorros G, Kelsey SF, Van Raden M, Detre K (to be published) Emergency coronary artery bypass surgery following coronary angioplasty. Am J Cardiol

Chapter 17. Coronary Angioplasty for Evolving Myocardial Infarction

JÜRGEN MEYER

Coronary Angioplasty for Unstable Angina

Coronary angioplasty was first used by A. Gruentzig for the treatment of chronic stable angina pectoris [1]. In 1980 we extended the indications for this method to include patients with unstable angina [2]. Since then, coronary angioplasty has become an established treatment for this potentially fatal form of coronary artery disease [3–7].

Indications

The patient's anginal symptoms must be severe and of recent onset (within the last 2 months) and increasing intensity and duration (Table 1). They may occur at rest and during the night. Some patients suffer from a sudden deterioration of their chronic anginal symptoms. During the attacks negative T waves and ST segment elevations or deflections may be recorded in the electrocardiogram.

The ideal indications are isolated, proximal stenoses of less than 2.0 cm in one of the main coronary arteries. Two adjacent stenoses in one vessel can easily be treated during the same intervention.

Two isolated stenoses in different arteries can also be treated successively within one session. Some physicians, however, prefer to postpone the treatment of the second stenosis to the next day. In any case, the most severe stenosis should be treated first ("worst first").

Stenoses of the main stem of the left coronary artery system can also be treated by angioplasty. This indication is no longer disputed among experienced operators. In case of a vessel occlusion, however, the patient will be in a critical condition [8, 9]. Therefore standby facilities for cardiac surgery are mandatory in such cases.

Occlusions of saphenous vein grafts may also cause increasing symptoms of unstable angina. Coronary angioplasty is indicated in proximal bypass stenoses

Table 1. Indications for angioplasty in unstable angina

Severe angina of recent onset
Isolated, proximal, short (<2.0 cm) stenosis in one or two coronary arteries
Subsequent tandem stenosis
Stenosis in bypass grafts
Main stem lesions
Recanalization of totally occluded vessels (occlusion time: days to weeks)

at the aortic insertion, in the body of the vein, and also at the distal insertion [10].

Some patients with unstable angina suffer from a total vessel occlusion without the clinical signs of acute myocardial infarction. Their coronary arterial system shows well-developed collaterals, which may not be large enough, however, to supply the jeopardized myocardium. Such total occlusions with a history of some days or weeks can also be recanalized with a balloon catheter [7, 11, 12].

Not only concentric hourglass-like stenoses but also eccentric ones, even with slight microcalcifications, can be treated successfully [7, 13]. In multivessel disease with primary indications for bypass surgery the main, or most critical, coronary stenosis can be dilated immediately after the coronary angiography to gain time for the total revascularization.

The operator's experience in selecting patients with stenoses suitable for angioplasty is the basis of the degree of success he/she can attain. The accuracy of his/her judgement as to when dilatation is possible and when it is too risky increases steadily with the accumulation of practical experience [14, 15]. In difficult cases the angiofilm should be analyzed not only by the operator but also by more experienced colleagues and by a cardiac surgeon.

Evaluation of the Method

Coronary angioplasty occupies a middle position in the treatment of unstable angina, between medical/conservative treatment and bypass surgery. Medical treatment with the aid of nitroinfusions, calcium antagonists, and beta blockers can stabilize the situation and lead to a chronic form of the disease. These drugs, however, do not modify the underlying atherosclerosis or the organic vessel stenosis. The coronary blood flow can be improved only slightly, if at all.

With the aid of a bypass operation, especially in multivessel disease, multiple segments of the coronary artery system can be supplied with an augmented coronary blood flow. Besides the complete revascularization, additional surgical corrections like aneurysmectomy, reconstruction of papillary muscles, or valve replacements may be performed within a single session. The disadvantages of the surgical procedure are the expensive and elaborate operation with the extracorporeal circulation, the risk of hepatitis, and the high costs incurred for the longer hospital stay and the subsequent rehabilitation phase [16, 17]. Many patients have difficulty in returning to their previous jobs after surgery. In the case of recurrent symptoms a second operation will not be easy.

Coronary angioplasty can be compared to cardiac catheterization. The whole procedure is performed under a local anesthetic within 45–60 min. The total duration of the hospital stay is only 4–5 days. No special rehabilitation program is necessary. The patient can return to work within 1 week. If there is a recurrence of the coronary stenosis the dilatation procedure can easily be repeated on the occasion of the control angiography.

The total expenses during the hospital phase are much lower than those of a bypass operation, since the costs for medical equipment, sterile goods, drugs, blood, anesthesia, personnel, intensive care, and hospital stay are lower [17]. Coronary angioplasty can also relieve the patient's symptoms much faster. In all cases of unstable angina we make preparations for dilatation before the coronary angiography. The patient is informed and the cardiac surgeon is on standby. If the situation in the coronary artery is suitable for dilatation we perform it within the same catheterization laboratory session. In this way, causal and immediate treatment of the symptom is provided. On the other hand, we save costs by using the catheterization laboratory equipment and occupying its staff only once. Especially in countries with long waiting lists for coronary angiography and for bypass operation, this is an important factor.

Initially it was estimated that about 10% of the candidates for surgery could be treated by angioplasty. Because of the improvements in the catheter material, the increasing experience of the operators, and the extended indications, at the moment about 20%–25% of these patients can be treated by this method as a first attempt. It will still be some years before experience and further development allow the indications to be stated definitively.

Prerequisites

For the Patient

The patient must agree to an emergency bypass operation in the case of a vessel occlusion during the dilatation procedure. This operation must be permissible from the aspect of the patient's general condition. Operable tumors are not a contraindication. We have performed angioplasty in one patient with operable carcinoma of the stomach, in one with a bronchial carcinoma, and in one with a melanoma [18]. Specific tumor therapy was started immediately afterward.

Nor is advancing age a contraindication. Older patients are particularly likely to benefit from this semioperative technique. In all cases, however, the problem of an emergency operation has to be discussed beforehand with the patient and the surgeon. Diffuse arteriosclerosis of the iliofemoral arteries is no problem: in such patients the transbrachial Sones technique can be used.

For the Cardiological Center

It must be possible to move the entire X-ray system through 180° around the patient to allow hemiaxial, angulated views. The high-resolution amplifier equipment must include a high-speed cinecamera and a videotape. Biplane systems with separately moving arches allow quick orientation within the coronary artery system. Because of their size, however, they may be somewhat inconvenient in use, especially for the Sones technique. Beside the three extremity leads at least one chest lead must be recorded on the electrocardiogram and displayed on a large screen. Two equally sensitive transducers will record the pressures at the balloon tip and at the guide catheter.

The emergency set must include an external stimulator, a defibrillator and a respirator system. Solutions of nitroglycerin, nifedipine, heparin, atropine, positive inotropic substances, streptokinase, and lidocaine ready for injection must be at hand. An adequate stock of guide and balloon catheters and of guidewires of different sizes and shapes must be available. After some training each operator will develop an individual technique with preferences for particular catheter systems. Some limitation to only a certain number of catheters enables economical stock control and saves money.

Normally the catheterization laboratory staff will consist of the operator and an assistant. One person is needed for the continuous ECG and pressure recording and monitoring. Two additional members of staff handle the X-ray equipment and the balloon pump. They may also pass sterile goods to the team.

Since in about 2%–3% of all cases even with an experienced operator a coronary occlusion occurs during the procedure, surgical standby must be guaranteed. It must be possible for an emergency bypass operation to be available within 90 min [8, 9]. It is appropriate to schedule the angioplasty procedure at about noon, when the first bypass operations are normally finished. It must be borne in mind, however, that emergency situations may also occur in the surgical program, which may delay an emergency operation in a dilatation patient.

For the Operator

The operator should be well trained in catheterization procedures and should regularly perform at least 100–150 routine catheterizations per year to gain and maintain sufficient manual skill and experience in the evaluation of cineangiograms. Experience in cardiac resuscitation and in the treatment of rhythm disturbances is essential. The operator who treats patients with unstable angina should be already well trained in coronary angioplasty in patients with chronic stable angina. This will enable him/her to concentrate on the patient's symptoms, the intracoronary situation, and the monitoring parameters.

Informed Consent

The operator explains the necessity of treatment in the unstable angina and the different possibilities to the patient, describing the pros and cons of balloon dilatation and of the bypass operation. It should be explained that angioplasty is still an investigatory method, despite the good results and the great progress since the first treatment in 1977. The patient is informed that contrast medium is used and that intensive care monitoring will be necessary for 24 h.

The operator should also inform the patient of the success rate and the actual complication rate of his team with reference to emergency bypass operation and to mortality. The patient must agree to an emergency operation in case of a vessel occlusion. Finally, a written informed consent must be obtained from the patient.

Preparation and Technical Procedure

Medication

Patients with unstable angina are normally treated with 3–4 × 20 mg nifedipine/day, oral nitroglycerin, or even a continuous infusion of nitroglycerin (3–10 mg/h). Additional therapy may consist of beta blockers. The evening before angioplasty and on the morning of the intervention 500 mg acetylsalicylic acid is given (Table 2) together with 20 mg nifedipine.

During the dilatation procedure the nitroglycerin infusion is continued. Before the first coronary angiography 20 mg nifedipine and 0.8 mg nitroglycerin are given. Prior to stenosis dilatation 0.2 mg nitroglycerin and 0.2 mg nifedipine are injected into the coronary artery affected. For anticoagulation 10000 IE heparin is given. An infusion of dextran (100 ml/h) is also maintained throughout the procedure. After the last balloon dilatation another 3000 IU heparin and 0.2 mg nitroglycerin are injected into the coronary artery directly in front of the treated stenosis via the balloon catheter.

During the following 24 h of intensive care monitoring the patients receive a continuous infusion of heparin (800–1500 IU/h) to extend the thrombin time to 80–120 s, plus 3 × 500 mg acetylsalicylic acid and 3 × 20 mg nifedipine.

Table 2. Medical treatment during angioplasty for unstable angina

Pretreatment	
Evening before:	Nifedipine 20 mg PO Acetylsalicyclic acid 500 mg PO
Morning before:	Nifedipine 20 mg PO Acetylsalicyclic acid 500 mg PO
Dilatation	
Before angiography:	Nifedipine 20 mg PO Nitroglycerin 0.8 mg PO Heparin 10000 IU IV
With probability of coronary spasm:	Nifedipine 0.2 mg Nitroglycerin 0.2 mg into coronary artery
During angioplasty:	Dextran, sodium free, 100 ml/h i. v.
End of angioplasty:	Nitroglycerin 0.2 mg Heparin 3000 IU into coronary artery
Coronary care unit (24 h)	Heparin 800–1500 IU/h i. v. Dextran 300 ml/h IV for 3–4 h Nifedipine 3 × 20 mg PO Acetylsalicyclic acid 3 × 500 mg PO
Followup treatment (6 months)	Nifedipine 3 × 20 mg/day PO Acetylsalicyclic acid 500 mg/day PO Nitroglycerin or beta blockers as needed

Technique of Coronary Angioplasty

In patients with stenoses of the left anterior descending artery a venous catheter is placed into the pulmonary artery, while in cases of circumflex or right coronary artery disease the tip of the catheter lies in the apex of the right ventricle. These catheters are used for orientation within the coronary artery system and as an emergency pacing device. With the transbrachial Sones procedure ventriculography of both arteries is performed with the routine catheter. The special guide catheter is advanced subsequently. Users of the Judkins technique will initially perform ventriculography and angiography of the vessel assumed not to be occluded. Angiography of the diseased vessel is performed via the guide catheter directly, preparatory to introduction of the prepared balloon catheter immediately afterward. All arterial catheters are introduced with the aid of a 16-cm-long, 9-F sheath, which because of its length reaches the common iliac artery and makes the advancement of catheters possible even in atherosclerotic arteries. Catheters are introduced and changed over Teflon-coated guidewires.

Selection of the guide and the balloon catheter is mainly influenced by the experience of the operator. Low-profile catheters are widely used at present. With the aid of flexible and steerable guidewires even very narrow, irregular stenoses and angulated vessel segments can be reached. We usually start with a balloon 3.0 mm in diameter. If the stenosis is too narrow to be passed we change to a thin 2.0-mm balloon. The use of a 3.7-mm or even of a 4.2-mm balloon may be necessary if after several inflations there is still significant residual stenosis and a pressure gradient.

The balloon is normally inflated five to eight times in the area of the stenosis (Figs. 1 and 2). Its exact position can be localized with the aid of the auxiliary catheter. If the stenotic area is more than 1.0 cm long or the localization is not

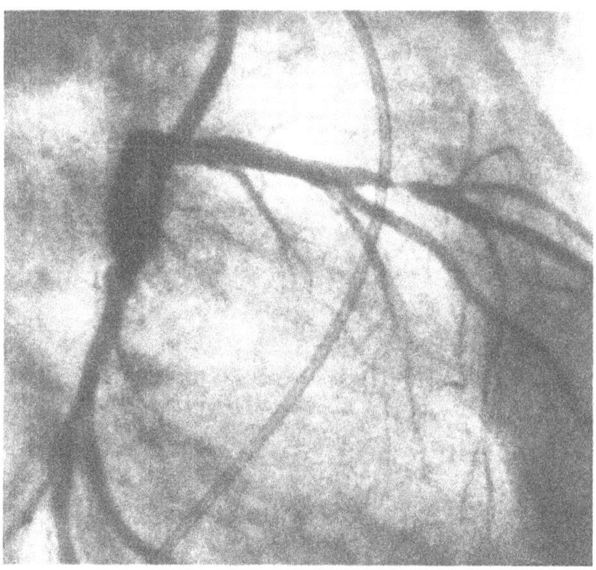

Fig. 1. High-grade stenosis of the left anterior descending artery before the bifurcation

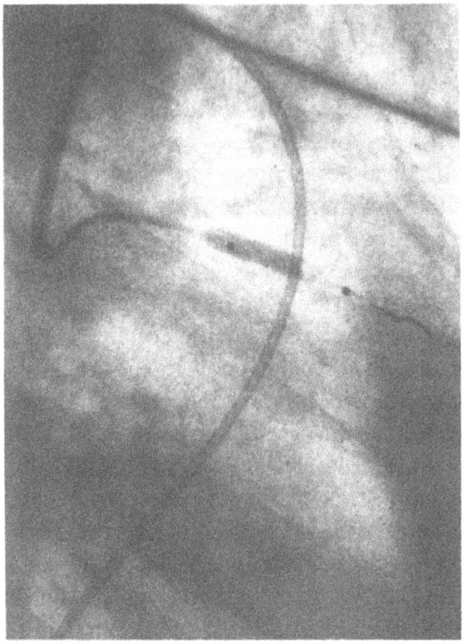

Fig. 2. Dilatation balloon (low profile, 3.7 mm diameter) inflated in the area of the stenosis

precisely known, several insufflations in slightly different positions are performed. Between two inflations a recovery period of 2–5 min should elapse.

The duration of the inflation depends on the occurrence of anginal symptoms, of ST segment changes, and of extrasystoles. The patient is instructed to give notice of new anginal symptoms during the procedure. Even in patients with severe unstable angina the balloon can be inflated for at least 15 s. Some patients tolerate inflation times of 60 s and more. The inflation pressure is specified by the manufacturer of the balloon catheter. It also depends on the outer diameter. Smaller balloons can stand higher pressures. Inflation pressures of at least 6 bar should be reached.

If there are two isolated stenoses in different vessels the more severe one is always treated first (worst first). The second stenosis can be dilated during the same session or during a second session the next day. Lesions of less than 50% diameter reduction are not treated. They are, however, noted for possible treatment during the control angiography after 6 months. Two narrowings close together within the same vessel are treated during a single procedure. The easiest way is to pass the balloon catheter over the guidewire through both stenoses and first to dilate the distal one and then to withdraw the catheter far enough to dilate the proximal one. In the case of very narrow segments, however, the more critical one should be treated first.

At the end of the procedure control angiography is performed in multiple views (Fig. 3). An injection into the contralateral artery is given only if collaterals have been visible before. The patient is monitored in the catheterization labora-

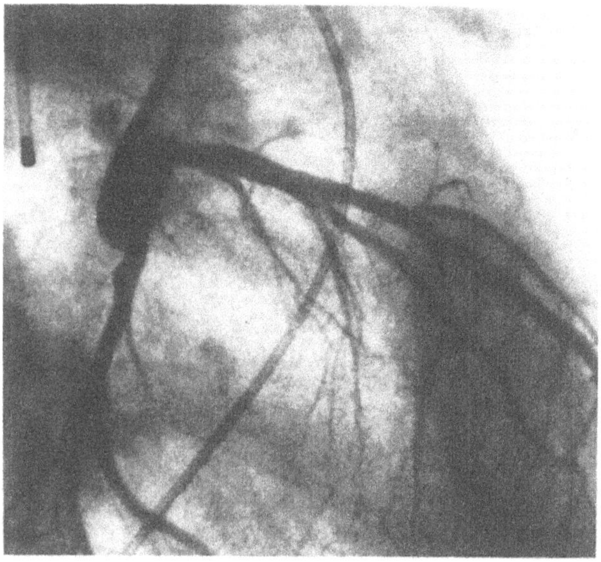

Fig. 3. Control coronary arteriography immediately after succesful dilatation without residual stenosis

tory for another 15 min before being transferred to the coronary care unit. With the Sones technique the cut is sutured immediately. When the Judkins approach is used the introducing sheath is left in the groin for 24 h and then replaced by a compression bandage. During the 24 h monitoring in the coronary care unit the ECG and the serum enzymes are monitored at 6-h intervals.

Followup Treatment and Study with Reference to Work Capacity

The followup treatment consists in 500 mg acetylsalicylic acid plus 3 × 20 mg nifedipin daily for 6 months (Table 2). Previous medication with nitroglycerin and/or beta blockers is discontinued. Such drugs are unnecessary after successful angioplasty. If anginal symptoms recur, however, these drugs can be given again. If medical treatment does not relieve recurring symptoms early reexamination is indicated.

Before hospital discharge control ergometry, including myocardial scintigraphy, is performed. The patient is unable to work for 5–7 days after the procedure, but after this the normal work and physical activity can be resumed. The patient is informed of this and encouraged to perform the same physical activity each day. In this way an early restenosis can be detected by a sudden change in the patient's previous work capacity. Three months later another ergometry is performed by the referring physician. After 6 months a complete coronary angiography, including ventriculography and scintigraphy, is performed in the center where the dilatation was done (Fig. 4). Restenosis or any new stenoses in other areas of the coronary artery system will be dilated during the control study. Pretreatment and surgical standby requirements are the same as for the regular angioplasty.

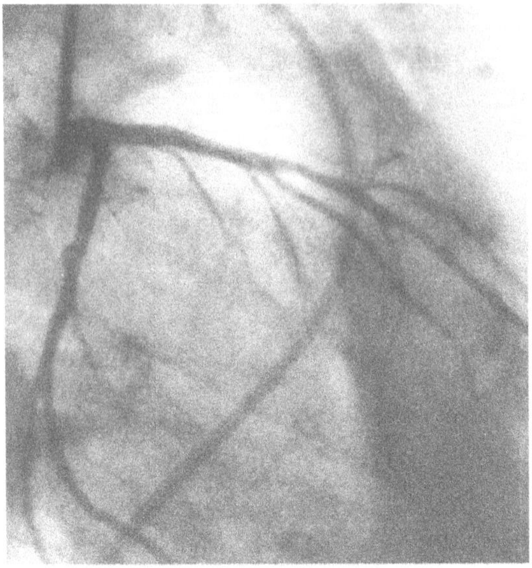

Fig. 4. Control coronary arteriography 6 months after successful dilatation with good late result

State of the Art: Results

With the aid of low-profile balloon catheters and steerable guidewires suitable coronary stenoses can be passed and successfully dilated in 90%–95% of all cases. The primary success rate is similar in stable and in unstable angina pectoris [5–7, 19]. In totally occluded arteries with a history ranging from some days up to 4–6 weeks the success rate is around 50% [7, 11, 12].

The luminal diameter of high-grade coronary stenoses can be improved by 20%–90% (mean approximately 50%) [7, 19]. In some cases no residual stenosis is detectable after the dilatation [7]. Improvements of less than 20% are insignificant and such results are regarded as unsuccessful.

The long-term efficacy of angioplasty seems to be somewhat lower and the restenosis rate to be higher in unstable than in stable angina [3, 5–7, 19–24]. The primary success rate and the long-term results seem to be influenced by several factors, such as balloon size, balloon pressure, inflation time, number of inflations, and followup treatment. The importance of the individual factors, however, has not yet been analyzed in detail.

Complications and Their Management

Surgical standby must be guaranteed for every dilatation procedure [8, 9]. It depends on the morphology of the coronary artery system how acute any emergency arising is likely to be. In cases with main stem stenoses, main stem equivalents, and stenoses proximal to the first septal branch in dominant left coronary arteries, the emergency operation should start within 30 min after any vessel occlusion. If this backup is not guaranteed the dilatation should be postponed to a more convenient date. Cardiological centers without such a surgical standby team should refrain from treating such cases.

In cases with stenoses in the middle part or in relatively small coronary arteries the likelihood of an urgent bypass operation becoming necessary is not so high, but in some of these patients the need for an emergency operation still has to be discussed. Even with an early operation there will be some localized myocardial infarction, because of the time that elapses between the vessel occlusion and completion of the bypass. Thoracotomy, with all its problems, including the risk of hepatitis, and followup treatment also cannot be neglected. Without an operation the patient will certainly experience an infarction, probably a small one. However, it will occur in the environment of a fully equipped cardiological center with all the facilities for treatment of acute infarct complications. Therefore, in each case of an acute vessel occlusion critical evaluation of the merits of an operation with a single bypass and the risks this involves should be carefully weighed against those of conservative treatment.

However, sudden vessel occlusion is not always a definite disaster [25]. Contact between the balloon catheter and the intima and overstretching of the coronary artery can cause severe vasospasms and even lead to total vessel occlusion. The first intervention is therefore injection of 0.2 mg nitroglycerin and 0.2 mg soluble nifedipine directly into the coronary artery via the dilatation catheter. If the occlusion persists the dilatation catheter is advanced to the area of the obstruction. In the majority of vasospastic occlusions these measures are successful. Once it is reopened we inject a further 0.2 mg nitroglycerin plus 3000–5000 IU heparin into the vessel. If occlusion still persists a fresh intracoronary thrombus may be responsible. The supraselective injection of 50000 IU streptokinase followed by a continuous infusion of 5000 units/min for 30–60 min may be tried. In our experience, however, definite occlusions are rarely caused by thrombi. Intimal dissections are more often the pathomechanism. A smooth hourglass-like obstruction of the vessel is indicative of a spasm, while irregular, bizarre contours of the prestenotic vessel segment suggest a dissection. In the case of a sudden vessel occlusion during angioplasty the whole range of intensive care measures must be at hand. Defibrillation, stimulation, and intubation sets and lidocaine, atropine, and positive inotropic drugs must be available in the catheterization laboratory. In cases of right or circumflex coronary artery occlusion a stimulation catheter should be inserted into the right ventricle. In cases of LAD disease a floating catheter in the pulmonary artery will allow left ventricular filling pressure and cardiac output to be monitored. The patient should be monitored continuously and should be accompanied to the operation theater or to the coronary care unit by an experienced physician.

The probability of a dissection of the intima with a vessel obstruction was 2.2% in our consecutive series of 500 cases. There were no sudden deaths during the procedure. The mortality rate was 0.4%, with one pulmonary embolus on the second day and one sudden death on the third day. In both cases autopsy showed patent coronary arteries at the site of the previous dilatation. A third patient died of septicemia several weeks after an emergency bypass operation.

Limitations and Perspectives

During recent years the spectrum of indications has continously been extended. Patients with triple-vessel diseases, however, are treated only in a few centers [26–28]. Stenoses more than 1.5 cm in length and with an irregular configuration and marked calcifications and those with diffuse, narrow vessel segments in the periphery are not very suitable for correction by this method. In patients with severe impaired left ventricular function and ejection fractions of less than 40% the risk in the case of a vessel occlusion is markedly elevated. Such patients and those with additional operable diseases such as papillary muscle dysfunction or ventricular aneurysms should be referred to the cardiac surgeon as a matter of policy.

Coronary Angioplasty in Acute Myocardial Infarction With and Without Thrombolysis

In about 90% of all cases, after selective intracoronary or intravenous thrombolysis and after the administration of tissue-type activators, significant coronary stenosis can be found at the site of the previous occlusion (Figs. 5 and 6) [29–33]. This residual stenosis, at a site which has already been the crystallization point of a thrombus because of its rough surface and because of the flow limitation, may be the origin of another clot formation despite anticoagulation [34–36]. The stenosis may also impede the coronary flow to the previously ischemic part of the myocardium and in this way delay the recovery of the myocardial metabolism [36–38]. Finally, such a stenosis may cause angina pectoris in the recovery phase and during subsequent months.

Indications for Angioplasty

As we have shown for the first time [39, 30], residual stenoses at the site of the previous occlusion of at least 60% of luminal diameter can be effectively treated with angioplasty (Figs. 7 and 8). Immediately after thrombolysis and after reperfusion of the artery there may be some clot material adherent to the intimal plaque (Fig. 6). Thrombolysis should therefore be continued for at least 30 min to dissolve this residual material, to be sure that only organic cholesterol parts form the obstruction. Two adjacent stenoses within the same coronary vessel can be dilated within the same session.

If further significant stenoses are present in one of the noninfarcted arteries angioplasty of these obstructions should be postponed until the end of the recovery phase from the acute myocardial infarction. Otherwise the patient would be in a critical condition, if during the angioplasty of such a vessel an infarction were to occur in another myocardial zone.

Stenoses of the main stem are very seldom found, since survival of infarctions caused by a main stem occlusion is rare. Dilatation of such critical central stenoses, however, would be of the utmost importance for the patient.

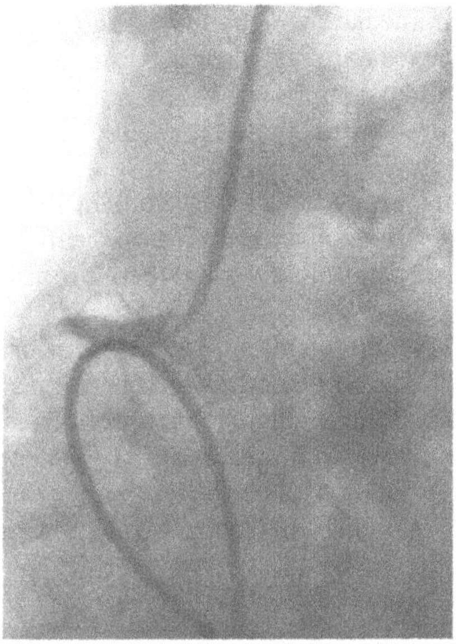
5

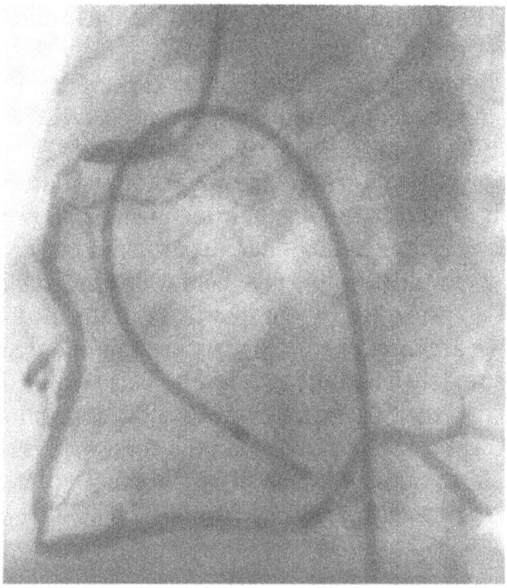
6

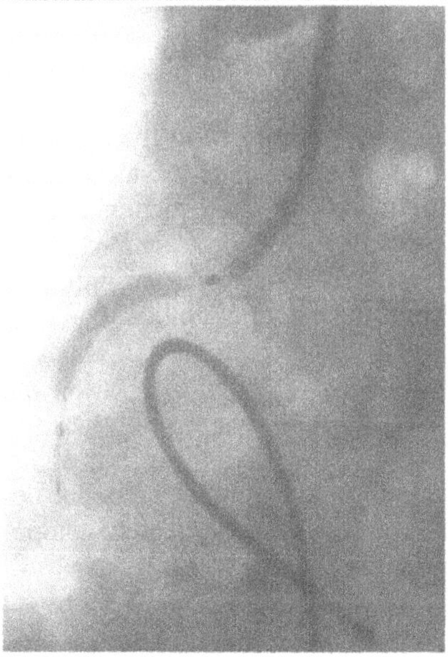
7

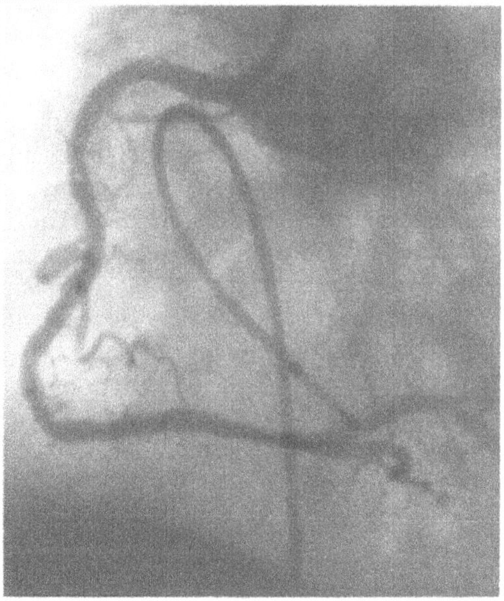
8

Fig. 5. Thrombolysis of an acute myocardial infarction: Occluded right coronary artery

Fig. 6. Right coronary artery immediately after successful thrombolysis. High-grade coronary stenosis at the site of the previous occlusion. Residual clot formation distal to the stenosis

Fig. 7. Angioplasty of the remaining stenosis after successful thrombolysis. (Balloon size 3.7 mm diameter)

Fig. 8. Final result after successful thrombolysis and angioplasty of the underlying coronary stenosis

If the patient is in a critical situation because a proximal part of a major artery is occluded, angioplasty may be performed immediately without waiting for the effect of the thrombolysis [11, 41]. By this means coronary flow is reestablished immediately. The remaining clot material will be compressed to the vessel wall. Subsequent thrombolysis regularly resolves the residual material within the next 30–60 min.

Patients with acute myocardial infarctions are older on average than those with stable and unstable angina. Age, however, is not a general contraindication, since older patients derive particular benefit from thrombolysis and therefore also from the flow improvement following angioplasty.

Angioplasty should only be performed in patients in whom the reopened coronary artery perfuses myocardium that is still vital. If thrombolysis is performed too late a definite scar is left. This part of the ventricle will no longer profit from the reperfusion nor from any additional angioplasty. If, however, the ST segment elevations normalize and the chest pain is relieved immediately after the reperfusion, vital myocardium can be expected. Such patients will certainly benefit from recanalization procedures.

Informed Consent

The operator explains to the patient the possibility of dissolving the coronary thrombus by means of thrombolytic agents. The advantages of the method are the early reperfusion of the ischemic myocardium and the consequent chance of diminishing the myocardial necrosis. The disadvantages are local hemorrhage at the puncture site and in rare cases also an allergic reaction to the thrombolytic substances. The head physician then explains that there is a possibility of dilating the underlying coronary artery stenosis with the balloon technique and that this method is still in an investigatory phase. The advantages are: better perfusion and probably a lower risk of reocclusion of the vessel. The disadvantage of the additional angioplasty essentially is the risk of reoccluding the vessel by an intimal dissection and in this way establishing the same situation as before the lysis. The operator should also in form the patient of the success rate and the actual complication rate of his team with both thrombolysis and angioplasty.

Preparations and Technical Procedure

Thrombolysis Technique

We prefer to combine intravenous and intracoronary administration of streptokinase or urokinase and additional mechanical maneuvers [42]. The time between the onset of symptoms and the start of the IV streptokinase infusion should be less than 6 h (Table 3). The chest pain typical for acute myocardial infarction must have lasted for more than 20 min. The electrocardiogram should show ST

Table 3. Prerequisites for thrombolysis of an acute myocardial infarction

Time lapse between onset of symptoms and thrombolysis <6 h
Chest pain typical of acute myocardial infarction for >20 min
ST segment elevation >0.3 mV in the chest leads in anterior wall infarctions
ST segment elevation >0.2 mV in the limb leads in posterior wall infarctions
No contraindications to thrombolytic therapy

Table 4. Medical therapy in thrombolysis of an acute myocardial infarction and after subsequent angioplasty

Before catherization	Streptokinase 500 000 IU/30 min i. v. Heparin 5000 IU i. v. Acetylsalicylic acid 1 g i. v. Prednisone 250 mg i. v.
During catheterization	Streptokinase 50 000 IU intracoronarily Streptokinase 5000 IU/min until reopening Streptokinase 10 000 IU/min for 30 min into coronary artery after reopening
Coronary care unit	Heparin 8–1500 IU/h for 5 days, starting 6 h after thrombolysis Coumadin starting on day 3, overlapping with heparin
Followup treatment	Coumadin for 6 months Nifedipine, nitroglycerin, beta blockers, digitalis, diuretics as needed

segment elevations of at least 0.3 mV in the chest leads in anterior wall infarctions and of at least 0.2 mV in the extremity leads in posterior wall infarctions. There should be no contraindications to thrombolytic therapy such as bleeding diseases or recent operation.

Once the diagnosis of infarction has been confirmed and informed consent obtained, an i.v. infusion of 500 000 IU streptokinase within 30 min is started (Table 4). In addition, 5000 IU heparin, 1 g acetylsalicylic acid, and 250 mg prednisone are given. While the infusion is running, the patient is transferred to the catheterization laboratory. Coronary angiography is performed by the Judkins technique using the 8-F or 9-F guide catheter (Fig. 5). This catheter is introduced via a 16-cm-long introducing sheath size 9 F.

After angiography of the vessel thought to be diseased a further 50 000 IU streptokinase is injected as a bolus and 5000 IU/min as a continuous infusion via a special catheter advanced directly into the occluded coronary artery up to the thrombus. In posterior wall infarctions both the right and the circumflex artery are injected, to make sure which is infarcted.

At 10 min after the start of the intracoronary infusion a control angiogram is performed. If the thrombolytic occlusion persists the special reperfusion catheter is advanced through the thrombus to make a hole in it to enable the streptokinase to reach the inside of the thrombus also.

This creates a marginal flow to the distal part of the vessel [42]. After recanalization the streptokinase infusion is continued for another 30 min at an infusion rate of 10000 IU/min to dissolve the residual clot material, which may adhere to the stenotic area or be embolized into peripheral parts of the vessel. Finally, several angiograms of the vessel in different views are performed.

Angioplasty Technique

If the final coronary angiogram after successful thrombolysis shows a proximal stenosis of more than 60% of the luminal diameter of the vessel at the site of the previous occlusion balloon angioplasty is performed subsequently within the same catheterization laboratory session [7, 11, 34, 39, 40] (Figs. 6 and 7).

In patients in a critical clinical condition because of the thrombotic occlusion of the left main stem or the proximal obstruction of a major coronary artery, we do not wait to see the effect of the intracoronary thrombokinase injection. In such cases we immediately advance the balloon catheter into the occluded artery, perforate the thrombus, and press the clot material to the vessel wall, by this means also dilating any underlying stenosis that may be present [11, 34, 41]. Continuous intracoronary infusion of streptokinase is then resumed for another 30–60 min.

In regular angioplasties after successful thrombolysis a low-profile balloon catheter is advanced via the guide catheter already in place, with the aid of a steerable guidewire. The balloon size is adjusted for the prestenotic vessel segment. We mostly start with a 3.0-mm balloon in the LAD and with a 3.7-mm balloon in the right coronary artery. If significant stenosis still persists after several balloon inflations we change to a larger size and repeat the procedure.

Normally the balloons are inflated five to eight times in the area of the stenosis. The duration of each balloon inflation depends on the new onset of anginal symptoms, recurring ST segment elevations, or extrasystoles. The inflation times vary between 30 and 60 s. Even in patients without collaterals inflation times of at least 15 s can be reached. The inflation pressure must be adjusted to the manufacturer's specifications, but at least 6 bar can and should be used.

At the end of the procedure another control angiography (Fig. 8) at different angulations and a ventriculogram are performed. The patient is monitored for another 15 min in the catheterization laboratory before being transferred to the coronary care unit.

Followup Treatment and Study

The patient is transferred to the coronary care unit and treated as is usual after thrombolysis with continuous electrocardiographic and hemodynamic monitoring with the aid of a floating catheter. Serum enzymes, coagulation parameters, and cardiac output are analyzed every 6 h within the first 24 h and every 12 h for the second and the third days (Table 4).

Heparinization starts 6 h after the end of the streptokinase infusion. At that time AT III and fibrinogen begin to normalize. Heparin treatment is strictly controlled to prevent a reocclusion. Thrombin time should be prolonged to 80–120 s. In uncomplicated cases Coumadin treatment is started on the third day, while heparin is successively withdrawn. The introducing sheath is left in place for the first 36 h to avoid bleeding. It is than withdrawn and replaced by a compression bandage.

Coumadin treatment is continued until the third week, when heparin is started again. At that time control angiography of both arteries and of the ventricle is performed. If a restenosis has occurred it will be dilated again during this session. If there is significant stenosis of another vessel it can also be treated at this time.

The long-term treatment for the next 6 months consists in Coumadin medication. Nifedipine, nitroglycerin, digitalis, diuretics, or beta blockers are given as required.

The followup studies after 3 and 6 months in the outpatient clinic include physical examination, bicycle ergometry, two-dimensional echocardiography, blood coagulation, and serum cholesterol analysis. Another control angiography is suggested to the patient 6 months after angioplasty, to analyze the final outcome of this combination of thrombolysis and angioplasty. It the patients are elderly or in a poor general condition, we may not insist on this. Therefore, the rate of restudy is not 100%.

State of the Art: Results

The success rate in angioplasty of residual stenoses after thrombolysis cannot be compared with that in stable and in unstable angina [5–7, 19, 21, 23, 40]. In our series, the mean age of patients with myocardial infarctions is approximately 6 years higher than that of those in stable angina [7, 40], and their coronary vessels are more often severely damaged, calcified, and contorted. The coronary stenoses are more bizarre in their contours, with longer stenotic and irregular parts. Moreover, angioplastic manipulations will always be performed much more cautiously in the situation of an acute myocardial infarction immediately after

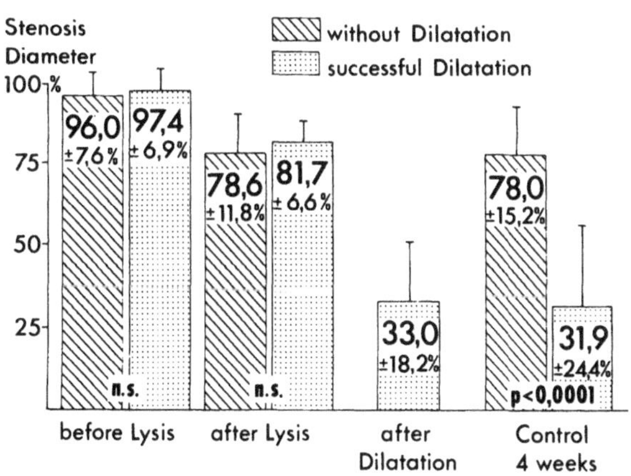

Fig. 9. Results of angioplasty in patients with successful thrombolysis compaired with non-treated patients

reopening of a coronary artery than during angioplasty in stable or unstable angina. Attempts to reach "success" at any price are inappropriate. If the procedure cannot be brought to a successful conclusion within 30 min we stop, postponing further manipulations to a second procedure some days later if necessary.

The luminal diameter of the stenoses can be enlarged in succesfully treated cases by the same amount as in normal cases of angioplasty [5, 7, 19, 40]. In our first series an average improvement of 50% of the luminal diameter of the coronary artery has been reached (range 20%–90%) (Fig. 9). As in regular angioplasty, the primary and the long-term results may be influenced by the character of the stenosis, the balloon size, pressure, and inflation time, the number of inflations, and the followup treatment. In about 25% of successfully treated patients restenoses occur within the next 6 months, which can be dilated during the control study [7].

Complications and Their Management

Principally the same complications can occur during angioplasty after thrombolysis as in dilatation for angina pectoris. The main problem in both patient groups is the intimal dissection, which in these sometimes severely narrowed and calcified vessels may occur more easily than during regular dilatations. In our series of angioplasty in infarctions the occlusion rate was 3%, as against 2.2% in stable and unstable angina [7]. The chance of a new thrombosis caused by formation of a fresh clot is very low, since the heparin and streptokinase treatment prevents it. In addition, regular flushing of the catheters with heparinized saline solution will also diminish this risk.

If a vessel occlusion occurs because of an iatrogenic intimal dissection the same situation of acute infarction as before thrombolysis is produced. In this situation an acute bypass operation can be discussed. This operation, however, is by no means mandatory or indicated in all cases. The cardiac surgeon would have to operate on a patient in the acute phase of a myocardial infarction. The occlusion time from the onset of symptoms is mostly more than 6 h. Therefore, the surgeon will certainly find a transmural infarction intraoperatively. It is not yet established whether such an emergency operation will be of much advantage to the patient in terms of final outcome and preservation of myocardium. The operation will rather involve a high risk for the patient. Up to now only a few centers have some initial experience of bypass surgery during acute myocardial infarction [43–45].

We therefore try to stabilize the patient's hemodynamic and rhythm situation in cases of vessel dissection during angioplasty. Generally the treatment of complications will be similar to that applied for those encountered in angioplasty of stable and unstable angina.

Limitations and Perspectives

In patients with rather tortuous coronary arteries and severe calcifications it can be quite difficult or even impossible to advance even very soft and thin balloon catheters into the stenotic area. In such cases, therefore, the success rate is low and the probability of an artificial vessel occlusion, significantly higher. In acute infarction it is dangerous to treat further stenoses in other branches of the coronary artery system during the same catheterization laboratory session. The occlusion of another vessel would lead to severe deterioration in the patient's status. Therefore, the treatment of multivessel stenoses should be postponed to another session several weeks later if necessary.

Stenoses that are more than 2.0 cm in length and severely irregular, diffusely calcified, distal vessel parts also limit the results that can be achieved with angioplasty. In such cases the success rate in terms of adequate enlargement of the vessel is quite low. Furthermore, a large, fresh wound of the intima and the media will be created by the extended angioplasty, which in the situation of acute myocardial infarction could give rise to a new thrombosis despite strict anticoagulation.

It is to be expected that the indications for and the merits of angioplasty in the acute phase of myocardial infarctions will be the subject of further scientific studies. The exact timing of a dilatation, the role of primary angioplasty even before lysis has become effective, the features distinguishing stenoses in which good results are likely from those in which they are not, and also technical details of balloon size, pressure, inflation time, and followup treatment have yet to be finally established. Further improvements of the catheter material can also be expected.

Angioplasty, and particularly its application in the situation of acute myocardial infarction, is still in a developmental phase. The possibilities and limitations of this application must therefore be considered and defined critically in the future.

References

1. Gruentzig AR, Senning A, Siegenthaler WE (1979) Nonoperative dilatation of coronary artery stenosis: Percutaneous transluminal coronary angioplasty. N Engl J Med 301:61
2. Meyer J, Böcker B, Erbel R, Bardos P, Messmer BJ, Effert S (1980) Treatment of unstable angina with transluminal coronary angioplasty (PTCA). Circulation 62/III:160
3. Meyer J, Schmitz H, Erbel R, Kiesslich T, Böcker-Josephs B, Krebs W, Braun BC, Bardos P, Minale C, Messmer BJ, Effert S (1981) Treatment of unstable angina pectoris with percutaneous transluminal coronary angioplasty. Cathet Cardiovasc Diagn 7:361
4. Williams DO, Riley RS, Singh AK, Gewirtz H, Most RS (1981) Evaluation of the role of coronary angioplasty in patients with unstable angina pectoris. Am Heart J 102:1
5. Meyer J, Schmitz HJ, Kiesslich T, Erbel R, Krebs W, Schulz W, Bardos P, Minale C, Messmer BJ, Effert S (1983) Percutaneous transluminal coronary angioplasty in patients with stable and unstable angina pectoris: Analysis of early and late results. Am Heart J 106:973

6. Faxon DP, Detre KM, McCabe CH, Fisher L, Holmes DR, Cowley MJ, Bourassa MG, van Raden M, Ryan TJ (1984) Role of percutaneous transluminal coronary angioplasty in the treatment of unstable angina: report from the National Heart, Lung, and Blood Institute percutaneous transluminal coronary angioplasty and coronary artery surgery study registries. Am J Cardiol 53:131 c
7. Meyer J, Erbel R, Schmitz HJ, Pop T, Meinertz T, Schreiner G, Henkel B, Henrichs KJ, Rupprecht HJ, Effert S (1984) Transluminale Angioplastik – unstable angina, frischer Infarkt. 50. Jahrestag der Deutschen Gesellschaft für Herz- und Kreislaufforschung. Mannheim. Z Kardiol
8. Williams DO, Gruentzig A, Kent KM, Myler RK, Stertzer SH, Bentivoglio L, Bourassa M, Block P, Cowley M, Detre K, Dorros G, Gosselin A, Simpson J, Passamani E, Mullin S (1982) Guidelines for the performance of percutaneous transluminal coronary angioplasty. Circulation 66:693
9. Cowley MJ, Dorros G, Kelsey SF, van Raden M, Detre KM (1984) Emergency coronary bypass surgery after coronary angioplasty: the National Heart, Lung and Blood Institute's percutaneous transluminal coronary angioplasty registry experience. Am J Cardiol 53:22c
10. Douglas JS Jr, Gruentzig AR, King SB III, Hollman J, Ischinger T, Meier B, Craver JM, Jones EL, Waller JL, Bone DK, Guyton R (1983) Percutaneous transluminal coronary angioplasty in patients with prior coronary bypass surgery. J Am Coll Cardiol 2:745
11. Erbel R, Meinertz T, Wessler I, Meyer J, Seybold-Epting W (1984) Recanalization of occluded left main coronary artery in unstable angina pectoris. Am J Cardiol 53:1725
12. Serruys PW, Heyndrickx GR, de Feyter PJ, van den Brand M (1984) Elective PTCA of totally occluded coronary arteries not associated with acute MI. Eur J Cardiol 5/I:57
13. Meier B, Gruentzig AR, Hollman J, Ischinger T, Bradford JM (1983) Does length or eccentricity of coronary stenoses influence the outcome of transluminal dilatation. Circulation 67:497
14. Meier B, Gruentzig AR (1984) Learning curve for percutaneous transluminal coronary angioplasty: skill, technology or patient selection. Am J Cardiol 53:65c
15. Kelsey SF, Mullin SM, Detre KM, Mitchell H, Cowley MJ, Gruentzig AR, Kent KM (1984) Effect of investigator experience on percutaneous transluminal coronary angioplasty. Am J Cardiol 53:56c
16. Holmes DR, van Raden MJ, Reeder GS, Vlietstra RE, Jang GC, Kent KM, Vetrovec GW, Cowley MJ, Dorros G, Kelsey SF, Detre KM, Mock MB (1984) Return to work after coronary angioplasty: a report from the National Heart, Lung and Blood Institute percutaneous transluminal coronary angioplasty registry. Am J Cardiol 53:48c
17. Jang GC, Block PC, Cowley MJ, Gruentzig AR, Dorros G, Holmes DR Jr, Kent KM, Leatherman LL, Myler RK, Sjolander SME, Stertzer SH, Vetrovec GW, Willis WH Jr, Williams DO (1984) Relative cost of coronary angioplasty and bypass surgery in a one-vessel disease model. Am J Cardiol 53:52c
18. Meyer J, Messmer BJ, Reifferscheid M (1981) Präoperative Behandlung hochgradiger Koronarstenosen mit der Ballontechnik bei Patienten mit operablen Karzinomerkrankungen. Dtsch Med Wochenschr 106:1366
19. Gruentzig AR (1984) Percutaneous transluminal coronary angioplasty: 6 years' experience. Am Heart J 107:818
20. Meier B, Gruentzig AR, Siegenthaler WE, Schlumpf M (1983) Long-term performance after percutaneous transluminal coronary angioplasty and coronary artery bypass grafting. Circulation 68:796
21. Kent KM, Bentivoglio LG, Block PC et al. (1984) Long-term efficacy of percutaneous transluminal coronary angioplasty (PTCA): Report from the National Heart, Lung, and Blood Institute PTCA registry. Am J Cardiol 53:27c
22. Kaltenbach M, Kober G, Schmidt-Moritz A, Scherer D (1983) Rezidivhäufigkeit nach erfolgreicher transluminaler Koronarangioplastik. Dtsch Med Wochenschr 108:1387
23. Holmes DR Jr, Vlietstra RE, Smith HC, Vetrovec GW, Kent KM, Cowley MJ, Faxon DP, Gruentzig AR, Kelsey SF, Detre KM, van Raden MJ, Mock MB (1984) Restenosis after percutaneous transluminal coronary angioplasty (PTCA): A report from the PTCA registry of the National Heart, Lung and Blood Institute. Am J Cardiol 53:77c

24. Schmitz HJ, Meyer J, Kiesslich T, Effert S (1982) Greater initial dilatation gives better late angiographic results in percutaneous coronary angioplasty (PTCA). Circulation 66/II:123
25. Ischinger T, Zack P, Aker U (1984) Acute coronary occlusion during balloon angioplasty due to intracoronary thrombus and coronary spasm: a reversible complication. Am Heart J 107:1271
26. Hartzler GO (1983) Percutaneous transluminal coronary angioplasty in multivessel disease. Cathet Cardiovas Diagn 9:537
27. Dorros G, Stertzer SH, Cowley MJ, Myler RK (1984) Complex coronary angioplasty: Multiple coronary dilatations. Am J Cardiol 53:126c
28. Ischinger T, Russ T, Zack PM, Aker UT, Kennedy HL (1984) Complex coronary angioplasty: angiographic and functional results. Eur Heart J 5/I:57
29. DeWood MA, Spores J, Notske R, Mouser LT, Burroughs R, Golden MS, Lang HT (1980) Prevalence of total coronary occlusion during the early hours of transmural myocardial infarction. N Engl J Med 303:897
30. Rentrop P, Blanke H, Karsch KR, Wiegand V, Köstering H, Rahlf G, Oster H, Leitz K (1979) Wiedereröffnung des Infarktgefäßes durch transluminale Rekanalisation und intrakoronare Streptokinase-Applikation. Dtsch Med Wochenschr 104:1438
31. Neuhaus KL, Köstering H, Tebbe U, Sauer G, Kreuzer H (1981) Intravenöse Kurzzeitstreptokinase-Therapie beim frischen Myokardinfarkt. Z Kardiol 70:791
32. Schröder R, Biamino G, von Leitner ER, Linderer T (1981) Intravenöse Streptokinase-Infusion bei akutem Myokardinfarkt. Dtsch Med Wochenschr 106:294
33. Van de Werf F, Ludbrook PA, Bergmann SR, Tiefenbrunn AJ, Fox KAH, de Geest H, Verstraete M, Collen D, Sobel BE (1984) Coronary thrombolysis with tissue-type plasminogen activator in patients with evolving myocardial infarction. N Engl J Med 310:609
34. Meyer J, Merx W, Dörr R, Lambertz H, Bethge C, Effert S (1982) Successful treatment of acute myocardial infarction shock by combined percutaneous transluminal coronary recanalisation (PTCR) and percutaneous transluminal coronary angioplasty (PTCA). Am Heart J 103:132
35. Merx W, Dörr R, Rentrop P, Blanke H, Karsch KR, Mathey DG, Kremer P, Rutsch W, Schmutzler H (1981) Evaluation of the effectiveness of intracoronary streptokinase infusion in acute myocardial infarction: Postprocedure management and hospital course in 204 patients. Am Heart J 102:1181
36. Harrison DG, Ferguson DW, Collins SM, Skorton DJ, Ericksen EE, Kioschos JM, Marcus ML, White CW (1984) Rethrombosis after reperfusion with streptokinase – importance of geometry of residual lesions. Circulation 69:991
37. Mates RE, Gupta RL, Bell AC, Klocke FJ (1978) Fluid dynamics of coronary artery stenosis. Circ Res 42:152
38. Poole-Wilson PA (1983) Angina-pathological mechanisms, clinical expression and treatment. Postgrad Med J 59/III:11
39. Meyer J, Merx W, Schweizer P, Erbel R, Dörr R, Halfenberg R, Messmer BJ, Effert S (1982) Advantages of combining transluminal coronary angioplasty (PTCA) with selective coronary thrombolysis in acute infarction. Circulation 66/II:261
40. Meyer J, Merx W, Schmitz H, Erbel R, Kiesslich T, Dörr R, Lambertz H, Bethge C, Krebs W, Bardos P, Minale C, Messmer BJ, Effert S (1982) Percutaneous transluminal coronary angioplasty immediately after intracoronary streptolysis of transmural myocardial infarction. Circulation 66:905
41. Hartzler GO, Rutherford BB, McConahay DR, Johnson WL, McCallister BD, Gura GM, Conn RC, Crockett JE (1983) Percutaneous transluminal coronary angioplasty with and without thrombolytic therapy for treatment of acute myocardial infarction. Am Heart J 106:965
42. Erbel R, Pop T, Meinertz T, Kasper W, Rückel A, Pfeiffer C, Schreiner G, Meyer J (1983) Rapid recanalization in acute myocardial infarction by combined mechanical and medical therapy. Circulation 68/II:326
43. Mathey DG, Rodewald G, Rentrop P, Leitz K, Merx W, Messmer BJ, Rutsch W, Bücherl ES (1981) Intracoronary streptokinase thrombolytic recanalization and subsequent surgical bypass of remaining atherosclerotic stenosis in acute myocardial infarction: complementary

combined approach effecting reduced infarct size, preventing reinfarction, and improving left ventricular function. Am Heart J 102:1194

44. Messmer BJ, Merx W, Meyer J, Bardos P, Minale C, Effert S (1983) New developments in medical-surgical treatment of acute myocardial infarction. Ann Thorac Surg 35:70
45. DeWood MA, Spores J, Berg R Jr, Kendall RW, Grunwald RP, Selinger SL, Hensley GR, Sutherland KI, Sheilds JP (1983) Acute myocardial infarction: a decade of experience with surgical reperfusion in 701 patients. Circulation 68/II:8
46. Walker WE, Smalling RW, Fuentes F, Gould KL, Johnson WE, Reduto LA, Sterling RP, Weiland AP, Wynnn MM (1984) Role of coronary artery bypass surgery after intracoronary streptokinase infusion for myocardial infarction. Am Heart J 107:826

Chapter 18. PTCA in Patients with Variant Angina

PAUL ROBERT DAVID and THIERRY CORCOS

Physiology of Coronary Artery Tone

The epicardial coronary arteries in man are now considered dynamic vascular structures rather than passive conduits. Recordings from ring segments of human coronary arteries placed in an isolated tissue bath have shown coordinated rhythmic periods of contraction and relaxation [1]. Calcium ions are the final common mediator of coronary tone, but regulatory mechanisms include vasoactive amines [2], biochemical environment, autonomic nervous system [3], circadian biorhythms [4], and local factors.

Local Factors in Coronary Artery Spasm

Coronary spasm, whether spontaneous or provoked, tends to occur repeatedly at the same vascular site in an individual patient. Therefore, there appears to be a hypersensitive target zone localized in a particular segment of the coronary vasculature. This zone is often associated with an organic atherosclerotic lesion [5, 6]. Local changes in intracellular calcium or pH, or in the synthesis of prostacycline may be associated with atherosclerosis [8, 9] and contribute to abnormalities of vessel contraction, but the atherosclerotic stenosis itself plays an important role in dynamic coronary occlusion.

Rationale for Coronary Angioplasty in Variant Angina

There is a wide spectrum of anatomic subsets in patients with variant angina, ranging from those with angiographically normal coronary arteries [9] to those with severe multivessel disease [10]. Organic lesions are found in most patients with variant angina, and when they are present coronary spasm is intimately associated with an organic stenosis in 90% of cases [5]. Different combinations of fixed and variable obstruction may produce myocardial ischemia (Fig. 1) [11]. At the site of a significant (i.e., >50%) coronary stenosis, a slight increase in coronary tone or even in coronary vasomotion within the physiological range could completely occlude the coronary artery (Fig. 2) [12, 13]. Thus, in patients with variant angina and significant organic stenosis, the coronary stenosis is not only an "irritative spine" but actually accounts for the major part of the occlusion. In these settings suppressing the organic stenosis would theoretically prevent inter-

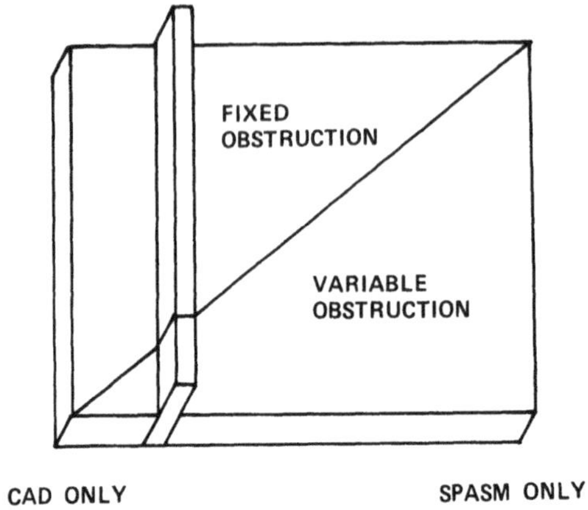

Fig. 1. Different combinations of fixed and variable obstruction can produce myocardial ischemia. The *vertical bar* represents a patient in whom both variable and fixed obstruction play significant roles in occluding a coronary artery

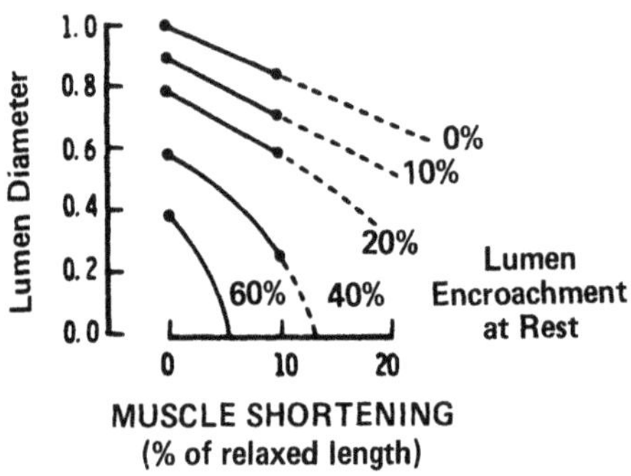

Fig. 2. Effects of transient acute shortening of coronary smooth muscle on lumen diameter in the presence or absence of coronary stenoses of variable severity. The same stimulus, resulting in a similar muscle contraction, will lead to different degrees of lumen reduction and impairment of flow in the presence of different degrees of coronary atherosclerosis. (From [13], by permission of Grune & Stratton, Inc.)

mittent vasocontrictive occlusion of the artery. Therefore, we considered PTCA as an alternative treatment for patients with variant angina and significant coronary artery stenosis.

Selection of Patients

Among the first 230 patients treated with PTCA between February 1980 and October 1982, variant angina was recognized before PTCA in 12 cases and discovered within 4 months after PTCA in 6 others.

All 18 patients had a coronary artery stenosis (single-vessel disease in all patients but 1) considered suitable for PTCA according to accepted criteria [14, 15].

Criteria for the diagnosis of variant angina were:

- Burning or squeezing restrosternal chest pain at rest
- Relief by sublingual nitroglycerin in less than 5 min

- ST segment elevation of at least 0.2 mV, not present during the baseline ECG but documented during pain and disappearing with relief of pain
- No subsequent evidence of myocardial infarction

Variant angina was also diagnosed when these events were provoked by ergonovine.

Evaluation Before PTCA

Efforts were made to record a 12-lead ECG during spontaneous attacks of angina at rest. When unstable angina was absent the patients underwent a graded treadmill exercise test with monitoring of 15 ECG leads, according to a modified Bruce protocol, and thallium-201 studies [16].

In all patients, coronary arteriography was a separate procedure performed before PTCA. In patients with suspected or documented variant angina an ergonovine test was performed, usually in the coronary care unit [17] or occasionally during coronary arteriography, but never during PTCA.

Premedication Before PTCA

All patients were premedicated with sulfinpyrazone 200 mg four times a day or dipyridamole 75 mg three times a day plus aspirin 650 mg per day the day before and on the morning of PTCA. Diltiazem, 90 or 120 mg, was given the evening before and on the morning of PTCA; patients with known variant angina were also given nifedipine 20–40 mg and isosorbide dinitrate orally 2 h before PTCA.

PTCA Technique

The PTCA technique used was no different for our patients with variant angina and other patients. The prior coronary artery angiogram was first viewed, and the diameter of the coronary artery at the site of, and proximal and distal to the stenosis was measured with a caliper in at least two views. True diameters were obtained by comparing these measurements with those of the coronary artery catheters, for which the actual diameters were known. The size of balloon catheter was chosen according to these measurements. After percutaneous femoral insertion of arterial and venous sheaths with obturators, low-molecular dextran was first infused IV. A polyethylene catheter was introduced through a percutaneous femoral approach and advanced to the left ventricle to measure left ventricular and aortic pressures and then removed. A pacemaker electrode was placed in the right ventricle. Nitroglycerin infusion at a rate of 10–30 µg/min was then started. Before PTCA a coronary arteriography was performed using preformed Bourassa polyethylene catheters [18]. Before injection of the stenosed coronary artery the other major artery was opacified to allow visualization of any collateral branches to the narrowed artery. The artery to be dilated was filmed in several

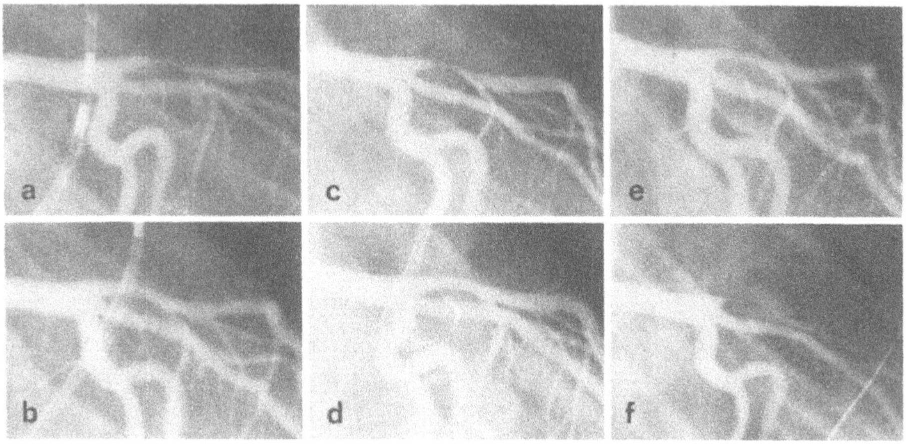

Fig. 3 a–f. Left coronary arteriogram in the right anterior oblique view from patient 4. **a** Before the first PTCA the arteriogram reveals an 85% proximal LAD stenosis. **b** Immediately after the first PTCA the LAD stenosis is reduced to 30%. **c** At 6 weeks after the first PTCA the proximal LAD stenosis graded at 80% has recurred at the site of PTCA. **d** After the second PTCA the 80% LAD stenosis has again been reduced to 30%. **e** Two months after the second PTCA an LAD restenosis graded at 60% is seen at the site of the previous PTCAs. **f** After ergonovine administration 2 months after the second PTCA. Angina and ST elevation in leads V_1 to V_3 accompanied the severe coronary spasm observed in this illustration at the site of PTCA. Coronary spasm disappeared promptly after the administration of nitroglycerin

craniocaudal and craniocaudal sagittally angulated views [19]. As soon as a stenosis was confirmed to be suitable for PTCA, a bolus of 10000 IU heparin was administered i.v. The PTCA technique was similar to that described by Gruentzig et al. using nonsteerable dilating catheters [14]. The pressure gradient accross the stenosis was measured before and after each balloon inflation. A USCI inflation device was used for balloon inflation; the inflation medium was Renografin 76 warmed and diluted to 30% of the usual concentration. The number of balloon inflations varied according to the value of the residual gradient across the stenosis and the appearance of the lesions during control angiography. Intracoronary boluses of nitroglycerin were given if coronary spasm was suspected during the procedure. The patients were brought back to their rooms with nitroglycerin and low-dose heparin infusions. Arterial and venous sheaths were removed at least 4 h after PTCA to allow for subsidence of the effects of the heparin bolus.

Post-PTCA Medication

All patients received platelet function inhibitors for 6 months after PTCA. Calcium antagonists (usually diltiazem 120 mg three times a day) were generally continued after PTCA when variant angina was diagnosed before the procedure.

Clinical, Noninvasive, and Angiographic Followup

All patients underwent clinical evaluations and graded treadmill exercise tests with 15 ECG leads at 1, 3, and 6 months after PTCA, including thallium-201 scintigraphy at the 1- and 6-month tests [20]. Coronary arteriography was performed in all patients 6–8 months after PTCA, unless recurrence of angina and/or results of the noninvasive tests indicated that it was necessary earlier [21]. The degree of coronary stenosis was defined according to the criteria of the Coronary Artery Surgery Study [22] in the view showing the greatest reduction in diameter for the vessel in question. All comparisons between pre-PTCA and post-PTCA films were made using the same view, taken after the administration of nitroglycerin.

Restenosis was defined as a 20% or more increase in the degree of stenosis compared with the coronary angiogram immediately after PTCA, resulting in a stenosis of more than 50% at the repeat angiogram.

Patients' Data Before PTCA

Table 1 is a description of the clinical and angiographic data before and after PTCA for the 18 patients in this study. Patients were classified into three groups according to the short-term results of PTCA.

Table 2 summarizes the clinical and angiographic data before PTCA. Among the 18 patients aged 36–69 years (mean $\pm$ SD = 48 ± 14 years), all but 4 were male, all had had angina at rest for less than 8 months (2 ± 2 months) and all but 4 had had angina on exertion for 1–48 months (7 ± 2 months).

Variant angina was documented before PTCA in two-thirds of the patients (12 of 18). In 8 of these, the ECG recorded during angina at rest demonstrated transient ST elevation. In the other 4, no attacks of angina occurred during hospitalization and the diagnosis was made after ergonovine administration. In these 4 patients and in 5 of the 8 patients in whom variant angina was documented during a spontaneous episode and who also had an ergonovine test, the result was positive in 7 patients at a dose of 0.1 mg or less, induced ST segment depression in another, and was negative in the last patient. Treadmill exercise tests were performed by 14 patients. The test induced ST segment elevation in 6 patients (in the same anterior ECG leads as during spontaneous or provoked attack), ST depression in 4 patients, and no ST abnormality in 4 patients. In 2 of these last 4 patients a reversible perfusion defect was demonstrated during the exercise thallium scan; in the other 2, exercise was stopped at 3 min or less because of fatigue. ST elevation before or after PTCA was located in the anterior ECG leads in all patients except patient 10, for whom ST elevation was in the inferior leads.

Each patient had a coronary artery stenosis graded at 60%–95%, which was located in all patients but 1 in the left anterior descending artery (LAD) and in all but 3 patients in the proximal third of that artery. Each patient had single-vessel disease with no additional coronary lesions elsewhere, except for patient 6, who had a 65% posterior descending artery stenosis.

Table 1. Clinical and angiographic data of patients before and after PTCA

Patients (age range 36–69; 3 F, 15 M)		Before PTCA: Duration of angina (months): Rest	Before PTCA: Duration of angina (months): Effort	Before PTCA: ECG during: Rest angina	Before PTCA: ECG during: Ergonovine test (mg)	Before PTCA: ECG during: Exercise test	Before PTCA: Diagnosis of VA before PTCA	During PTCA: Vessel	During PTCA: % sten. pre/post
Failures	1	8	None	↑ST	↑ST (0.025)	↑ST	Yes	Prox. LAD	80[a]
	2	1	1	–	↑ST (0.05)	Th. pos.	Yes	Prox. LAD	90/80
Reste-nosis	3	2	None	↑ST	↑ST (0.025)	↑ST	Yes	Prox. LAD	70/20
	4	2	2	–	–	↓ST	No[b]	Prox. LAD	85/30
	5	1	1	↓ST	–	–	No	Prox. LAD	60/40
	6	1	48	↓ST	–	–	No	Prox. LAD	65/25
	7	3	3	–	neg	↓ST	No[b]	Prox. LAD	60/30
	8	1	7	–	–	–	No	{ Prox. LAD	60/50
								{ 1st diag.	80/60
	9	1	None	↑ST	↓ST (0.025)	↑ST	Yes	{ Mid-LAD	80/30
								{ Mid-LAD	50/35
	10	3	13	↑ST	–	↓ST	Yes	Mid-RCA	85/35
Con-tinued sucess	11	4	4	↑ST	–	Neg[d]	Yes	Mid-LAD	70/30
	12	4	4	–	–	Th pos.	No	Prox. LAD	90/25
	13	1	4	–	↑ST (0.1)	↑ST	Yes	Prox. LAD	95/50
	14	1	1	↑ST	↑ST (0.05)	↓ST	Yes	Prox. LAD	90/60
	15	1	1	↑ST	↑ST (0.1)	Neg[d]	Yes	Prox. LAD	90/10
	16	1	1	–	↑ST (0.1)	↑ST	Yes	Prox. LAD	85/10
	17	1	None	–	–	↑ST	Yes	Prox. LAD	80/10
	18	2	2	↑ST	–	–	Yes	Prox. LAD	85/35

[a] Unable to cross stenosis
[b] Variant angina diagnosed after second PTCA
[c] Plus new 75% left main coronary artery stenosis →CABG →MI
[d] Exercise test duration less than 3 min

Abbreviations: LAD, left anterior descending artery; 1st diag, 1st diagonal branch; RCA, right coronary artery; Cx, left circumflex artery; Prox, proximal; ↑ST, ST segment elevation; ↓ST, ST segment depression; Th pos, positive thallium exercise scan without ST changes; Neg, negative; CA, calcium antagonist drug; EL/EM CABG, elective/emergency coronary artery bypass grafting; MI, myocardial infarction; VA, variant angina; EL, elective; EM, emergency

Table 1 (continued)

Patients (age range 36–69; 3 F, 15 M)		After PTCA: CA after PTCA	Immediate outcome: Angina: Rest	Immediate outcome: Angina: Effort	ECG during: Angina Rest	ECG during: Exercise test	ECG during: Ergonovine test (mg)	At time of diagnosis of restenosis: Angina: Rest	At time of diagnosis of restenosis: Angina: Effort	Repeat angiogram or second PTCA % sten. pre/post	Late outcome: Clinical followup: Duration (months)	Clinical followup: Angina	Clinical followup: Currently receiving on CA	Coronary angiography: Duration (months)	Coronary angiography: % stenosis	Coronary angiography: Ergonovine test: % stenosis (mg)
Failures	1		Yes	No	–	–	–			– (EL CABG)	39	No	No	–	–	
	2		No	Yes	–	↑ST				80/100 (EM CABG, MI)	24	No	No	–	–	
Restenosis	3	No	No	No	–	Neg	Neg	No	Yes	70/25	40	No	No	25	25	→ 70 (0.4) Clinically Neg
	4	No	No	No	–	Neg	–	Yes	Yes	80/30	37	No	No	21	100	
	5	No	Yes	Yes	–	Neg	↑ST (0.05)	No	Yes	75[c] (EL CABG, MI)	36	No	No	–	–	
	6	No	No	No	–	↓ST	–	Yes	No	75/40 (MI)	6	–	–	–	–	
	7	No	No	No	–	–	–	Yes	Yes	70/40	35	No	No	21	40	Neg
	8	No	Yes	Yes	–	Neg	–	Yes	Yes	60 80	31	No	No	15	{55 {70	Neg
	9	Yes	No	No	–	–	Neg	Yes	No	70 40	29	No	Yes	22	{70 {40	95 (0.2)
	10	Yes	No	No	–	–	–	Yes	No	70/50	26	No	No	22	20	→100 (0.4)
Continued success	11	Yes	Yes	No	↑ST	Neg	–	–	–	10	36	No	No	18	10	Neg
	12	Yes	No	No	–	Neg	↑ST (0.1 mg)	–	–	25	35	No	No	19	20	Diffuse narrowing (0.3)
	13	Yes	No	No	–	Neg	Neg	–	–	40	34	No	No	19	30	Neg
	14	Yes	No	No	–	Neg	Neg	–	–	50	33	No	No	18	50	Neg
	15	Yes	No	No	–	Neg	–	–	–	35	17	No	No	6	35	
	16	Yes	No	No	–	Neg	–	–	–	10	13	No	No	6	10	Neg
	17	Yes	No	No	–	Neg	–	–	–	20	12	No	No	6	20	
	18	Yes	No	No	–	Neg	–	–	–	30	12	No	No	12	30	

Table 2. Summary of clinical and angiographic data of the 18 patients before PTCA

Age (years)	48 ± 14	(range 36–69)
Sex (*n*)		
Male	14	
Female	4	
Angina (*n*)		
Rest and effort	14	
Rest only	4	
Diagnosis of variant angina (*n*)		
Before PTCA	12	
After PTCA	6	
Single-vessel disease (> 50%) (*n*)	17	
Diseased artery (*n*)		
Anterior descending artery	17	
Right coronary artery	1	
Degree of stenosis (%)	78 ± 13	(range 60–95)

Results

Immediate

PTCA was successful in all but two patients.

Failures

In patient 1 the catheter did not cross the stenosis; variant angina persisted in spite of maximum medical therapy and the patient underwent uncomplicated coronary artery bypass grafting associated with plexectomy 12 days later. In patient 2 the results of PTCA were mediocre; a second PTCA attempt 1 month later resulted in a coronary dissection with complete coronary occlusion complicated by myocardial infarction, which was not prevented by emergency coronary artery bypass surgery associated with plexectomy.

Primary Success

PTCA was thus successful in 16 of the 18 patients (88%). None of the first PTCA attempts was complicated by coronary artery spasm during the procedure.

Immediate Outcome

Soon after successful PTCA (16 patients), all but 3 patients were free of symptoms. In all 4 asymptomatic patients who underwent an ergonovine test after PTCA the test was positive before PTCA and became negative after PTCA. Patient 11 had infrequent attacks of variant angina after PTCA, which were easily controlled by calcium antagonists. Except for this patient, all patients who had persisting or recurring angina after successful PTCA developed restenosis.

Persistent Coronary Spasm Preceding Restenosis

In 2 patients (nos. 4 and 5) who developed restenosis documented at 4 months after PTCA, a spontaneous or provoked coronary spasm superimposed on 35% and 40% residual stenoses was demonstrated at control angiography and 2 months after PTCA, respectively.

Restenosis

Restenosis was invariably associated with persistent or recurrent angina and developed within 4 months after PTCA in 8 patients, i.e., half those in whom PTCA was successful. In 3 of them, variant angina was still demonstrated during an episode of angina at rest. Of these 8 patients, 7 underwent an exercise test, which was negative in 1 patient and induced ST segment depression in the others. In 4 of these patients, an ergonovine test induced chest pain associated with ST segment elevation.

Continued Success

In patient 11, for whom calcium antagonists were restarted 3 days after PTCA, and in the 7 other patients who continued to receive calcium antagonists for a few months after PTCA, the repeat coronary angiogram at 6 months after PTCA showed no restenosis. All these patients were asymptomatic, except for patient 14 who developed recurrent angina at rest and during exertion 4 months after PTCA while taking nifedipine and became free of symptoms when diltiazem was added to nifedipine. This patient had a poor angiographic result of PTCA (residual stenosis = 60%).

Management of Restenosis

Except for patients 4 and 7, in whom variant angina was not diagnosed until after the second PTCA, patients with restenosis were treated with calcium antagonists for several months, usually in addition to a second PTCA attempt. Repeat PTCA was attempted in 5 patients. The immediate results were good except in patient 6, in whom coronary spasm occurred during the procedure, completely occluding the LAD and requiring nitroglycerin for relief. An acute anterior infarction developed 6 h later, which was complicated by two episodes of ventricular fibrillation and by transient heart failure. This patient died suddenly 1 month later. Autopsy revealed a hemorrhage under a plaque associated with a 95% stenosis of the

Table 3. Summary of clinical and angiographic data of the 18 patients after PTCA

Duration of clinical followup (months)	28 ± 11	(range 12–40)
Status (*n*)		
Alive	17	
Without MI or surgery	14	
After MI	2	
Uncomplicated surgery	1	
Dead	1	
Symptoms (angina) (*n*)	0	
Current medical treatment (*n*)		
More	16	
Calcium antagonists	1	
Duration of angiographic followup (months) (14 pts)	16 ± 6	(range 6–25)
Status (*n*)		
No more stenosis >50%	11	
Restenosis (>50%)	3	
Ergonovine test (*n*)		
Negative	7	
Positive	3	

MI, myocardial infarction

LAD, an anteroseptal infarction, and a mural thrombus. In patient 5, a new 75% left main coronary artery stenosis, which was not present at PTCA or at repeat angiography 1 month after PTCA, developed and was associated with 75% restenosis of the LAD. Double coronary artery bypass grafting the day after angiography was complicated by an acute myocardial infarction. Lastly, 2 patients received only calcium antagonists.

Of the 4 patients with successful repeat PTCA long-term success was obtained in the 2 patients who continued receiving calcium antagonists after PTCA, but in the 2 others angina at rest recurred 1 and 6 weeks after repeat PTCA. These 2 patients became symptom-free when calcium antagonists were restarted 4 and 6 weeks after PTCA (when variant angina was diagnosed using an ergonovine test), but one of them developed a complete occlusion at the site of PTCA without evidence of myocardial infarction.

Restenosis and Calcium Antagonists

In the 20 successful PTCA attempts (16 primary successes and 4 successful repeat PTCAs) the restenosis rate was 17% (2 of 12) when patients received calcium antagonists soon after PTCA and 88% (7 of 8) when calcium antagonists were not administered soon after PTCA. This difference is statistically significant ($P<0.01$, Fisher's exact probability test).

Late Outcome

Duration of clinical followup was 28 ± 11 months (range 6–48 months). One patient died and all the others are currently free of symptoms. Three of them had coronary artery bypass surgery and no longer receive antianginal therapy. Only 1 patient (patient 9) is still receiving calcium antagonists. In the remaining 13 patients it is more than 6 months since calcium antagonists were discontinued (mean $= 19 \pm 9$ months), and they remain free of symptoms.

Calcium antagonist administration was discontinued 7 ± 5 months after PTCA in patients with continued success and 12 ± 3 months after repeat PTCA in patients who had restenosis.

Repeat angiography was not performed in the 4 patients who had myocardial infarction and/or surgery, but was carried out in each of the remaining 14 patients. One of them had a complete coronary artery occlusion at the site of PTCA and only 2 still have significant (>50%) coronary stenosis. Ten patients underwent an ergonovine test, which was usually performed during the last repeat angiography. The test was negative (according to criteria described above) in 7 patients (but induced a 70% spasm in patient 3) and positive in 3 patients (with a diffuse narrowing of the arteries without spasm at the site of PTCA in patient 12) at a high dose level of ergonovine (0.2 mg or more).

Discussion

Spasm associated with significant atherosclerotic coronary lesions is a relatively frequent clinical problem: among 162 consecutive variant angina patients undergoing coronary arteriography at our institution, 61% had organic lesions $\geqq 70\%$ [23].

Recent studies have shown that the single most important prognostic factor in medically treated patients with variant angina is the presence or absence of fixed obstructive coronary artery disease [23, 24] and that in patients with variant angina the probability of death and myocardial infarction is higher than in those with nonvariant angina coronary artery disease [24].

Thus, cardiac catheterization is required for identification of variant angina patients with significant atherosclerotic lesions, because these patients may need a more aggressive approach than other subsets of patients [25].

Coronary bypass surgery has been advised for these patients, but the results are not so good as in patients with fixed coronary artery disease [26–28].

Coronary spasm is a known complication of PTCA, occurring in 2% of patients undergoing this procedure, and in some cases it has been associated with infarction [24] or the need for emergency bypass surgery [29]. Until recently, patients with preexisting coronary spasm were believed to be at a higher risk for development of coronary artery spasm and potential complications during PTCA.

This study gives an answer to several questions about PTCA in patients with variant angina. First, as shown in a preliminary study [30], PTCA is technically feasible in such patients. The high success rate is probably due to the fact that most of our patients fulfilled the ideal criteria for selection for PTCA: single-vessel disease and discrete proximal noncalcified stenosis in a major coronary artery suitable for coronary artery surgery. This pattern is more frequent in patients with variant angina [30] than in the global population of patients undergoing coronary arteriography [31].

Second, PTCA is relatively safe in patients with variant angina. In 23 PTCA attempts, coronary spasm (complicated by myocardial infarction) occurred only once. The other PTCA-related myocardial infarction was due to coronary dissection. Thus, the incidence of complications, and particularly of those related to coronary spasm, does not appear to be much higher in these patients than in other patients who undergo PTCA [14, 19, 31] or in patients with active variant angina [33, 34].

Third, restenoses are very frequent in patients with variant angina. They may be due to persistence of coronary spasm during the recovery period after PTCA, and can sometimes be prevented by calcium antagonists. The possibility of variant angina should thus be considered in patients with angina at rest who are referred for PTCA, because they may need specific medical therapy after PTCA [30], as do variant angina patients undergoing coronary bypass surgery [35]. In 6 patients the diagnosis of variant angina was not made until after PTCA, usually before or at the time of restenosis. We believe that these patients, like those recently reported by the Atlanta group [36], had variant angina which had been overlooked before PTCA.

Lastly, although our long-term results must be interpreted with great caution, because spontaneous remission is a frequent outcome of variant angina [37], PTCA appears to be an effective treatment for this syndrome, since we achieved a very high rate of patients who are currently free of symptoms and have received no medical treatment for more than 6 months.

We do not yet have any experience of PTCA in other anatomic subsets of patients with variant angina, such as patients with multivessel disease (who have been shown to have the worst prognosis and for whom coronary artery bypass surgery has been advised) or patients with insignificant organic coronary artery stenoses or none at all, in whom it could be hypothesized that scarring of the coronary artery media after overstretching of smooth muscle cells may prevent coronary artery spasm. These patients may provide a future field of application for this new revascularization technique.

References

1. Ginsburg R, Bristow MR, Harrison DC, Stinson EB (1980) Studies with isolated human coronary arteries. Some general observations, potential mediators of spasm, role of calcium antagonists. Chest 78:180
2. Zuberbuhler RC, Bohr DF (1965) Response of coronary vascular smooth muscle to catecholamines. Circ Res 16:431
3. Feigl EO (1967) Sympathetic control of coronary circulation. Circ Res 20:262

4. Yasue H, Omote S, Takizawa A, Nagao M, Miwa K, Tanaka S (1979) Circadian variation of exercise capacity in patients with Prinzmetal's variant angina: role of exercise-induced coronary arterial spasm. Circulation 59:938
5. Prinzmetal M, Kennamer R, Merliss R, Wada T, Bor N (1959) Angina pectoris. 1. A variant form of angina pectoris. Am J Med 27:357
6. MacAlpin RN (1980) Relation of coronary arterial spasm to site of organic stenosis. Am J Cardiol 46:143
7. Dembinske-Kiek A, Gryglewski T, Zunde A, Gryglewski RJ (1977) The generation of prostacyclin by arteries and by the coronary vascular bed is reduced in experimental atherosclerosis in rabbit. Prostaglandins 14:1025
8. Angelov C, Villa S, Mysliewic A (1978) Defective fibrinolytic and prostacyclin like activity in human atheromatous plaques. Thromb Haemost 39:535
9. Cheng TO, Bashour T, Kelser GA, Weiss L, Bacos L (1973) Variant angina of Prinzmetal with normal coronary arteriograms. A variant of the variant. Circulation 47:476
10. Théroux P, Waters DD, Latour JG (1982) Clinical manifestations and pathophysiology of myocardial ischemia with special reference to coronary artery spasm and the role of slow channel calcium blockers. Prog Cardiovasc Dis 25:157
11. Muller JE (1980) Prinzmetal's angina. A model for the role of spasm in ischemic heart disease. J Cardiovasc Med 5:19
12. MacAlpin RN (1980) Contribution of dynamic vascular wall thickening to luminal narrowing during coronary arterial constriction. Circulation 61:296
13. Maseri A, Chierchia S (1982) Coronary artery spasm: demonstration, definition, diagnosis and consequences. Prog Cardiovasc Dis 25:169
14. Gruentzig AR, Senning A, Siegenthaler WE (1979) Nonoperative dilatation of coronary artery stenosis. Percutaneous transluminal coronary angioplasty. N Engl J Med 301:61
15. Rapaport E (1979) Percutaneous transluminal coronary angioplasty (editorial). Circulation 60:969
16. Waters DD, Szlachcic J, Bourassa MG, Scholl JM, Théroux P (1982) Exercise testing in patients with variant angina: results, correlation with clinical and angiographic features and prognostic significance. Circulation65:265
17. Waters DD, Théroux P, Szlachcic J, Dauwe F, Crittin J, Bonan R, Mizgala HF (1980) Ergonovine testing in a coronary care unit. Am J Cardiol 46:922
18. Bourassa MG, Lespérance J, Campeau L (1969) Selective coronary arteriography by the percutaneous femoral artery approach. AJR 107:377
19. Lespérance J, Saltiel J, Petitclerc R, Bourassa MG (1974) Angulated views in the sagittal plane for improved accuracy of cinecoronary angiography. AJR 121:565
20. Scholl JM, Chaitman BR, David PR, Dupras G, Brévers G, Guiteras Val P, Crépeau J, Lespérance J, Bourassa MG (1982) Exercise electrocardiography and myocardial scintigraphy in the serial evaluation of the results of percutaneous transluminal coronary angioplasty. Circulation 66:380
21. Dangoisse V, Guiteras Val P, David PR, Lespérance J, Crépeau J, Dyrda I, Bourassa MG (1982) Recurrence of stenosis after successful percutaneous transluminal coronary angioplasty (PTCA). Circulation 66 [Suppl II]:331 (abstract)
22. Coronary Artery Surgery Study Investigators (1981) National Heart Lung and Blood Institute. Coronary artery surgery study. Circulation [Suppl I]:14
23. Waters DD, Miller DD, Szlachcic J, Bouchard A, Méthé M, Kreeft J, Théroux P (1983) Factors influencing the long-term prognosis of treated patients with variant angina. Circulation 68:258
24. Mark DB, Califf RM, Morris KG, Harrel FE, Pryor DB, Hlatky MA, Lee KL, Rosati RA (1984) Clinical characteristics and long-term survival of patients with variant angina. Circulation 69:880
25. Shubrooks SJ, Bette JM, Hutter AM, Block PC, Buckley MJ, Daggett WM, Mundth ED (1975) Variant angina pectoris: clinical and anatomic spectrum and results of coronary bypass surgery. Am J Cardiol 36:142
26. Gaasch WH, Lufschanowski R, Leachman RD, Alexander JK (1974) Surgical management of Prinzmetal's variant angina. Chest 66:614

27. Grondin CM, Limet R (1977) Sympathetic denervation in association with coronary artery grafting in patients with Prinzmetal's variant angina. Ann Thorac Surg 23:111
28. Bertrand ME, Lablanche JM, Rousseau MF, Warembourg HH Jr, Stankowtak C, Soots G (1980) Surgical treatment of variant angina: use of plexectomy with aortocoronary bypass. Circulation 61:877
29. Myler RK (1980) Percutaneous transluminal coronary angioplasty. Arch Inst Cardiol Mex 50:401
30. David PR, Waters DD, Scholl JM, Crépeau J, Szlachcic J, Lespérance J, Hudon G, Bourassa MG (1982) Percutaneous transluminal coronary angioplasty in patients with variant angina. Circulation 66:695
31. Hamby RI, Katz S (1980) Percutaneous transluminal coronary angioplasty: its potential impact on surgery for coronary artery disease. Am J Cardiol 45:1161
32. Vliestra RE, Holmes DR, Smith HC, Hartzler GO, Orszulak TA (1981) Percutaneous transluminal coronary angioplasty. Mayo Clin Proc 56:287
33. Maseri A, Severi S, DeNes M, L'Abbate A, Chierchia S, Marzilli M, Ballestra AM, Parodi O, Biagini A, Distante A (1978) "Variant" angina: one aspect of a continuous spectrum of vasospastic myocardial ischemia. Pathogenetic mechanisms, estimated incidence and clinical and coronary arteriographic findings in 138 patients. Am J Cardiol 42:1019
34. Waters DD, Szlachcic J, Miller D, Théroux P (1982) Clinical characteristics of patients with variant angina complicated by myocardial infarction or death within one month. Am J Cardiol 49:658
35. Endo M, Kanda I, Hosada S, Hiyashi H, Hirosawa K, Konno S (1975) Prinzmetal's variant form of angina pectoris. Re-evaluation of mechanisms. Circulation 52:33
36. Hollman J, Austin GE, Gruentzig AR, Douglas JS Jr, King SB III (1983) Coronary artery spasm at the site of angioplasty in the first 2 months after successful percutaneous transluminal coronary angioplasty. J Am Coll Cardiol 2:1039
37. Waters DD, Bouchard A, Théroux P (1983) Spontaneous remission is a frequent outcome of variant angina. J Am Coll Cardiol 2:195

Subject Index

www.ingramcontent.com/pod-product-compliance
Lightning Source LLC
Chambersburg PA
CBHW061159240926
51846CB00006B/1056
* 9 7 8 3 6 4 2 7 0 8 1 7 6 *